THERAPEUTIC RECREATION AND THE NATURE OF DISABILITIES

THERAPEUTIC RECREATION AND THE NATURE OF DISABILITIES

KENNETH E. MOBILY
RICHARD D. MACNEIL

VENTURE PUBLISHING, INC.

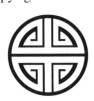
Production Manager: Richard Yocum
Manuscript Editing: Valerie Paukovits, Richard Yocum
Cover Design by Echelon Design

Library of Congress Catalogue Card Number 2002103088
ISBN 1-892132-22-2

DEDICATION

This book would not have been possible without the love, support, and encouragement of my family—Paula, Michelle, Matthew, Vesta, and Paul. Thanks for being there.

—Kenneth E. Mobily

This book is dedicated to Stella and Ray, who inspired me to dream; to Mary, whose endless support has allowed me to reach for my dreams; and to Adam, Leslie, and Jessica, who are so much better than anything I could have ever dreamed possible! I love you all!

—Richard D. MacNeil

TABLE OF CONTENTS

LIST OF TABLES AND FIGURES

CHAPTER 1
INTRODUCTION AND ORGANIZATION OF THE TEXT

Changing Nature of Therapeutic Recreation

Therapeutic recreation (TR) is an often misunderstood profession. From the day the student declares TR as a major in college and tries to explain it to his or her parents and relatives, and for the balance of the person's professional career, he or she will have to answer numerous questions about the field from professional colleagues and consumers alike. However, TR is slowly making progress as a credible healthcare profession.

Healthcare reform favors efficiency and effectiveness. More research now confirms TR's usefulness as a palliative technique for treating symptoms and conditions secondary to a variety of primary diagnoses, as well as a method of addressing long-term impairment associated with chronic conditions. Other factors that illustrate TR's efficiency include its ability to offer:

- Day, night, and weekend service
- Delivery to groups instead of one-to-one
- Services also offered by physical therapy or occupational therapy at lower costs
- Additional services under the rubric of "health promotion"

TR's image is evolving because of the changing scene of healthcare delivery. More healthcare services traditionally offered on an inpatient basis are now being offered through other venues, such as outpatient, community-based, at home delivery, or patient education. TR is uniquely positioned among healthcare professions insofar as it has long been offered at the community level. Hence, much of the infrastructure necessary for effective service delivery is already in position and under the direction of the municipal recreation departments that have programs in community-based TR. Similarly, clinical TR departments usually make ample use of existing municipal recreation resources, and are

accordingly well networked for the delivery of outpatient and community-based programming. This also makes the professional profile of TR more attractive because of the efficiency associated with not admitting the client to a hospital and containing healthcare expenses as a result. Therefore, TR cannot be characterized in terms of traditional inpatient treatment.

Likewise, TR cannot be characterized as a healthcare discipline that limits itself to patients customarily treated on an inpatient basis. There is no longer a prototypical patient seen on an inpatient basis. The types of patients now seen in healthcare across the board cannot be completely cured or rehabilitated. The chronic condition (an affliction that is managed but usually not cured) is now the norm in healthcare. Chronic conditions are also the type associated with the aging process (e.g., arthritis, osteoporosis, hypertension), and thus will likely increase for the foreseeable future because of the aging U. S. population. Many of the interventions for chronic impairments pertain to the treatment of symptoms (e.g., pain management), self-management by the patient (e.g., perceived control), lifestyle change (e.g., stress management), patient education (e.g., teaching alternative leisure activities), and quality of life initiatives (e.g., personal empowerment).

Purpose of this Book

One of the major competency areas tested on the examination for certification as a therapeutic recreation specialist is *diagnostic groupings and populations served*. Yet few curricula give this competency the attention it deserves. Most professional curricula treat the topic of special populations as a part of an introductory course or within the greater context of courses such as anatomy and physiology. In the latter case, impairments and disabilities are only used to illustrate a point about normal function. In both cases, rarely are the symptoms, functional limitations, implications for treatment, and overall impact of the disability on the person considered.

Common sense suggests that if a profession is to treat, design interventions for, and plan programs for persons with disabilities, then a complete working knowledge of disabilities, their impact on the individual, and the implications for treatment should be an expected prerequisite. Therefore, this book delivers pertinent information about working with persons with disabilities. Without a working knowledge of impairments and their functional implications students will not be prepared to plan and design programs in TR.

In addition, a common culture exists among the healthcare professions with its own expectations and language. One of the expectations among the healthcare culture is a common understanding of the basic concepts that surround disability and impairment. Much of this common understanding is part of the language of the rehabilitation and healthcare community. This book attempts to disseminate the content of the healthcare culture and the language necessary to provide effective and accurate communication among professionals and across disciplines. The TR profession must start to expect more of itself. Mastering the content of this book speaks to the credibility of the future professional and the self-respect that comes with setting high standards for the profession.

This book also focuses on the populations served rather than TR programming. It emphasizes the distinct nature of each impairment, with particular attention to details that bias the person as a good candidate for one intervention, but not another. Only through acquiring a complete knowledge of the normal function of a system and what happens to the system when it is impaired can the professional avoid the pitfalls associated with well-intended but errant programming.

Finally, this book emphasizes research. Relevant literature has been reviewed for each impairment with respect to pertinent interventions that may be employed by the TR specialist, the effectiveness of each intervention, and any specific precautions that practitioners should be aware of when programming for a specific type of impairment. This provides the reader with the confidence that comes with research-based interventions.

Organizational Framework

This book explores the wide range of illnesses, conditions, and disorders that therapeutic recreation specialists (TRS) commonly encounter as they provide professional services. While it is impossible to include every disorder to which TRS may be exposed, the authors have drawn from their combined 40 years of professional experience to select the conditions and disorders most relevant to the TR profession. TR personnel must possess a basic understanding of these disorders to function as competent, respected members of the health service community. This text examines a large number of disabilities and includes the following information:

- General overview focusing upon distinct symptoms and characteristics related to each condition

- Relevant variations of the condition and levels of severity that would impact the course and treatment of the disorder
- Information about the etiology (cause) of the disorder
- Statistical data related to prevalence, incidence, and risk
- Variations of disorders that may be attributable to the individual's cultural setting, gender, or developmental stage (e.g., infancy, childhood, adolescence, adulthood, or late life)
- Information about the expected course of the disorder (e.g., age of onset, mode of onset, patterns of recurrence and duration)
- General trends related to the expected progression of the condition over time
- Common treatment approaches used by healthcare professions to improve or restore health or to minimize functional deficits.
- Implications for TR intervention
- TR goals, programs strategies, and precautions for the conditions reviewed

Three Domain Approach

The disabilities surveyed in this text compromise the overall health of affected individuals. The concept of health is an admittedly elusive idea that cannot be defined in simple terms. Although health has traditionally been associated with physical well-being, increasingly people have come to agree with the World Health Organization's (WHO) description of health as a state of complete physical, mental, and social well-being. This view suggests that health is not merely the absence of disease and infirmity, but a harmonious interrelationship of all the elements that make us human—physical, social, emotional, and intellectual.

A useful way to explore this view of health is to conceive of human beings as comprised of three broad behavioral domains (see **Figure 1.1**), each with different behavioral characteristics but all tied together to form a unique individual. The *cognitive domain* includes all the mental processes used to obtain knowledge or to become aware of the environment. It includes perception, imagination, judgment, memory, learning, thinking, and language. The *affective domain* focuses on personality and social development. Emotional development is primarily included in this domain, as is the impact of the family and the larger society on the individual. This domain references terms such as self-esteem, self-concept, life satisfaction, and adaptation. The *psychomotor domain* includes all the growth and change that occurs in a person's body. Changes in height, weight, bone, muscle, the brain and sense organs, and physical appearance are part of this domain. In addition, motor skills and voluntary actions, including everything from learning to walk to writing and feeding oneself, are also part of the psychomotor domain.

The three-domain approach increases our understanding of the concept of health and serves as a useful conceptualization for categorizing diseases and disorders. Each of the three main sections of this text will begin with a brief review of one of the behavioral domains. First we provide an overview of the nature and parameters of each domain, discuss what aspects of normal functioning are associated with this domain, and discuss how processes in the domain relate to broader issues of health and independent functioning. Next, we review relevant theories related to development and expected behavior in the domain (e.g., in the cognitive domain we will explore Jean Piaget's theory of intellectual development). Third, we review the various components that make up each domain, including physical structures (e.g., brain, muscles) and psychological constructs (e.g., self-esteem, personality). We discuss how these components work together to produce normal functioning in this domain. Finally, we explore various problems identified with the domain, which constitute the conditions and disorders that are the focus of this text.

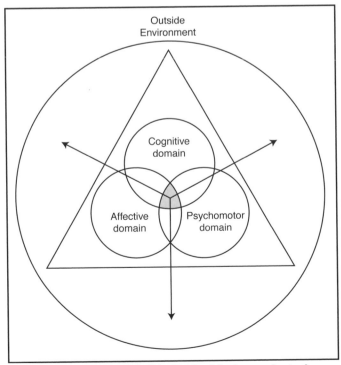

Figure 1.1 The "healthy" individual is the product of the interaction of all three behavioral domains

Before we leave the topic of the three-domain approach, we must provide an important word of caution: While it is convenient to discuss each domain as if it were a separate entity, in reality every individual is the sum product of the interaction of all three domains. Thus a disorder that may be identified primarily with one domain inevitably influences functioning in the other domains as well. Congenital blindness serves as an example of this point. While blindness is categorized as an impairment in the psychomotor domain, it is also known to effect development in the cognitive and affective domains of the individual. For instance, the congenitally blind child, when compared to sighted peers, is usually slower in developing gross and fine motor skills (e.g., psychomotor domain), typically produces lower scores on measure of knowledge, judgment, and language (e.g., cognitive domain), and generally exhibits developmental lags on measures of social and emotional development. However, once individualized learning strategies and alternate modes of communication are developed, the otherwise healthy child who is blind will typically overcome early developmental lags and perform at similar levels to their nonimpaired peers on most measures of healthy development.

Overview of Text

Chapter 2 examines the cognitive domain. It explores concepts such as intelligence and cognition and presents a model of normal cognitive functioning. Much of the chapter examines mental retardation, the condition most directly related to this domain. An overview of this condition, emphasizing its primary characteristics and functional expectations, is provided. The chapter closes with a discussion of the use of therapeutic recreation services for individuals with mental retardation.

Chapter 3 provides an introduction to the affective domain. This domain refers to those aspects of human behavior related to feelings, emotions, attitudes, and personal-social behaviors. Disorders associated with this domain are classified by the general term mental illness. The chapter presents an historical overview of the social attitudes toward and the treatment of people who have mental illness. The chapter also presents a variety of theories that have been developed to explain the nature and causes of mental illness. A classification system used to differentiate various categories of mental disorders concludes the chapter.

Chapter 4 presents an overview of mental disorders associated with excessive levels of anxiety. The disorders discussed include panic disorder, phobias, obsessive compulsive disorder, posttraumatic stress disorder, and generalized anxiety disorder. As with all the chapters in this section, relevant information related to the characteristics, cause, and possible treatments of each disorder are discussed.

Chapter 5 offers a discussion of affective disorders, conditions characterized by disturbances in moods and emotions. These intense disturbances produce significant disruption in the lives of people affected by them. The types of mood disturbances presented in this chapter include major depressive disorder, dysthymic disorder, bipolar disorder, and cyclothymic disorder.

Chapter 6 examines perhaps the most severe and puzzling form of mental illness: schizophrenia. Individuals with this disorder display symptoms that make it difficult for them to separate real from unreal experiences. This chapter discusses how the concept of schizophrenia has evolved over time, the essential features and symptoms of the illness, and different treatments used for the disorder.

Chapter 7 explores a wide variety of disorders associated with the use and abuse of substances. Substances such as alcohol, opium, and cannabis are used in the hope of reducing pain, relieving stress, or altering states of consciousness. Unfortunately, for some individuals the use of such substances causes disturbances in their ability to function in their everyday lives. After explaining the distinctions between substance use disorders and substance-induced disorders, we explore seven classes of substance-related disturbances: alcohol, central nervous system stimulants (e.g., amphetamines and cocaine), opioids, hallucinogens, cannabis, phencyclidine (PCP), and inhalants.

Chapter 8 concludes our review of the affective domain. In this chapter we discuss a variety of disorders identified either early or late in life. Among the disorders discussed are a series of disturbances marked by inattentiveness and impulsivity and usually diagnosed during the childhood years. These include attention-deficit/hyperactivity disorder, oppositional defiant disorder, and conduct disorder. Autism is a pervasive developmental disability usually diagnosed in infancy or early childhood. Anorexia nervosa and bulimia nervosa are two common varieties of eating disturbances usually identified during adolescence or early adulthood. In contrast, dementia is a disorder associated with later life—rarely is it diagnosed in individuals younger than 50. In this chapter we focus upon Alzheimer's disease, now recognized as the leading cause of dementia.

Chapter 9 begins the second half of the book. This chapter emphasizes physical impairments by reviewing

the psychomotor domain. The psychomotor domain pertains to physical acts of a skilled or unskilled nature. The taxonomy of behaviors in the psychomotor domain is useful in planning, assessing, and evaluating observable behaviors and dysfunction that present observable, physical markers. The chapter closes with a caveat to the reader: While we can theoretically discuss discrete areas of behavior, real human behavior is much more complex. Nevertheless, the behavioral domains remain useful for instructive purposes and assessment and evaluation of clients.

Chapter 10 reviews the skeletal and joint systems. These two systems are treated together because knowledge of the skeleton is prerequisite to the study of movement at joints. The skeletal and joint systems are of particular importance because of the frequency with which each is affected by the "new" disease of the post-industrialized world—the chronic condition (e.g., arthritis and osteoporosis).

Chapter 11 addresses the system of muscles, which attach to bones and produce movements at joints. The infrastructure of muscles is briefly examined to give the reader a sense of how muscles produce actions through contractions. The reader is also oriented to the concept of muscle tone—a contraction that produces no observable movement. Chapter 11 covers another important chronic condition, low muscle strength (frailty), which like arthritis and osteoporosis is increasing in incidence and relevance.

Chapter 12 explores the nervous system, the instigating force behind movement. The nervous system directs human activity and behavior through sensory and motor capabilities. Many of the disorders common to contemporary rehabilitation present physical signs that appear to be disorders of muscular or skeletal systems, but instead are primarily neurological in etiology. In other words, many of the impairments in the ability to move using muscular, skeletal, and joint systems are because of nervous system damage.

Chapter 13 covers special sensory systems, which abound in several areas of the body. Most people know of the sensory importance of the eyes, ears, taste buds and sense of smell; however, the sensory tissues in the skin are often overlooked. Sensory systems usually develop from nervous tissue and therefore remain tethered to it by way of a sensory neuron. This chapter primarily discusses vision and hearing, but briefly covers other sensory systems.

Chapter 14 discusses the cardiopulmonary system. Cardiovascular disease is the number one cause of death for both men and women in the United States. However, the risk factors for developing serious cardiac, vascular, or pulmonary impairments can be drastically reduced through lifestyle changes. This marks cardiac and pulmonary disease as one of the leading areas of initiative for TR-delivered health promotion programs. Modifiable lifestyle habits such as smoking, exercise (or lack thereof), weight, and stress level number among the behaviors that can be changed to lower the risk of cardiac, vascular, or pulmonary diseases.

Chapter 15 explores the remaining systems found in the anterior body cavity (chest and abdomen). The word "viscera" is commonly used to refer to the digestive, urinary, and reproductive systems collectively. These systems carry on functions vital to life at a subconscious level, such as maintaining blood pressure, fluid balance, and acid-base balance.

This book emphasizes the diagnostic groupings of populations commonly served by the therapeutic recreation profession. Before proceeding, we offer two explanations.

First, it is imperative to understand that each individual is the sum product of the interaction of all of our behavioral domains—cognitive, affective, and psychomotor. In the following chapters, however, we highlight conditions and disorders from the perspective of the primary domain in which they occur (e.g., cognitive domain for mental retardation, affective domain for depression, psychomotor domain for cerebral palsy). For convenience of explanation it is easier to discuss each domain (and associated disabilities) as if it were a separate entity. As a result of this emphasis upon only one domain at a time, it may appear that we are discounting the importance of the other two domains upon each individual, but this is not the case.

Second, many general statements will be made about disorders and how they affect individuals who are afflicted with them. While it is true to say that different individuals diagnosed with the same disorder often share characteristics associated with the disorder, it is certainly not true to say that they are alike in other ways as well. For instance, two people diagnosed with Down syndrome may be similar in terms of level of retardation or physical appearance. But it should not be assumed that their personalities, their creativity, their interests, or their likes and dislikes are the same. Few situations are as dehumanizing as being identified by only one trait or characteristic, especially if that trait tends to be viewed negatively by society. Consequently, it is important that the reader recognize that general statements about aggregates of people who experience a similar condition are only that: general statements. The principle that each person is unique and special is the guiding principle upon which this book is based.

We believe that a recognizable void exists within TR literature with respect to the systematic study of the populations we commonly serve. We hope that this book begins to fill this void by helping future TR professionals understand how illnesses and disabilities affect the lives of their clients and how TR can improve quality of life for all individuals.

CHAPTER 2 COGNITIVE DOMAIN

Most people define cognitive ability as thinking and intelligence—"using your head." In the psychological literature it is frequently associated with intelligence, reasoning, perception, creativity, problem solving, memory, attention, meditation, and imagery. For the purposes of this text, we view the cognitive domain as a general set of constructs dealing with those aspects of behavior centered around the ability to think, reason, and conceptualize.

Cognitive functioning is difficult to assess and evaluate. Most people have specific areas of strengths and weaknesses in terms of cognitive abilities. For some individuals, however, deficiencies in cognitive functioning are so pronounced that they compromise their ability to lead healthy, independent lives.

This chapter begins with a discussion of intelligence and cognition and presents a model of cognitive functioning. Next, we utilize the work of famous Swiss psychologist and educator Jean Piaget to explain the course of development in the cognitive domain. This is followed by an introductory discussion of mental retardation, the primary disorder in this domain. As part of this discussion we will highlight the evolving definition of the condition, theories as to its cause and diagnosis, classification of levels of retardation, and general characteristics associated with the disorder. Then we will examine therapeutic recreation protocol with respect to mental retardation. Before continuing we recommend you complete Exercise 2.1 (p. 8).

Intelligence

Of all the desirable social attributes, few are as highly valued as intelligence in most societies. But what constitutes intelligence? What does it mean to say someone is intelligent? Can intelligence be measured?

Compare your answers to Exercise 2.1 with the correct responses listed at the end of this chapter (see page 32). Most likely every reader has seen an exercise like this one. Conventional wisdom suggests that because each of the items listed is so common it does not require much intelligence for someone to come up with the "right" answers. Could an exercise like this one be used to measure intelligence? As you look at this exercise ask yourself what skills are required to correctly identify the objects in each box. It would seem that at a minimum one must:

- Be familiar with popular symbols in our culture
- Evaluate common terms and symbols to see them in an "out-of-the-ordinary" manner
- Draw conclusions from incomplete sources of information
- See new relationships between common objects

It could be stated that the ability to score "well" on this exercise is reflective of intelligence. While we do not suggest that this exercise be used as an intelligence test, it does raise questions about how we define intelligence.

Before we offer our own definition we will review some definitions advanced in the past. Louis Terman, an American psychologist, offered this explanation of intelligence in 1916: "An individual is intelligent in proportions as he is able to carry out abstract thinking." Typical of many early definitions, Terman's view characterized intelligence as a one-dimensional concept—in this case abstract reasoning. Terman conceived abstract reasoning as thought apart from direct application, such as the ability to answer questions like, what if the world were square instead of round? or respond appropriately to directions, such as define the word "honesty." Terman felt that intelligence is an inherited trait which remains stable over time (Terman, 1916).

David Wechsler, author of a popular Intelligence Quotient (IQ) test, provided another definition of intelligence. According to Wechsler (1958) "intelligence is the aggregate or global capacity of individuals to act purposefully, to think rationally, and to deal effectively with his environment." In contrast to Terman, Wechsler's definition suggests that intelligence is multidimensional. Important to his view is the idea of an applied dimension to intelligence—an aspect that is reflected in one's daily interactions within one's environment. The IQ tests developed by Wechsler include subtests designed to measure verbal and performance skills as well as several different dimensions of functioning. Whereas verbal skills tend to emphasize cultural or learned aspects of intelligence, performance skills are more directed toward abilities such as finding missing parts, solving special problems, and constructing objects from models.

Most contemporary theorists advocate acceptance of the notion of intelligence as a range of abilities rather than a general ability. Much of the recent research on

DIRECTIONS: Identify the object or phrase located in each box using the clues provided.

1 SAND	2 MAN ――― BOARD	3 STAND ――― I	4 R|E|A|D||I|N|G
5 WEAR ――― LONG	6 R R O A D S A D S	7 T O W N	8 CYCLE CYCLE CYCLE
9 LE 　　VEL	10 0 ――― M.D. Ph.D. B.S.	11 KNEE LIGHTS	12 SUNNY
13　　CHAIR	14 DICE DICE	15 T O U C H	16　　GROUND ――――― FEET FEET FEET FEET FEET FEET
17 MIND ――― MATTER	18 HE'S/HIMSELF	19 ECNALG	20 DEATH/LIFE
21 GI ――― CCC CC C	22 ―――― PROGRAM	23 L B O U S E	24 J YOU U ME S T

adult intellectual functioning has utilized the distinction made between fluid intelligence and crystallized intelligence (Cattell, 1963). *Fluid intelligence* is an innate set of abilities involved in seeing and processing abstract relationships and patterns, such as building a boat from a blueprint. It may be considered "native" intelligence since it involves processing information that is not embedded in a context of existing information for the individual. *Crystallized intelligence* refers to the ability to use a body of accumulated general information to make judgments or solve problems. It is thought to be acquired through education and life experiences. It may range from recalling facts like the names of the 50 states to recognizing signs of danger on the street.

For purposes of this text we adopt this definition:

Intelligence is a hypothetical construct that refers to an individual's ability to perceive, understand, and adapt to his or her environment.

By referring to intelligence as a hypothetical construct we acknowledge that much of our understanding of this trait is assumed to be true but exists without empirical proof. Our definition also implies the multidimensionality. Finally, we perceive intelligence to be the product of both heredity and environment. Our genes provide us with cognitive potential and our environment allows this potential to develop.

The Measurement of Intelligence

Nineteenth-century French educator Alfred Binet is usually identified as the founder of intelligence testing. Binet developed a method to measure intelligence to diagnose and assist students who needed extra help for learning. His original IQ test produced a single score based on responses to a series of age-based questions and tasks.

From this modest beginning, intelligence testing has grown into a multimillion dollar industry. Efforts to measure both what an individual may know at any given time as well as his or her aptitude for future learning have led to the use of intelligence testing in educational, governmental, and business settings. Test results have been used for a wide variety of purposes, many only marginally related to Binet's goal of helping students learn. Scores on intelligence tests have contributed to decisions about who to admit to a certain college, who to hire for a certain job, and who to send to officer's training.

The most commonly used IQ tests for children are the Stanford-Binet Intelligence Scale and the Wechsler Intelligence Scales for Children. The *Stanford-Binet Intelligence Scale* tests children older than two years of age. The scale uses 15 tests to assess four areas of intelligence: verbal abilities, abstract and visual thinking, quantitative reasoning, and short-term memory. The *Wechsler Intelligence Scales* are the preferred tests for children over 4 1/2 years of age. The *Wechsler Preschool and Primary Scale of Intelligence* (WPPSI) is used for children with mental ages of 3–7 years; the *Wechsler Intelligence Scale for Children* (WISC-III) is used for children who function above a 6-year-old level. Both scales contain subtests of verbal and performance skills.

The most widely used measure of adult intelligence is the *Wechsler Adult Intelligence Scale* (WAIS). It consists of 11 subtests, six verbal scales (which measure crystallized intelligence) and five performance scales (which measure fluid intelligence). Verbal scales measure the test taker's ability to define words, explain common societal symbols, interpret proverbs, complete comprehension tasks, and explain similarities between words and concepts. Performance scales focus on an individual's ability to manipulate unfamiliar objects and words. These include tests of spatial relations and abstract reasoning and may require an individual to complete a puzzle, match pictures with symbols or numbers, or arrange pictures in a predetermined pattern.

While IQ testing is a popular method used to differentiate between individuals in our society, it is not a procedure without controversy. Questions persist about the accuracy and usefulness of IQ testing. Some critics of testing are concerned about the test maker's ability to isolate questions and/or tasks that are representative of intelligence at a particular age. For example, a test taker may be able to define a triangle as a figure with three straight lines and three interconnected angles, but does this knowledge necessarily imply intelligence? Does it mean the test taker could pick out a triangle in a complex figure? Is there any correlation between the ability to define a triangle and using the figure creatively to solve a problem? Because intelligence is a multidimensional trait, can a score on any one test (or series of tests) accurately reflect all of the previously mentioned dimensions of intelligence?

Critics have also raised concerns over cultural biases they claim are inherent in IQ tests. They suggest that because these tests often require familiarity with culturally based terms and experiences, scores produced may be a better reflection of knowledge of one's culture rather than overall intellectual ability. Furthermore, even within the same culture, racial, or ethnic differences may affect the interpretation of questions and ultimately one's score. The bottom line is that a test taker may have a very intelligent reason for producing a wrong answer, but the answer is still wrong in terms of test results.

Another area of criticism concerns the use of the results produced by IQ tests. Whereas the original IQ tests were used for diagnostic purposes in educational settings, in recent years these tests have been used for many other purposes. For example, during both World Wars and the Korean conflict an enlisted man's score on an IQ test often determined whether the individual served in the infantry (front lines) or in an office. During the early part of the twentieth century IQ scores helped determine immigration quotas. Additionally, the eugenics movement, a social movement popular at the turn of the twentieth century, was concerned with the improvement of hereditary qualities of human beings. Many in the eugenics movement felt that the continued breeding of humans of lower intelligence would lead to a gradual decline in the general public's overall intelligence. Supporters advocated the sterilization of institutionalized women who were declared mentally impaired based on an IQ test.

Although IQ tests are not without inherent problems, and although abuses have occurred with respect to measuring intelligence, IQ testing remains an accepted scientific procedure. Its value lies in its ability to help make general distinctions with respect to intellectual functioning. As a result, IQ scores play a significant role in distinguishing the potential functional capacities of individuals with mental retardation, a point we will return to later in this chapter.

Cognition and Cognitive Functioning

At one time or another all of us have all been admonished by a parent, teacher, or coach to "c'mon and think!" This admonition carries with it the command to begin a process that requires engagement of our cognitive capacities. *Cognition* refers to our attempts to make sense of incoming information and plot a course of action. In short, cognition is the process of thinking.

According to one prominent set of theorists (Anderson & Bower, 1973; Gagne, 1977; Greeno & Bjork, 1973) thinking or cognitive functioning may best be viewed according to an information-processing model. The information-processing theories postulate that a number of internal structures in the human brain are responsible for the processes corresponding to "thinking." A version of this model is presented in **Figure 2.1**.

As Figure 2.1 shows, receptor organs (i.e., senses) receive stimulation from the environment. Receptor organs are located throughout the body and are specialized in terms of sensations to which they are sensitive. For instance, receptors in the retina are sensitive to light, receptors located under the surface of the skin are sensitive to heat and touch. Since the brain cannot respond directly to environmental stimuli, the receptor organs must transform incoming information into neural impulses. Thus the retina not only collects visual stimuli from the environment, but also transcribes light rays into neural information that can be processed by the brain. This assembled information is then collected

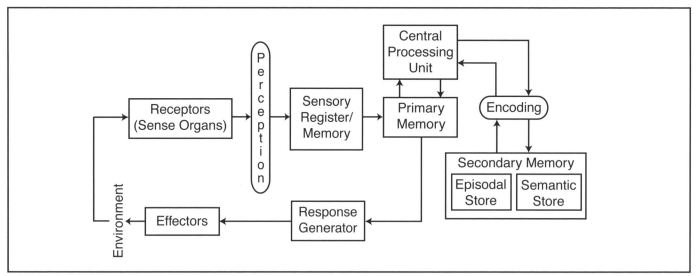

Figure 2.1 Information-processing model representing cognitive functioning (Adapted from Gagne, 1977 and Kaulser, 1982)

in the sensory memory of the brain. The sensory memory is thought to have several sections, one postulated for each sensory modality. Information received in the sensory memory is believed to reside very briefly, stored for perhaps less than a second. Most of the information in sensory memory is lost due to nonuse, but some may pass on to the primary/short-term memory.

Not all information obtained by the senses is recorded in the sensory memory. Some sensory stimuli are unconscious and unperceived. *Perception* consists of consciously appreciated sensory stimuli. It functions like a filter, allowing selected information to pass onto the sensory memory and ignoring other pieces of incoming data. Thus instead of random arrays of stimuli, we perceive patterns of stimulation. This process, known as selective perception, depends on the individual's ability to focus on certain features of the contents of the sensory register while ignoring others (Lindsay & Norman, 1972). Perception may also adjust incoming stimuli to accommodate preconceived ideas or beliefs. For example, perception allows two people cheering opposing basketball teams to see a particular play in an entirely opposite fashion.

Selected pieces of information are transferred to the primary memory (short-term memory) where they persist for only a minimal time. *Primary memory* is theorized to be a temporary stage of holding and organizing information and not necessarily a storage area in the brain. Despite its temporary nature, primary memory is critical for our ability to process new information. Everyone has experienced situations in which they have received a bit of information, such as someone's name or address, used that information immediately, then quickly forgot it. It is believed that the capacity of our primary memory is small, perhaps about seven (plus or minus two) pieces of information (e.g., numbers, words, symbols) at any time. Once this capacity has been reached, old items are pushed out as new ones are added.

When information is received in the primary memory, three options are available. First, if the information must be acted upon, it is passed to the central processing unit that quickly activates an appropriate response. Responding to the question, what is your academic major? would be an example of this option. Second, if no immediate response is required, the information may be temporarily stored. For example, you probably noticed the front page headline if you read this morning's paper, but you may have trouble recalling it now. It was pushed out of the primary memory and forgotten as new stimuli were received. The third option pertains to long-term storage. Information that we deem as important to remember is passed on to our *secondary*

memory and stored for later use. In the transfer from primary to secondary memory, the process of encoding takes place. *Encoding* is the transformation of information into a meaningful, conceptual mode. Data are not stored as sounds or shapes, but as concepts whose meaning is clear and can be easily referenced. We seldom try to memorize every specific detail of new information, rather we try to isolate main themes that enable us to "fill in the details" at a later date.

Kausler (1982) postulated that information within the secondary memory may be stored in either the episodal or semantic store. The *episodal store* contains personal, dated information (e.g., What did you do last Saturday evening? When did you last call your parents?) This is in contrast to the *semantic store* that contains general information (e.g., How much is five times five? What are the six New England states?).

Some researchers have suggested that once information is stored in encoded form in the secondary memory, it is permanently retained (Adams, 1967). While it is presently impossible to determine the actual retention level of stored information, it seems evident that what is stored may eventually become inaccessible. Gagne (1977) believes that at least two factors are responsible for stored data becoming inaccessible: interference between new and old memories and ineffectiveness of the search and retrieve process. When stored information becomes inaccessible, we call the phenomenon forgetting. The opposite of forgetting is, of course, remembering. The process of remembering is essential to learning and depends on the ability to retrieve data from the secondary memory.

> It is generally supposed that the process called retrieval requires certain cues be provided, either by the external situation or by the learner (from other memory sources). The cues are employed to match or "link" what is learned, in a process of search. The entities so located are considered to be "recognized," and may then be retrieved. (Gagne, 1977, p. 55)

Once retrieved, information is returned to primary memory where it becomes readily accessible for use. This use may be either combining the information with other entities to form new concepts to be encoded or activation of the response generator to facilitate bodily performance.

The basic purpose of the response generator is to ensure organized physical performance. To do this, the response generator must first determine the appropriate form of response (e.g., speech, head movement, movement of small or large muscle groups). Second, it must decide on the pattern of movement—the sequence and timing of muscle contractions. After these decisions have been made, the information passed from the response generator activates the effectors that produce externally observed behavior. **Figure 2.2** depicts the process viewed from an input-output perspective. According to the information-processing school, normal cognitive functioning is defined as the ability to:

- Receive accurate information about the environment
- Encode received information in an organized fashion
- Store information in a systematic pattern in the secondary memory
- Initiate an efficient and effective search and retrieval system to recall stored information
- Activate necessary effector organs to produce desired and appropriate motor responses

Factors Affecting Cognition

The process of cognitive functioning described in Figure 2.2 does not operate in isolation. A variety of factors affect the normal process of cognition. We will briefly describe three such factors—attention, expectation, and curiosity/creativity—and highlight the relationship of each to the process of thinking and learning.

Attention

Seldom does a day pass where a teacher does not say to a class, "pay attention to me" or "listen to me" or "look at me." These statements request that learners disregard competing stimuli and concentrate their attention solely on the teacher. The notion of single-mindedness is inherent in the word *attention,* which we will define as the phenomenon in which the sense organs are placed in a state of readiness to be effectively stimulated.

The ability to attend selectively is the most fundamental skill necessary for learning. Intuitively we understand that we are able to concentrate more intently on some task when distracting stimuli are removed from our environment. The more difficult the task, the greater need for selective attention. Consequently, an individual unable to focus his or her attention selectively will have difficulty in terms of cognitive functioning.

Expectations

Expectations may be described as our estimate of the probability of some occurrence based on *experience.* Psychological research has demonstrated that when we expect to have some control over the outcome of a situation, this influences our motivation to affect the outcome (Seligman, 1975). For example, most college students believe they have both strengths and weaknesses in terms of coursework in various fields. A student who had difficulty in math courses in high school would probably approach college-level math requirements with the expectation of mediocre grades in math classes. This expectation would be associated with a mind-set like this: Even if I study very hard in this course I'm probably not going to get a good grade since I'm not good at math. Thus, I will work hard enough to pass the course, but I'll work harder in other courses in which I have a better chance of getting an A.

Julian Rotter (1954) explored the association between expectations and learning outcomes. He theorized that two extremes of learning styles exist based on expectations. *Success-strivers* expect to succeed in most learning situations. These individuals seem undaunted by occasional failure and are highly motivated to do well. In contrast, *failure-avoiders* are uncertain about their ability to succeed but are motivated to enter into situations with the intent of avoiding failure or the appearance of failure.

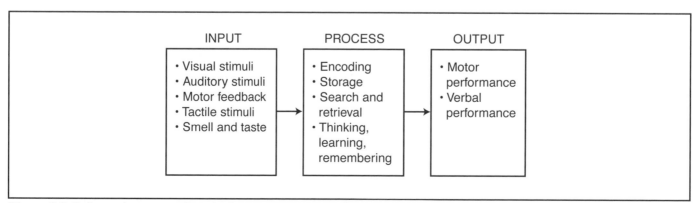

Figure 2.2 Information processing: An input-output perspective

In summary, our expectations can influence the process of cognition. The expectancy of success contributes to our motivation and the cognitive effort we put forth. Conversely, the expectancy of failure leads to diminished motivation and the increased likelihood of poor performance.

Curiosity and Creativity

We will deal with these two forms of behavior together. *Curiosity* is a form of exploratory behavior directed toward seeking more information about a stimulus field. An infant fingering a block, rolling it in his hand, rubbing it through his hair, and attempting to chew on it, displays curiosity. *Creativity* is a form of exploratory behavior marked by efforts directed toward changing and/or interpreting a stimulus field. Professional photographers view the same sunset as the average individual, but they are often able to film the sunset in a way which is more appealing than the photo taken by you or me. Due to their creative instincts the photographers have altered the stimulus field (the sunset) by shading, the use of light, and the incorporation of other details to interpret the scene in a unique fashion.

Curiosity and creativity relate in an important way: Curiosity fosters creativity by providing information about objects that cannot be gathered without exploration. Furthermore, both curiosity and creativity relate to cognitive functioning—they impact the quantity and quality of information processed.

Development in the Cognitive Domain

The process of development in the cognitive domain has attracted the attention of psychologists and educators for well over 100 years. Although a number of theories explaining this process have been advanced, the work of the Swiss educator Jean Piaget usually receives the most attention.

Piaget (1952) viewed development as an inherent, evolutionary process that varies little from culture to culture. Piaget believed that cognitive development may be divided into a series of distinct phases marked by a homogeneous cognitive pattern for the entire period. Each of the phases can further be divided into subphases in which smaller steps toward the final pattern are achieved. The completion of the one phase creates an imbalance that then begins a new phase. For example, once an infant realizes that his or her mother

exists even when she is out of sight, this leads to questions about where she is when she cannot be seen. Piaget believed in absolute continuity between all developmental phases and that each level of development is rooted in the previous phase.

Piaget perceived cognitive development as a continuous process of generalization to differentiation. He used the terms assimilation and accommodation to describe this process. *Assimilation* refers to the incorporation of a new object, experience, or concept into a child's existing perception. For instance, the first time a child views a small, flying creature a caretaker may identify it as a bird. The child is said to have assimilated that concept (bird) if it is retained in his or her memory. *Accommodation* is the process by which a child changes his thoughts or actions to manage new objects or situations. Thus, once the concept of bird is assimilated in a child's mind, he or she would likely identify all flying creatures as birds. Eventually, however, he or she realizes that small creatures other than birds may also fly (e.g., insects) and he or she also learns to distinguish between different species of birds. The incorporation of these new concepts into an existing perception requires the modification of the old perception (accommodation).

Piaget divided the process of intellectual development into four phases:

- Sensorimotor (birth to 2 years)
- Preoperational (2 to 7 years)
- Concrete operations (7 to 12 years)
- Formal operations (12+ years)

While chronological ages are used in reference to each phase, Piaget suggested that they only be used as general markers of progress. More meaningful with respect to cognitive development was the level of progress a person demonstrated through the identified phases.

Sensorimotor Phase (Birth to 2 Years)

This early phase is characterized by the use of one's senses and motor abilities to learn about the world. Being told that an object is round, soft, or smooth does not mean anything to an infant. Infants learn about their world by experiencing it through their senses and motor skills. During the sensorimotor stage, primitive forms of intelligence are evident. Even before a child is able to use language well, he or she exhibits some complex behavior. The child begins to coordinate activities to reach certain goals, such as pulling a string to reach a brightly colored ring attached to it. In addition, the child gradually becomes more interested in the world and less self-absorbed. In exploring the environment, the child, through experimentation, finds ways of acting and relating to achieve goals. For example, an 18-month-old child may want something out of reach. To do this, he or she finds a chair or stool and climbs on it to reach the desired object. The child is beginning to find solutions to concrete problems. However, the child still cannot generalize what is learned to new situations. Most discoveries are made through trial and error. The three major cognitive acquisitions of the sensorimotor phase (Piaget, 1952) include the ability to:

- Coordinate and integrate information from all five senses
- Exhibit goal-directed behavior
- Recognize the world as a permanent place (Piaget called this *object permanence* and said that without this ability concepts such as space, time, and causality would not be possible.)

Preoperational Phase (2 to 7 Years)

The preoperational phase is characterized by the use of meaningful language. In the sensorimotor phase, the child deals with visible objects. With the use of language the child can use symbols to represent objects that are not present. For example, at this age, a child may pretend a mud pie is a chocolate bar and may also pretend to eat it. A child at age three can make up a story and may reconstruct the recent past and project into the very near future. Even with the use of language and the ability to think in more abstract terms, the preoperational phase of development remains a relatively primitive type of intelligence. Although the child is beginning to be able to classify and group objects, he or she is not yet proficient at it. Also, while the child can distinguish between certain quantities— for example, big versus little—he or she is not yet able to perform the operation of conservation. A child of four, for example, believes that when water is poured from a tall, thin glass into a widemouthed, shorter glass, there is less water. He or she is taken in by the appearance of more water. The ability to understand that quantity cannot be judged by appearance alone is refined during the phase of concrete operations. Individuals with more severe forms of mental retardation seldom move beyond this level of development. The two major cognitive acquisitions of the preoperational phase (Piaget, 1952) include the ability to:

- Think symbolically and use symbols (language) as the primary means of communication.
- View actions sequentially

Concrete Operations Phase (7 to 12 Years)

During the stage of concrete operations, a child becomes better able to order and classify objects and to see relationships between different items. For example, a 9-year-old can speak of one object as being wider than another and shorter than something else. A child at this point also can arrange objects according to size or weight and can divide something into its parts. Children in this stage of development are able to solve some mathematical problems and to read well. They also are able to generalize learning to new situations and to begin to appreciate another person's point of view. However, these children still have difficulty dealing with hypothetical problems. In addition, although children in this stage are better able to understand the concept of past and future, this understanding is somewhat limited. Individuals with mild retardation usually remain at this level of development. The three major cognitive acquisitions of the concrete operations phase (Piaget, 1952) include the ability to:

- Move from the actual, present, and concrete to other places and times
- Perform adult activities like classifying, serializing, and looking at various aspects of a situation
- Diminish egocentrism as thoughts become more logical

Formal Operations Phase (12 Years and Beyond)

Piaget's final stage of intellectual development proceeds from age 12 throughout one's life. During the stage of formal operations, individuals are able to project themselves into the future and to think about long-term goals. They also develop sensitivity to the feelings of others and become increasingly self-conscious. They develop the ability to reason using hypotheses. For example, if Jim is taller than Tom and shorter than Fred, who is the shortest of all three? To solve this problem, a child must be able to form a system that includes all possible combinations of each element. As another example, a child may be asked to determine how many combinations can be formed with three colors. Once again, the child must be able to figure out all the possible combinations of the three colors to arrive at an answer. The use of higher mathematics is also possible. Development of formal thought involves the ability to isolate a problem, to review it systematically, and to figure out all possible solutions to that problem.

Thus, Piaget's perspective on intellectual development involves the addition of more complex and abstract abilities with each stage. The child progresses from one stage to another. A person who is unable to progress through all the stages is limited in his or her ability to adapt as an adult (Piaget, 1952).

Developmental Disabilities

The term *developmentally disabled* first appeared in federal legislation of 1970—the Developmental Disabilities Assistance Bill of Rights Act (Public Law 94-103). The act brought three major disorders under a single federal legislative umbrella: mental retardation, cerebral palsy, and epilepsy. It also included all other neurological conditions occurring before age 18 that produce similar consequences (i.e., compromised ability to function independently). The legislation intended to bring together under one law disability groups that have comparable service needs. Following enactment of the law, however, there continued to be discussion as to the usefulness of the designation and whether other disabilities also should be included. Subsequently, both autism and severe dyslexia were added. This was soon followed by a decision to give up a categorical definition (one that identified the disabilities by their traditional names) and to substitute for it a functional definition (one that focused on their common adaptive problems). This was accomplished with the enactment of the Rehabilitation, Comprehensive Services, and Developmental Disabilities Amendments of 1978 (Public Law 95-602). Disavowing any reference to specific conditions, the current definition directs our attention exclusively to the effects of these and related disabilities, especially when they are severe and chronic in nature. A *developmental disability* is now defined as a severe and chronic disorder involving mental and/or physical impairment that originates before age 22. Such a disorder is likely to persist indefinitely and cause substantial functional limitations in at least three of seven areas of major life activity, including self-care, receptive and expressive language, learning, mobility, self-direction, capacity for independent living, and economic self-sufficiency. Developmental disability is a broad term that incorporates a variety of different conditions. In this chapter our focus will be limited to mental retardation.

Mental Retardation

The concept of mental retardation has undergone many changes over the past half century. Such changes have been motivated by the desire to improve our understanding of the condition and avoid dehumanization of individuals afflicted by the condition. Terms such as *moron*, *imbecile*, and *idiot* are no longer used to classify individuals with mental retardation. According to Schalock and colleagues (1994) current thinking emphasizes:

> the conception of mental retardation not as an absolute trait expressed solely by the person, but as an expression of the functional impact of the interaction between the person with limited intellectual and adaptive skills and that person's environment. (p. 81)

This perspective suggests that the condition of mental retardation is most appropriately viewed as only one characteristic that affects an individual in terms of his or her functional interaction with his or her environment. Such a view helps to avoid stereotypic generalizations about retardation and respects the dignity of individuals who may be affected by this condition.

The definition of mental retardation as advanced by the American Association on Mental Retardation (AAMR) in 1992 reads:

> Mental retardation refers to substantial limitations in present functioning. It is characterized by significantly subaverage intellectual functioning, existing concurrently with related limitations in two or more of the following applicable adaptive skill areas: communication, self-care, home living, social skills, community use, self-direction, health and safety, functional academics, leisure and work. Mental retardation manifests before age 18. (p. 1)

A careful reading of this definition reveals emphasis being place on three characteristics:

1. Significantly subaverage intellectual functioning

2. Impairments in at least two adaptive skill areas

3. Manifestation before age 18 (during the developmental period)

Intellectual Functioning

Identification of significantly subaverage intellectual functioning occurs when a person receives a score on standardized IQ test that is below the average score to such a degree (two standard deviations) that society has determined this person requires assistance beyond what is typically provided by the family and community. The average intelligence quotient has been determined to be a score of approximately 100. A score below approximately 70–75 results in significantly subaverage intellectual function.

Adaptive Skills

The ability of an individual to adapt to the demands of his or her environment has long been associated with retardation. This 1992 definition helped to refine the concept of adaptive behavior by identifying 10 specific skill areas, which may be considered a collection of individual competencies. Specific adaptive limitations often coexist with strengths in other adaptive skills or personal capabilities. Recognition of individual strengths or limitations may help identify the person's individual needs for appropriate community support.

Leisure was identified as adaptive skill area. According to the AAMR (1992) leisure as an adaptive skill area is described as:

> the development of a variety of leisure and recreational interests (i.e., self-entertainment and interactional) that reflect personal preferences and choices and, if the activity will be conducted in public, age and cultural norms. Skills include choosing and self-initiating interests, using and enjoying home and community leisure and recreational activities alone and with others, playing socially with others, taking turns, terminating or refusing leisure or recreational activities, extending one's duration of participation, and expanding one's repertoire of interests, awareness, and skills. Related skills include behaving appropriately in the leisure and recreation setting, communicating choices and needs, participating in social interaction, applying functional academics, and exhibiting mobility skills. (p. 41)

Manifestation

The developmental period refers to the time after conception when growth and change occur at a rapid rate. This rate of development typically begins to slow as the person enters adulthood. For legislative purposes (e.g., the Developmental Disabilities Act), the oldest a person can be to receive a diagnosis of mental retardation is 18 years (AAMR, 1992). According to the AAMR (1992, p. 9) mental retardation begins in childhood when "limitations in intelligence coexist with related limitations in adaptive skills. In this sense, it is a more

specific term than developmental disability because the level of functioning is necessarily related to an intellectual limitation."

The AAMR (1992) has made it clear that the application of its definition of mental retardation rests upon several assumptions, including:

- Intelligence as defined by tests has limited use
- Valid assessment (of retardation) considers cultural and linguistic diversity, as well as differences in communication and behavioral factors
- Mental retardation is most meaningfully conceptualized as a phenomenon existing within the society which can only be observed through the depressed performance on measures of cognitive functioning by some of the individuals of that society
- With appropriate supports over a sustained period, the life functioning of the person with mental retardation will generally improve

The label *mental retardation* is simply that, a label. It is one characteristic that may be used to describe an individual. Appropriate and effective human services should be based on the profile of cognitive, affective, and psychomotor characteristics, not a single trait or condition.

Prevalence of Mental Retardation

Prevalence refers to the total number of cases of a disorder existing within a population at a particular place or at a particular time (*Dorland's Medical Dictionary,* 1957). Prevalence rates are usually expressed as percentages. While prevalence statistics are helpful in determining the need for services, variations in estimates of the prevalence of mental retardation have been found across studies and populations. Some of the factors that influence prevalence estimates are described here.

Definition and Method Variations

Prevalence figures vary in part due to the imprecision in defining mental retardation. Most prevalence surveys are conducted by reviewing case files, analyzing agency referral data, or counting tabulated census data. Few studies actually locate the subjects for testing or interviewing. As can be expected, prevalence figures differ markedly, based on the method used to calculate them. If IQ were the only criterion for defining this condition, approximately 3% of the population could be considered mentally retarded (Beirne-Smith, Patton & Ittenbach, 1994). However, the validity of the often-cited figure of 3% prevalence has been repeatedly challenged. Tarjan, Wright, Eyman, and Keeran (1973) have convincingly argued that the assumptions upon which the 3% figure is based are not supported by clinical evidence. They suggest that many individuals who score significantly low on psychometric tests of IQ do not show major impairment in general adaptation, which must appear concurrently with subaverage intellectual functioning for the diagnosis of mental retardation to be made. Moreover, the researchers argued that mortality in individuals with mental retardation is inversely related to IQ (i.e., the lower the IQ score, the higher the mortality). Consequently, although 3% of the newborn population may be diagnosed as mentally retarded at some time during its life, it is incorrect to assume that at any given time 3% of the overall population can be diagnosed as retarded (p. 370).

Gender Variations

Males are consistently identified as mentally retarded at higher rates than females. These sex differences in prevalence may be explained by at least two factors. First, biological defects associated with the X chromosomes have a greater probability of being manifested by males than by females. Second, it appears that differences in societal expectations and child-rearing practices are associated with sex differences in prevalence rates. This is particularly true of aggressive behavior that is typically reinforced in males but not in females. Acting upon aggressive impulses in social situations (especially in school settings) often leads to a perception of general behavior problems. A child identified as a behavioral problem has a greater chance of also being identified as retarded (Musland, Sarason & Gladwin, 1958).

Socioeconomic Variations

Socioeconomic conditions within communities also relate to differences in prevalence rates. Children born and reared in deprived, lower socioeconomic groups are 15 times more likely to be labeled mentally retarded than children from the suburbs (Tarjan et al., 1973). Prevalence figures indicate that as the severity of retardation increases cultural and socioeconomic factors become less pronounced. In other words, just as many wealthy families as poor families have children with severe retardation.

To summarize, in terms of prevalence accurate estimates are extremely difficult to determine. Definition, method, gender, and socioeconomic factors influence estimates. When all evidence is considered, most professionals believe prevalence rates to be less than 1%, not the commonly cited 3% (Bierne-Smith et al., 1994).

Causes of Mental Retardation

Mental retardation may arise from either biological or psychosocial causes. Biological causes involve damage to the brain and may be due to heredity, chromosomal abnormalities, or events occurring during pregnancy, at birth, or in early childhood. Damage to the brain after early childhood tends to produce specific rather than general impairment, such as paralysis and speech disorders following a stroke. If the brain damage is massive, however, there is often widespread loss of previous mental functioning and the creation of states either characterized as mental retardation or equivalent to it. Psychosocial causes refer to retardation in nonorganically impaired children, generally from impoverished families in which retardation is also found in parents and siblings (Grossman, 1983).

Biological Causes

Genes and Chromosomes

From conception events can occur that will adversely affect brain development. Some forms of retardation are hereditary, transmitted from parents to children through the genes in the reproductive cells. Most often the mode of transmission is recessive, which means that carrier parents are not affected and the children have a one in four risk of inheriting the disorder. Recessive disorders have been clearly tied to gene-caused biochemical abnormalities. Phenylketonuria is one of the best-known forms.

Phenylketonuria (PKU), an amino acid disorder, is the most common genetic-metabolic disorder associated with retardation. The condition of PKU develops when the body is unable to metabolize phenylalanine in high-protein foods such as dairy products. It is frequently associated with aggressiveness, hyperactivity, destructiveness, and other disruptive behaviors. Treatment for PKU involves diet control, which has produced positive results in a number of studies (Koch et al., 1988).

Since first described in the 1930s, PKU has been virtually eliminated as a causative factor in severe retardation, despite its incidence of one in every 12,000 to

15,000 births (Beirne-Smith et al., 1994). Menolascino and Egger (1978) noted that PKU has played a significant role in the field because it was the first inborn metabolic anomaly proven to cause retardation. Its discovery led to both increased research into etiology and a pronounced change in hopelessness that once surrounded retardation (Beirne-Smith et al., 1994).

Apart from gene-determined disorders, abnormalities of the chromosomes (structures on which genes are found) may themselves cause retardation. The best known chromosomal disorder is _Down syndrome_, a condition caused by the presence of an extra chromosome number 21. This condition is by far the most prevalent and most frequently researched type of biologically caused retardation. For many laypersons, the concept of a person with mental retardation is virtually synonymous with a Down syndrome child. A reasonable estimate of the prevalence of the syndrome is 5% to 6% of all persons diagnosed as having retardation.

Down syndrome is frequently associated with specific physical characteristics, including:

- Short stature
- Flat, broad face
- Small ears and nose
- Short, broad hands with incurving fingers
- Upward slanting of the eyes with folds of skins (epicanthic folds) at the inside corner of the eye
- Small mouth and short roof (may cause the tongue to protrude and contribute to articulation problems)
- Single crease across the palm
- Reduced muscle tone (hypotonia)
- Hyperflexibility of joints
- Heart defects (in about one third of instances)
- Increased susceptibility to upper respiratory infections
- Incomplete or delayed sexual development

These traits vary greatly from one individual to another. Contrary to popular opinion, the number of physical characteristics present does not predict the level of intelligence (Belmont, 1971). Many of the behavioral characteristics traditionally associated with Down syndrome have generally not been documented in research. In particular, the stereotype of the child with Down syndrome who is cheerful, affectionate, rhythmic, and unusually dexterous has not been empirically established (Belmont, 1971). Traditionally, the syndrome had been assumed to result most often in moderate retardation, with a ceiling IQ of 70. However,

it has been speculated that with successful early intervention many Down syndrome children can function at a higher IQ level (Rynders, Spiker, & Horrobian, 1978).

A second chromosomal abnormality associated with mental retardation is _fragile X syndrome_. This syndrome is caused by the loss of a small part of the X chromosome. After Down syndrome, fragile X syndrome is likely the most common clinical type of retardation (de la Cruz, 1985) and the most common hereditary cause of retardation (Lachiewicz, Harrison, Spridigliozzi, Callahan & Livermore, 1988). Because fragile X is associated with the X chromosome, it is typically more common in males than in females.

Common characteristics of fragile X include prominent jaw, macro-orchidism (large testes), long thin face, long and soft ears and hands, prominent forehead, and enlarged head. The syndrome has been associated in males with severe and profound levels of retardation, although reports of its occurrence in individuals with various levels of retardation suggest the need for caution in making such generalizations (Rogers & Simensen, 1987).

Normal cells have 46 chromosomes—44 autosomes (which determine an individual's inherited characteristics) and 2 sex chromosomes (which determine if an individual is male or female). Abnormalities in the sex chromosomes (as opposed to the autosomes) have also been found to affect development adversely and sometimes cause mental retardation. One example of this situation is _Klinefelter syndrome_, a condition in which males receive an extra X chromosome, so they have an XXY arrangement. The clinical pattern of the syndrome includes social retardation, sterility and underdevelopment of the male sex organs, and the acquisition of female secondary sex characteristics. The syndrome is often association with borderline or mild levels of intellectual retardation.

Congenital Factors

This category of factors includes a wide variety of harmful agents—_teratogens_—known to cause malformations in a developing embryo. Teratogens can significantly affect the development of a child at prenatal or postnatal levels and result in mental retardation in some cases. Factors proven to have teratogenic effects may be subdivided into several broad categories: maternal health, substance exposure, prematurity and perinatal concerns, and postnatal biological concerns.

Maternal Health

The first three months of pregnancy are critical to future development. During this time the fetus's developing brain is very susceptible to malformation. Infection of the mother by *rubella* (German measles) early in pregnancy has been found to result in fetal defects (including retardation) in up to 50% of all cases (Beirne-Smith et al., 1994). *Congenital syphilis* (as well as other venereal diseases) can damage the central nervous system and cause severe retardation in an offspring. A third known cause of retardation, although not a disease, is blood-group incompatibility. Commonly referred to as *Rh incompatibility,* this condition is caused by antibodies in a mother's blood attacking the central nervous system of the developing fetus. Rh incompatibility causes an estimated 10,000 stillbirths and 20,000 babies born with epilepsy, cerebral palsy, hearing impairments, and/or retardation each year (Menolascino & Egger, 1978).

Substance Exposure

Exposure to substances such as industrial chemicals, alcohol, lysergic acid (LSD), and other related drugs has also been linked to mental retardation. Of these teratogens, the best-studied association is between alcohol and retardation. The condition known as *fetal alcohol syndrome* results from a fetus being exposed to alcohol from a mother's heavy consumption. The alcohol's toxic effect on the fetus's brain results in a recognizable pattern of brain malformation and developmental disability.

Prematurity and Perinatal Concerns

An established link exists between prematurity and mental retardation. The greater the deviation away from normal term pregnancies (37 to 41 weeks) and normal birthweight (5.5 pounds and above) the greater the risk of mental retardation. Oxygen deprivation (anoxia) at birth can result from such difficulties as knotted umbilical cord, extremely short or long labor, or breech birth, and has been identified as a causative agent in more than 18% of cases of mild retardation (McLaren & Bryson, 1987).

Postnatal Biological Concerns

A variety of traumatic events occurring after birth may also cause retardation. Among the most common of these events are head injuries, child abuse, lead poisoning, and severe nutritional deprivation. In each situation damage to the brain either directly or indirectly impairs its ability to respond in an appropriate cognitive manner resulting in the diagnosis of mental retardation.

Psychosocial Causes

The Environment and Cognitive Development

Although there is no doubt that biological damage to the brain can cause mental retardation, one could ask whether a child's psychological environment also can produce a similar effect. While the research that relates to this question is less explicit than its biological counterpart, the evidence from a number of lines of study indicates that it can. The strongest evidence for the effect of environment on intelligence is found in studies of twins, especially identical twins separated in childhood and reared in different homes. The rationale of twin research is that differences between identical (monozygotic) twins, products of a single fertilized egg, must be nongenetic or environmental in origin because the twins are genetically identical. On the other hand, differences between fraternal (dizygotic) twins, products of two different fertilized eggs, may be genetic or environmental. Fraternal twins are not more alike genetically than ordinary single-born siblings; they just happened to have been conceived at the same time. Studies of IQ differences among identical twins reared apart reveal that they are greater than among identical twins reared together, evidence of an environmental effect (Erlenmeyer-Kimling & Jarvik, 1963; Jensen, 1971). However, if only the environment influenced intelligence, fraternal twins reared in the same home would be more similar than identical twins reared apart. This is not the case. Identical twins reared apart are actually more similar in IQ than fraternal twins reared together, evidence for a genetic effect. Both heredity and environment influence mental development.

Environmental Correlates

A child's environment can either enhance or depress intelligence, and that may make the difference between normal ability and mental retardation. Environmental causes have most often been associated with mild retardation. Psychosocial retardation has been closely linked to a number of variables that can occur in an environment of poverty. The common estimate that approximately 25% of all American preschoolers belong to families with incomes below the poverty level highlights the immensity of this problem (Beirne-Smith et al., 1994).

Many variables associated with poverty may place children at risk for school failure and identification with mental retardation. Within the poverty environment a lack of stimulation or excessive or inappropriate stimulation may interfere with cognitive development. Kagan

(1970) focused on several key psychological differences between children of lower socioeconomic class and those more privileged. He asserted that these differences emerge during the first three years of life and are stable over time. He identified seven major psychological differences between the two groups: language, mental set, attachment, inhibition, sense of effectiveness, motivation, and expectancy of failure. Garber (1988) draws attention to the poverty-bound mother with low IQ and limited verbal skills who cannot effectively mediate the environment for her child. All the variables may directly or indirectly influence school performance, and deficits in them can also limit a child's problem-solving skills.

In a lower socioeconomic environment, one parent (frequently the father) is often absent and the child rearing falls more heavily on the mother. The large number of children in many of these families aggravates the problem, and the potential result is a decrease in each child's direct, individual contact with adult role models.

Children born to teenage mothers run an especially high risk of subsequent difficulties. As Berg and Emanuel (1987) noted in their review:

> Teenage mothers as a group are at elevated risk for producing low birth weight babies: the younger the mother, the higher the risk. . . . A number of studies have found lower IQs among the offspring of teenage mothers and have attributed this association primarily to social disadvantages . . . Even if there is no biological factor, the multiple social and personal problems associated with teenage pregnancy indicate the need to discourage reproduction in this age group. (pp. 50–51)

The practical problems of making ends meet for persons living in poverty are often overlooked. The time and effort that middle-class parents spend to motivate and stimulate children may, in a lower-class home, need to be devoted to finding a job, finding suitable housing, and arranging childcare. Where poverty is the overriding concern, other priorities may mean that getting a child to preschool on time or following through on school lessons at home may be problematic.

Health problems can compound the detrimental effects of poverty. Particular concerns include nutritional deficiencies, lack of resistance to disease, exposure to toxic substances, and inadequate medical care. Although these are biological concerns, they tend to appear with a host of psychosocial factors and may jeopardize mental development.

One final consideration concerns variations in educational opportunities. In *Savage Inequalities: Children in America's Schools* (1991), Kozol concluded that vast differences exist between educational resources and opportunities in the nation's most affluent communities and its poorest. Poverty increases the likelihood of school failure. It becomes a vicious cycle as educational failure increases the risk of poverty.

In summation, evidence suggests a linkage between poverty and retardation. However, it is essential to clarify that the overwhelming majority of individuals reared in lower socioeconomic class homes *do not* experience mental retardation. More research is needed to help identify the specific factors that underscore this general linkage.

Classification Systems for Mental Retardation

Mental retardation has been classified in a number of different ways. In the past, *idiot* was used to refer to people of all levels of mental retardation. Idiocy derives from the Greek word *idiotes,* meaning a layman or unskilled worker, and was used to describe untrained or ignorant people until the 17th century. One of the first classification systems, developed in France in the 1830s by Esquirol, was based upon the individual's ability to use language. This system used two levels of classification: an *imbecile* could verbally communicate, albeit at an immature level; an *idiot* could use only single words and grunts and never developed adult speech patterns (Beirne-Smith et al., 1994).

J. Langdon Down developed a classification system in the 1850s based upon etiology. According to Down's system retardation could be divided into three categories:

- Congenital idiocy (retardation evident at birth or soon after)

- Developmental idiocy (appeared normal during infancy but retardation developed during childhood)

- Accidental idiocy (retardation as a result of an accident)

During the 1920s, the American Association for the Study of the Feebleminded (which later became the American Association on Mental Deficiency and is now known as the American Association on Mental Retardation) used IQ scores to classify retardation into three levels:

- Moron (IQ score 50–75)

- Imbecile (IQ score 25–49)

- Idiot (IQ score 24 or below)

Another classification system, popular in school settings, developed with the expansion of special education programs during the 1960s. This system attempted to assess educational potential based upon one's measured IQ. The terms used in this system included:

- Educable—could profit from an academically oriented curriculum (IQ score 50–75)
- Trainable—programs emphasized training in basic functional skills (IQ score 25–40)
- Custodial—would likely not benefit from educational training at any level (IQ score 24 and below)

Lately, these terms have fallen into disfavor with most professionals; however, they remain in use in some locations.

The system of terminology that remains in most common use classifies levels of retardation using the following categories:

- Mild (IQ score 52–68)
- Moderate (IQ score 36–52)
- Severe (IQ score 20–36)
- Profound (IQ score 20 and below)

The American Association on Mental Deficiency first adopted this classification system in 1961, and it dominated the literature on mental retardation until its revision in 1992. Concerned over the consequences of classifying individuals using inherently negative terminology, the American Association on Mental Retardation (AAMR) moved away from this classification system in that year.

The AAMR manual published in 1992 abandoned the system based on IQ levels and instead focused upon classifying the services or supports needed by individuals. The ninth edition of the AAMR manual suggests adoption of a system describing levels of support as a function of the different adaptive skill areas. The levels of support have been defined and described by the AAMR (1992, p. 26) as:

- Intermittent—Support on an as needed basis. Characterized by episodic nature, person not always needing the support(s), or short-term supports needed during life span transitions (e.g., job loss or an acute medical crisis). Intermittent supports may be high or low intensity when provided.
- Limited—Intensity of support characterized by consistency over time, time-limited but not of an intermittent nature. May require fewer staff members and less cost than more intense levels of support (e.g., time-limited employment training or transitional supports during the school to adult provided period).
- Extensive—Support characterized by regular involvement (e.g., daily) in at least some environments (such as work or home) and not time-limited (e.g., long-term support and long-term home living support).
- Pervasive—Support characterized by their constancy, high intensity, and potential life-sustaining nature. Pervasive supports typically involve more staff members and intrusiveness than do extensive or time-limited supports.

This system explains a person's functional limitations in terms of the degree of support he or she needs to achieve personal growth and development. It represents "a shift toward understanding mental retardation as a multidimensional concept that requires comprehensive assessment, rather than reliance on intelligence tests as a primary indicator of mental retardation" (Datillo, 1996, p. 133).

Whether this newest classification system will achieve acceptance remains to be seen. Without question, it will take some time for it to be used formally, especially by governmental agencies and professionals used to the familiar classification levels. For the remainder of this chapter we will integrate the two systems to address the recreation implications of working with people who have mental retardation. After first describing some general characteristics associated with all levels of retardation, we will next subdivide mental retardation into two broad categories that we shall discuss in more detail: mild and severe.

General Characteristics Associated With Mental Retardation

The accepted definition of mental retardation (AAMR, 1992) clearly points to deficiencies in two general areas of functioning: cognitive abilities and adaptive behavior. While deficiencies may vary by level of retardation, most individuals with mental retardation demonstrate a quality of thinking and mode of behavior characterized by similar traits.

Deficiencies in Cognitive Abilities

Individuals who experience mental retardation are more *suggestible* than nonretarded individuals; they are more easily influenced by external factors (Zigler, 1966). This vulnerability has at least two bases. First, retarded individuals have particular difficulty in considering more than one factor at a time in complex situations—they tend to center attention on only one aspect. Piaget referred to this as *egocentric thought*, which happens to be characteristic of the normal preschool-age child

(Piaget, 1952). A second source of greater suggestibility relates to the usual life experience of the average person with mental retardation. The chronic frustration in coping that people with retardation usually experience is bound to diminish self-confidence and to cause a great reliance on others. This is particularly true in unfamiliar situations where there is reduced confidence in one's own abilities (Balla, Styfco & Zigler, 1971).

In addition to suggestibility, individuals with retardation often demonstrate *passivity of thought* (Baroff, 1986). When a nonretarded person is confronted with a problem, he or she "sizes it up" and decides what will help to solve it. Such a person may seek more information, call on others for assistance, or even try to modify the problem to make it less complex. People with mental retardation, however, seem to lack awareness that they might create ways in which to help themselves. This has been shown in studies of memory in which there is an apparent lack of understanding of how material to be remembered might be organized to facilitate retention. Although persons with mental retardation know that they will be asked to recall something on a test, for example, they seem to be unaware that rehearsal or repetition of the material that will aid retention (Baroff, 1991).

Persons with mental retardation seem to lack *critical judgment* in their thinking. They may appear careless and indifferent to inconsistencies (Baroff, 1986). Perhaps this quality, too, is a reflection of a history of difficulty with thinking kinds of activities. Any solution, irrespective of quality, becomes a way of terminating an anxiety-arousing situation.

Individuals with mental retardation display *situation-specific thinking*. They often have difficulty generalizing or applying what has been learned in one setting to a different but comparable one. They are unable to ignore surface differences and to recognize underlying similarities. When asked how a fish and a bird are alike, a child diagnosed as mildly retarded may insist that they are not alike since "a fish swims in the water, and a bird flies in the air." The difference in the environment, rather than their underlying similarities as animals, dominates his or her thinking.

Another aspect of this *concreteness* is seen in the way that individuals with mental retardation interpret proverbs. Persons with retardation do not recognize that the language of a proverb is not to be taken literally, but rather understood at a symbolic level. Thus "a stitch in time" is likely to be understood as relating to the maintenance of clothing rather than a general warning about the value of prevention.

The future has no current reality—it is only hypothetical, to be imagined. Planning and foresight deal with the future; they are concerned with possibilities rather than realities. They are also affected by one's ability to consider multiple possibilities. We have already mentioned the tendency of people with retardation to focus upon only one aspect of a situation at a time. All this has the effect of limiting the person's capacity to think and plan ahead.

Another consequence of concreteness of thought is to limit imagination, the faculty that enables individuals without retardation to go beyond that which is directly given to the senses and to create something new. Although some people with mental retardation show true creative talents in music and art (the so-called idiot savant) as a rule these abilities are also diminished (Hill, 1974).

Deficiencies in Adaptive Behavior

The definition of mental retardation includes a reference to adaptive behavior as well as subaverage intelligence. Adaptive behavior refers to the degree to which one's behavior reflects the standards of personal and social responsibility expected for one's age and cultural group (Grossman, 1983). Measures of adaptive behavior give particular weight to age-related expectations in personal independence and self-sufficiency, traditional hallmarks distinguishing persons identified as mentally retarded from those who are not. The inclusion of adaptive behavior as a criterion for classification as mentally retarded also implies that not all persons with subaverage intelligence will show a major impairment in adaptive behavior. This is a distinction that particularly applies to socioeconomically disadvantaged individuals who test in the mildly retarded intelligence range but who are free of any organic basis for their intellectual impairment. Their primary adaptive behavior deficit will be in the academic realm; in other areas of general functioning they will perform much like their peers, although such people are more likely to be followers than leaders and to be perceived as "slow" (Baroff, 1991).

Forms of Mental Retardation

Persons with mental retardation demonstrate tremendous variability with respect to individual traits and characteristics. It is reasonable, nonetheless, to generalize about characteristics of persons with retardation if we distinguish between two groups: those with milder forms of retardation and those with more severe retardation. The primary difference between these two groups is the degree of deficiencies possessed (i.e., the degree of deviation from societal norms). We will first identify some basic characteristics of those with milder forms of retardation and then discuss people with more severe forms of retardation.

Characteristics of Mild Retardation

Using the classification system developed by American Association on Mental Retardation in 1961, the category of mild retardation referred to an individual with a measured IQ range of 52 to 68. Under current (1992) AAMR guidelines, the term mild has been replaced by intermittent, which refers to the provision of support as needed. Individuals who have milder forms of mental retardation can function independently most of the time and when support is needed, it tends to be episodic and short-term. Nonetheless, these individuals tend to have some general characteristics that distinguish them from both the more severely mentally retarded and their nonretarded peers. In this section we will describe some of the basic characteristics of persons who require intermittent care.

Socioeconomic Characteristics

The higher prevalence of milder forms of mental retardation among low-income families has been acknowledged for some time (Westling, 1986). In contrast, socioeconomic conditions do not seem to affect the prevalence of those with more extensive forms of retardation.

Environmental deprivation is recognized by the AAMR in its inclusion of "psychosocial disadvantage" as an etiological category. Individuals who experience impoverished environmental conditions involving poor housing, inadequate nutrition, or inadequate medical care are at greater risk of being identified with mental retardation. Lack of a stimulating, learning-oriented home environment may contribute to educational deficits associated with retardation.

A study conducted by the U. S. Department of Education (1992) associated the following variables with increased likelihood of being diagnosed with mental retardation among secondary school youth: living in a single-parent home, lower socioeconomic status, and lower household income.

Motivational Characteristics

Persons with milder forms of mental retardation have the same basic emotional needs as do all individuals; however, they experience failure far more often (especially in academic settings) than their nonretarded peers. As a consequence, they are much more likely to view new situations as threats rather than challenges. When a situation is viewed as threatening, one is usually motivated by the basic instinct to survive. A challenging situation, on the other hand, usually motivates individuals to overcome perceived obstacles and thrive.

A significant body of research (e.g., Iso-Ahola, 1980; Seligman, 1975) has established the idea that human behavior is largely motivated by perceived control over the expected outcome of such behavior. deCharms (1968) stated, "man's primary motivational propensity is to be effective in producing changes in his environment" (p. 269). We are motivated to put forth an effort when we feel that our effort will have an impact upon an outcome. Without the expectation of having some control over an outcome, we are less likely to be motivated to try to accomplish some goal.

Rotter (1954) tied such motivation to an anticipated expectancy associated with a given behavior. As you will recall, he suggested two broad categories of individuals: *success seekers*, who are confident of their ability to overcome new and challenging situations due to their past success in such experiences, and *failure avoiders*, who believe that their ability to succeed in challenging situations is tied more to environmental factors rather than personal qualities. Persons with milder forms of retardation may be described as failure avoiders. This would seem to be especially true in regard to academic situations. This may lead to a cycle in which past failure may have led to an identification with retardation, which leads to a perceived expectancy of failure, which leads to motivational deficits, which result in failure.

Behavioral Characteristics

With maturity comes the expectation of assuming greater control over one's life. For people to do so, they must develop self-regulation of many behaviors across different settings. For individuals who are mentally retarded, the process of self-regulation often contributes to a variety of other sociobehavioral problems. Some of the specific problem areas identified with milder forms of retardation include disruptiveness, attention deficits, low self-esteem (Polloway, Epstein, Patton, Culliman & Luebke, 1986), distractibility, and other attention-related problems (Epstein, Polloway, Patton & Foley, 1989).

Since individuals with retardation may exhibit inappropriate behaviors, they may be rejected by their peers and consequently have difficulty in establishing and maintaining interpersonal relationships and/or friendships (Polloway et al., 1986). The degree of peer rejection is associated with the degree of inappropriateness of behavior they display.

Speech and Language Characteristics

Speech and language problems occur with greater frequency among the population identified as mentally retarded. This is not unexpected, since cognitive ability and language development are closely related. The speech problems most often seen are difficulties in articulation or the pronunciation of words (Dunn, 1973). Common articulation errors include the substitution, omission, addition, or distortion of sounds, which makes speech less intelligible. Language disorders that commonly accompany mental retardation include delayed development of language and a restricted or limited vocabulary (Beirne-Smith et al., 1994).

Physical Characteristics

The physical characteristics of individuals with milder forms of mental retardation do not differ dramatically from their nonretarded peers. When health concerns are present, however, they tend to be more severe and occur with other problems. As the severity of retardation increases so do problems in physical health.

Motor skill development may be delayed and less accomplished among individuals with mental retardation. Common motor deficits include problems in balance, locomotion, and manipulative dexterity (Bruininks, 1974). Their physical growth may be slower, and these individuals are generally shorter and lighter than their normal peers (Bruininks, 1974).

Sensory defects, especially visual and auditory problems, are more common among individuals who are retarded. Convulsive disorders and major neuromuscular disturbances such as cerebral palsy are also more prevalent.

While not directly responsible for general health problems, the physical deficits associated with mental retardation tend to place individuals with this condition

at greater risk. For example, children with developmentally disabilities tend to be more poorly coordinated than their nonretarded peers. Add to this the poor judgment and impaired reasoning often associated with subaverage intellectual ability and a higher than average accident and injury rate can be predicted. Conditions accompanying the retardation—sensory deficits, muscle weakness, and seizures—add to increased injuries. Moreover, poor nutrition and inadequate healthcare increase the susceptibility to disease and illness among children from lower socioeconomic classes.

Characteristics of Severe Mental Retardation

Traditionally, the classification of severe mental retardation was based upon intelligence test scores. According to the American Association on Mental Deficiency's 1983 standards, persons who score below 50–55 on an IQ test have a severe disability (Grossman, 1983). In 1992 the AAMR revised its definition by placing less emphasis on the IQ guidelines and more emphasis on the intensity and pattern of care needed by individuals. In this section we will describe some of the basic characteristics of those individuals who require limited, extensive, or pervasive care.

Demographic Characteristics

The total number of individuals with severe disabilities is relatively small. While specific estimates vary, most place the total number of individuals in the United States who have severe disabilities in the range of approximately one third to one half million persons (Beirne-Smith, 1994). It is predicted that 0.13% of the total population of the United States has severe mental disabilities. Earlier we discussed the fact that the overall prevalence estimate for mental retardation is about 1%. Thus, it is clear that persons with severe retardation represent a very small percentage (perhaps 1 in 10) of the total population of persons with mental retardation.

Unlike milder forms of retardation no evidence exists that environmental and socioeconomic variables increase the likelihood of being diagnosed with this condition. Severe forms of mental retardation occur at approximately equal rates at all socioeconomic levels.

Behavioral Characteristics

Challenging behaviors often accompany severe forms of retardation. These behaviors may include verbally or physically aggressive acts, self-injurious acts (e.g., head banging), noncompliance, and self-stimulatory behavior (e.g., rocking or repetitive vocalizations). The presence of such behaviors often inhibits efforts by professionals to work with such individuals. In recent years efforts to deal with such behaviors have produced an approach called applied behavior analysis (behavior management), which has improved the ability to handle challenging behaviors. The underlying assumption of this approach is that behavior problems are learned. As with all behaviors, a problem behavior is largely a function of its immediate antecedents (events that trigger a behavior) and consequences (events that follow a behavior). Applied behavior analysis is the systematic study of behaviors and the application of reinforcement to encourage positive (desired) behaviors and to discourage negative (undesired) behaviors.

Communication Characteristics

Persons with severe mental retardation have extensive deficiencies in communication. Communication skills vary widely among this group. Some speak, others do not. Those who speak may do so in single words, short phrases, whole sentences, or complex conversations. For those who do speak, articulation difficulties often make understanding difficult for inexperienced listeners. Since communicating needs, thoughts, and ideas is a vital component of the cognitive domain, deficits in communicative abilities also accentuate cognitive differences between persons with severe forms of retardation and others.

Physical and Motor Characteristics

Many individuals with severe levels of retardation have physical limitations as well. The severity of involvement varies greatly, from minimal impairments to interference with basic daily activities such as eating, dressing, and toileting.

The most common causes of motor disabilities associated with severe retardation include cerebral palsy, epilepsy, and scoliosis. Adaptive equipment and devices allow these individuals to better perform functional life skills. Ambulation may be improved by using leg braces, scooter boards, wheelchairs, or crutches. Ma-nipulation of objects may be possible by adapting utensil handles to allow an individual to grasp them more easily or equipping shoes with Velcro straps to eliminate the need for tying laces. Such adaptation can enhance the abilities of persons with severe motor involvement to participate more fully in normal activities.

More severe forms of mental retardation are also often associated with extensive medical conditions. In addition to some of the physical problems already identified, some additional medical concerns include restricted movement, skeletal deformities, lung and breathing control difficulties, and disorders of the ears, bladder, skin, or digestive tract (Orelove & Sobsey, 1987). Any of these conditions may require extensive interventions throughout the individual's life and complicate the problems directly associated to mental retardation.

Issues across the Life Span

A common myth regarding mental retardation is that people who have this condition are eternal children. This perception results in part because the majority of individuals labeled as mentally retarded have difficulty with tasks involving self-management and personal responsibility. Delays in developing such skills lead to difficulties in many daily living activities and cause the individual to appear to be immature and act much younger than his or her chronological years. This is especially pronounced in those with more severe forms of retardation.

This situation becomes increasingly problematic in the case of the person who is no longer chronologically a child. Whether the person is an adolescent or an adult, the perception of him or her as an eternal child leads to expectations and activities that often strengthen the image of immaturity and preclude further growth. This scenario suggests that an understanding of the experiences of the life cycle as it relates to those with mental retardation is essential to providing experiences and services which are as similar as possible to their nondisabled peers. We now provide a brief sketch of some of the significant issues of the life span and their implications for individuals who are mentally retarded.

Infancy and Early Childhood (Birth to 6 Years)

During infancy and early childhood we begin to learn fundamental self-care skills such as feeding, dressing, and toileting. We also begin to use language for communication and develop basic motor and social skills. Retardation results in a slower rate of development in all of these areas, which causes the child to appear immature. For those individuals with more severe forms of retardation developmental deficits are usually recognized very early. However, for milder forms of retardation developmental lags in essential skill areas are often not recognized because they deviate only slightly from the norm.

The early years are also important in personality development and how the child comes to feel about himself or herself and relates to others. In large measure this will be the result of the degree to which parents and/or caregivers provide experiences that foster self-esteem, such as intimacy, success, and autonomy. Unfortunately, a child's disability may interfere with normal parental bonding or attachment and thus threaten the child's need for intimacy and growth of self-esteem.

The rearing of a seriously mentally retarded child does create stresses unknown to parents of nonretarded children (Gabel, McDowell & Cerreto, 1983). These include psychological stresses associated with the grief and guilt of having an offspring who deviates from societal norms as well as stresses related to practical concerns such as prolonged periods of dependency, possible health problems, and financial and educational concerns.

School Age (Approximately 6 to 18 Years)

The school years are particularly significant in the life of a child with mental retardation because the extent of the cognitive disability becomes the most pronounced. The child with retardation will not make normal school progress. Among children with mental retardation, usually only those with mild forms will achieve basic reading and arithmetic skills. Reading a newspaper requires about a sixth-grade achievement level, while at least fourth-grade arithmetic competency is required for even the simplest daily money-management activities. Unfortunately, the average level of attainment for the mildly retarded may be only about the third-grade level (Gunzberg, 1968). Individuals identified with a moderate form of retardation usually do not achieve much beyond the first-grade level, although some may acquire functional reading skills. The education of individuals with more severe forms of retardation is nonacademic in emphasis and stresses development of self-help, language, social, and motor skills.

The school years are also very important to a child's social development. School provides a time for loosening ties with caretakers and intensifying ties with same-sex and opposite-sex peers. The same pattern is seen in children with retardation, although at a slower rate. During adolescence in particular, efforts by the individuals with retardation to achieve greater autonomy, to define themselves, and to express sexuality can be particularly troublesome (Zetlin & Turner, 1985). For the parent of a child with a cognitive disability that interferes with the capacity for age-appropriate decision making, loosening the reins is bound to be unnerving.

A central feature of adolescence is the clarification of who one is, or as Erikson (1968) called it, "the defining self." In a study of 25 mildly retarded adults, the majority (84%) reported that is was during adolescence that they became aware of their differences and the effect of the social identity of "retarded" on their lives (Zetlin & Turner, 1985).

Adolescence represents a coming to terms with school learning difficulties. For the first time the adults in the study began to identify themselves in terms of their disability. For the subjects of Zetlin and Turner's study this realization was naturally damaging to their self-esteem. Some saw themselves as failures, as a disappointment to their parents, or as being held in lower regard than their siblings. Rejection by peers was also very common. Most reported experiences of being teased and taunted by schoolmates or neighborhood children (Zetlin & Turner, 1985).

During the later part of the school years, vocational consideration becomes a primary focus. The serious academic limitations of many individuals with mental retardation reduce the possibilities for postsecondary education as well as for formal vocational training. Many trades require reading and arithmetic skills that may be beyond the capacity of the person with cognitive disabilities. Nevertheless, most mildly and moderately retarded young people are employable, the former in regular though unskilled jobs and the latter in sheltered employment (Kiernan, McGaughey & Schalock, 1988). Moreover, the intensive employment thrust of recent decades has demonstrated that with support, even some severely retarded individuals are capable of working in regular jobs (Wehman & Kregel, 1989).

Adulthood (20+ Years)

In our culture we measure adjustment in adulthood by the degree to which we can live independently, work, use our free time, fulfill roles as spouse and parent, and conform to community mores. As in the school-age years, the quality of this adjustment is affected by the degree of retardation, as well as by the availability of support services.

Individuals with milder forms of mental retardation have the capacity to meet most normal standards for an adequate adult adjustment. They are capable of living independently, working, marrying, using leisure time, and presenting no special behavior problems (Edgerton, & Bercovici, 1976; Richardson, 1978; Zetlin & Turner, 1985). Major adaptive obstacles pertain to managing money, job vulnerability during periods of economic hardships, and social isolation. Social isolation relates to the likelihood of fewer friends and a lower rate of marriage—a more socially isolated existence.

Zetlin and Turner (1985) studied the adjustment of a group of young adults with milder forms of retardation. The researchers observed that for most of the people, achieving independent living, acquiring possessions, managing their daily affairs, working, and maintaining heterosexual relationships contributed to their self-esteem. Such individuals saw themselves as functioning in the world pretty much like everybody else.

Although the ranges of moderate to profound retardation cover a wide span of abilities and adaptation, they have in common the probability that fully independent adjustment will not be attained. Some degree of dependency, at least in the residential domain, is typical.

Within the range of moderate to profound retardation, striking differences in adaptation are found. Adults with moderate mental retardation are often employed, typically in sheltered workshops or day activity programs, although the supported employment thrust of the 1980s increased their access to jobs in regular work settings. Social relationships are also sought, although these usually do not include marriage and parenthood. Like their mildly retarded counterparts, however, these individuals can be expected to eventually acquire relatively complete self-care skills—feeding, dressing, bathing, and toileting.

At the levels of severe and profound retardation, the degrees of dependency are proportionately greater. Sufficiency in self-care is reduced, and there may appear to be little interest in peer relationships, especially for profoundly retarded individuals. Communication skills are very limited, especially in speech, and capacities for productive work are absent without special training.

Baroff (1991) claims that for this group "recreation tends to be the most neglected of services" (p. 98). According to Baroff, the life of an adult with moderate to profound retardation may be inordinately dominated by the mental, emotional, or physical impact of the disability. Daily experience may be limited to the place of residence and the day program, and evenings may be restricted to solitary activities or television. In some settings there may be little or no opportunity for leisure experiences

with peers. Baroff (1991) strongly advocates the provision of recreational opportunities to help enrich "the necessarily narrowed lives" of these individuals.

Implications for Therapeutic Recreation

Baroff's comments are based upon the premise that recreational involvement can enrich an one's life. The relationship between recreation involvement and healthy living has strong empirical support (Siegenthaler, 1997). Studies have provided evidence that leisure can assist in maintaining physical and mental health by helping people resist stress-induced illness (Coleman, 1993), boost morale during times of trauma (Patterson & Carpenter, 1994), and rebuild personal identities after traumatic life events (Klieber, Brock, Lee, Datillo & Caldwell, 1995).

While all individuals may share the benefits of recreation participation, the condition of mental retardation presents some special challenges to the recreation and parks professional. Therapeutic recreation helps individuals "to develop and use their leisure in ways that enhance their health, independence, and well-being" (National Therapeutic Recreation Society, 1994). Three specific areas of professional service provide the comprehensive approach needed to help attain this goal: recreation participation, leisure education, and therapy.

Recreation Participation

Participation in leisure and recreation activities is an important aspect of life for all members of society. Most individuals welcome time away from work, school, or other responsibilities and carefully plan ways to use their free time in a personally satisfying manner. Kraus (1997) maintains that the potential benefits derived from leisure involvement include the reduction of stress, emotional satisfaction, physical health, enjoyable social contacts, and feelings of achievement. Leisure seems to be a primary contributor to both personal and community well-being.

Persons with mental retardation are no different in their need for leisure and recreation. Unfortunately, this population has historically been excluded from leisure programs and services. The consequences of exclusion have been widely discussed in recent years. Efforts to integrate persons with disabilities into community leisure services are generally regarded as an outgrowth of the normalization principle and the resulting movement toward community placement. *Normalization*, a concept defined by Nirje (1969), involves making the societal patterns and conditions of everyday life available to persons with disabilities. Wolfensberger (1972) expanded upon the concept to include "the utilization of means which are as culturally normative as possible in order to establish or maintain personal behaviors or characteristics which are as culturally normative as possible" (p. 28).

Normalization is governed by the belief that persons with disabilities should be accepted as equal members of society and should be permitted to participate in the norms and patterns of the community. One of the patterns of mainstream community life recognized by Wolfensberger (1972) is recreation. Elaborating on this idea, he wrote:

> In a normalizing program scheme, there is a need not only for meaningful work, but also for recreation, each to be conducted at appropriate places and appropriate times. (p. 86)

In addition to being consistent with the principles of normalization, involvement in recreation and leisure programs contributes to the development of skills needed for independent functioning by individuals with mental retardation. Research has shown that improvements in language, cognition, and physical fitness can be realized by this population during participation in leisure-related experiences (Schleien & Wehman, 1986). Green and Schleien (1991) have convincingly argued that the development of friendships between individuals with developmental disabilities and their nondisabled peers may be fostered by skills developed during recreational activities. Moreover, factors such as self-concept (Van Andel & Austin, 1984), social skill development (Novak & Heal, 1980), and successful transition from school to adult life (Bedini, Bullock & Driscoll, 1993) may be enhanced through participation in recreational activities.

Unfortunately the majority of persons with disabilities participate in segregated recreation services if they participate at all. Studies conducted in the United States (Rynders & Schleien, 1991), in Hungary (Gollesz, 1994), and in the United Kingdom (Moss, 1994) lend support to this claim. In Australia, Suttie and Ashman (1989) found that less than 30% of people with a mild or moderate level of disability participate in general community recreational activities on a regular basis. Likewise, investigators in western Canada claimed that leisure and recreation activities that promote social and community involvement are not encouraged by agencies or homes concerned with the care of individuals with disabilities (Brown, Brown & Bayer, 1994).

The time has come to adapt a new way of thinking, one founded on the premise that the community belongs to everyone—regardless of level and type of ability. Inclusive community leisure services can be powerful vehicles for promoting this ideal (Schleien, 1993). The term *inclusive leisure services* captures the full acceptance and integration of individuals with developmental disabilities into the recreation mainstream. "Diversity is valuable—not just a reality to be tolerated, accepted, or accommodated, but a reality to be valued" (York, 1994, p. 11).

Inclusive leisure services benefit all community members (Dattilo, 1994). For people with disabilities, inclusive recreation can help to:

- Cultivate friendships
- Develop of a sense of affiliation
- Enhance social skills
- Provide positive role models
- Develop lifelong skills

For the nondisabled, inclusive recreation can help to:

- Develop positive attitudes
- Encourage understanding and acceptance of people with differences
- Promote personal growth

Two benefits in addition to those listed above—empowerment and self-determination—are integral to normalization and will be discussed in more detail. *Empowerment* refers to the transfer of power and control over values, decisions, choices, and directions of human services from external entities to the consumers of services (West & Parent, 1992). Empowering consumers provides them with the freedom (and responsibility) to make decisions with respect to the conduct of their lives. This freedom leads to self-determination. As described by Ward (1988), *self-determination* refers to attitudes and abilities that lead individuals to define goals for themselves, and their ability to take the initiative to achieve their goals. Self-determination is associated with personal dignity and increased motivation to participate and succeed. When self-determination is achieved, increased learning and perceptions of competence results (Dattilo, 1994). People who perceive themselves as capable and self-determining effectively deal with the challenges of day-to-day life (Iso-Ahola & Weissinger, 1984; Shary & Iso-Ahola, 1989).

A person's individuality emerges partly through the choices he or she makes. For those identified as mentally retarded, personal choices are often very limited. While opportunities for personal choice in some areas of life (e.g., work, education) may be extremely difficult to equalize for everyone, providing equal opportunities for leisure involvement should not be difficult (MacNeil & Anderson, 1999).

Given the desirability of inclusive leisure services, one may ask why they remain rare. An individual's own limitations may contribute to some obstacles. These are referred to as *intrinsic barriers* and include factors such as lack of knowledge about leisure opportunities, skill deficiencies (e.g., activity skills, social skills, decision-making skills), social ineffectiveness, and deficits in leisure decision making.

Many persons with mental retardation do not realize their maximum leisure functioning because they lack necessary information about community recreation resources. Pollingue and Cobb (1986) and Bedini, Bullock, and Driscoll (1993) identified a lack of awareness of recreational opportunities among individuals with developmental disabilities and their guardians. With insufficient knowledge of recreation resources or support services, the ability to make informed choices about leisure opportunities will obviously suffer.

Closely related to lack of knowledge as a barrier to leisure participation are deficiencies in skills necessary for recreation involvement. Sometimes the nature of their impairment limits individuals from developing appropriate skills; however, often persons with mental retardation do not get the opportunity to develop skills necessary to succeed in leisure. As a result, they correctly perceive that many recreation activities are too challenging for their present skill level and a sense of helplessness develops. With this perception comes fewer attempts to participate. As attempts decrease, opportunities to experience enjoyment also decline. The result is usually nonparticipation (Dattilo, 1994).

Another intrinsic barrier to leisure experienced by many persons with special needs relates to social ineffectiveness (Dattilo, 1987). This may be particularly true for individuals with mental retardation. Parental overprotection and segregation from people without disabilities account for deficiencies in interpersonal skills. As a consequence, persons with mental retardation often lack the ability to meet the social demands required for positive engagement in many community leisure settings (Heyne, Schleien & McAvoy, 1993).

An additional barrier to leisure involvement concerns identified deficiencies among individuals with mental retardation to make appropriate leisure-oriented decisions. One of the most significant ways in which society can empower individuals with mental retardation to become more self-advocating is through enabling them to make decisions for themselves (Mahon & Bullock, 1992).

Leisure Education

An appropriate response to deal with lack of knowledge or deficient skills would be the implementation of a leisure education program. The term *leisure education*, first used by Chinn and Joswiak (1981), describes the application of comprehensive models focusing on the educational process to enhance an individual's leisure lifestyle. While a variety of leisure education models exist, they all share the common goal of "exposing all people to the possibilities that leisure may hold for them to live creatively and give expression to the wide assortment of their capabilities" (Bucher, Shivers & Bucher, 1984, p. 290).

Leisure education programs typically employ a variety of components that directly address barriers associated with lack of knowledge or deficient skills, including:

- Awareness of self in leisure—knowledge of one's own preferences relative to leisure involvement, as well as a realistic understanding of one's skills, abilities, values, and attitudes toward leisure and participation in leisure activities
- Leisure appreciation—development of a sense of appreciation relative to leisure and its potential contribution to quality of life
- Self-determination—development of a perception of leisure competence and a sense of responsibility to make appropriate leisure choices
- Leisure decision making—encouraging the acquisition of decision-making skills
- Knowledge and utilization of leisure resources—learning about and using leisure resources
- Social integration skills—development of skills and abilities that facilitate integration into social groups and the community
- Recreation activity skills—development of recreation skills having the most potential to provide individuals with enjoyment and satisfaction (Dattilo & Murphy, 1991)

Empirical support for the effectiveness of leisure education in broadening participation of persons with mental retardation has been increasing in recent years. For example, researchers have identified that leisure education programs may contribute to the following:

- Increased activity and social interaction (Anderson & Allen, 1985)

- Increased leisure awareness and leisure decision-making skills (Mahon & Bullock, 1992)
- Improved ability to engage in recreational activities with peers without disabilities (Schleien, Meyer, Heyne & Brandt, 1995)
- Increased positive affect during free time (Williams & Dattilo, 1997)
- Increased leisure awareness, activity initiation, participation, and leisure appreciation (Bedini, Bullock & Driscoll, 1993)

Therapy

The word *therapy* refers to a healing or curing process used to help to remediate the effects of illness or disease. Because one cannot be "cured" of mental retardation, the traditional meaning of therapy must be modified in reference to therapeutic recreation (TR) intervention. Rather than imply a protocol designed to heal or cure an individual, the therapy component of TR intervention most often focuses on the development of functional skills and abilities that may enhance the overall quality of life for persons with this condition. Dattilo and Schleien (1991) identified four theoretical foundations that may serve as broad-based goals for developing TR interventions: leisure skill repertoires, autonomy, community integration, and social skill development.

Leisure Skill Repertoires

Engagement in meaningful recreational activities has long been considered a contributor to an individual's sense of health and well-being (Iso-Ahola & Weissinger, 1984). However, for many individuals with mental retardation, the ability to engage in recreation experiences is severely limited. A major factor limiting leisure development is the serious skill deficit often associated with mental retardation (Schleien, 1991). People with mental retardation often require systematic training in order to develop leisure repertoires (Wehman & Schleien, 1981). Clearly, a primary goal for TR intervention with this population should be to assist individuals to develop an appropriate recreational skills repertoire. Guidelines for achieving this goal have been developed by many authors (e.g., Wehman, 1979; Voeltz, Wuerch & Wilcox, 1982; Smith, Austin & Kennedy, 1996; and Dattilo, 1994).

Autonomy

Recreation provides opportunities for individuals to experience a sense of control. This sense of perceived control has consistently been identified with psychological health (Iso-Ahola, 1994; Iso-Ahola & Weissinger, 1984). Yet, persons with mental retardation have limited opportunities to express choice and may lack the ability to make decisions regarding a variety of aspects of their lives, including the area of leisure (Dattilo & Schleien, 1991). Given that research has demonstrated that leisure decision-making skills among individuals with mental retardation can be improved by means of systematic training (Mahon & Bullock, 1992), it would seem that developing autonomy should be a focus for TR intervention for this population.

Community Integration

In addition to providing feelings of pleasure and entertainment, recreation activities can enhance a wide variety of other skills that can help promote community integration. For purposes of our discussion concerning the therapy component of TR, we will address the issue of community integration in terms of the development of collateral skills. Development of any of these skills would constitute a legitimate goal for a TR treatment program. The collateral skills which researchers have suggested may be enhanced by leisure involvement include:

- Body image (Verhoven, Schleien & Bender, 1982)
- Communication and language skills (Bates & Renzaglia, 1982; Trader & MacKinnon, 1998)
- Cooperation and sharing (Schleien & Wehman, 1986)
- Enhanced self-concept and expression of emotions and feelings (Dattilo & Rusch, 1985)
- Improved leisure choices and time management (Bullock & Howe, 1991)
- Decline in undesirable or inappropriate behaviors (Wehman & Schleien, 1981)
- Improved manipulation of materials and motor skills (Kraus & Shank, 1992)
- Improved participation with nondisabled peers (Schleien et al., 1995)

Social Skill Development

The development of social interaction skills and leisure skills are mutually enhancing. Social development may be facilitated by engagement in leisure-oriented activities (Schleien & Wehman, 1986) and the development of leisure skills can enhance social skill development (Dattilo & Schleien, 1991). Appropriate, goal-directed leisure activities lead to increased social skill development. Inappropriate leisure activities result in decreased social skill development (Schleien, Kiernan & Wehman, 1981).

Delayed social skill development was previously identified as a characteristic common among persons with mental retardation. Because social development can be facilitated by recreation and play activities, individuals who fail to develop necessary skills to engage in such activities often experience problems in developing relationships (Green & Schleien, 1991). Development of cooperative play behavior and participation in recreation activities often leads to making friends, learning to share and cooperate with others, and more satisfactory social adjustment (Dattilo & Schleien, 1991).

Due to the complementary nature of leisure and social skills, TR programs should consider social development as a principal focus for intervention. With this in mind, the following two resources are recommended:

- *Making Friends: Using Recreation Activities to Promote Friendship Between Children With and Without Disabilities* (Heyne et al., 1993)
- *Community Recreation and People With Disabilities: Strategies for Inclusion* (Schleien, Ray & Green, 1997)

Programming Considerations

The development and implementation of effective recreation programs has been the subject of numerous textbooks (e.g., Farrell & Lundegren, 1991; Rossman, 1995; DeGraaf, Jordan & DeGraaf, 1999). For the most part the basic strategies for recreation programming promoted are applicable for individuals with mental retardation. However, persons with this condition often present special challenges for the recreation professional. Many of the challenges result from the deficiencies in cognitive abilities and adaptive behavior highlighted earlier in this chapter. We will now present several considerations to facilitate recreation programming for persons with mental retardation.

Individualized Activities

The wide range of behaviors and functional abilities of people with mental retardation necessitates careful consideration of each individual's abilities and interests when selecting recreational activities. Personalizing activities also enhances a sense of personal control and positive self-esteem. Individualized activities allow the TRS to accommodate the needs of individuals with different levels of mental retardation.

Limited Attention Spans

The ability to attend selectively is a prerequisite for learning. Lack of attention is a major limitation experienced by many individuals with mental retardation. Strategies which may be employed to help increase attention span include:

- Maximize the involvement of all participants
- Provide structured activities with numerous opportunities for repetition
- Keep rules and verbal instructions simple and direct
- Provide opportunities for participant feedback
- Vary the stimuli and equipment used in recreation programming
- Reduce extraneous stimuli
- Limit the quantity of materials, direction, and suggestions given at any one time
- Change activities frequently when participant interest is peaking

Conceptual Deficits

People with mental retardation have difficulties conceptualizing and utilizing stimuli in the environment. Some suggestions for dealing with these deficits include:

- Divide activities into manageable parts
- Sequence activities to offer a progression of skills
- Provide opportunities to learn by doing
- Provide a demonstration so participants may model desired behaviors
- Keep safety precautions in mind (Persons with mental retardation often place loose objects into their mouths, often have no fear of sharp or extremely hot objects, and may not understand dangers associated with height or moving objects.)

Low Self-Esteem

Avoid a sense of "progressive failure" by providing activities for which failure cannot be inferred (e.g., noncompetitive games, arts and crafts). The leader should ensure that the challenges of an activity correspond with the skills of the participants, allow time for task completion, and provide praise and reinforcement. When group activities are being used, the leader should be sure to equalize groups in terms of ability levels.

Age-Appropriateness

Interests and behavioral expectations based upon chronological age are often meaningless to individuals with mental retardation. Recreation professionals should assist participants in selecting age-appropriate activities. For instance, a popular activity for developing hand–eye coordination among children is the beanbag toss. A game of darts (rubber-tipped) can develop the same skills, but is age-appropriate for adolescents or adults.

Social Ineffectiveness

It is important for individuals to develop leisure skill repertoires that facilitate successful integration into the community. Individuals with mental retardation often lack the ability to meet the social demands required for positive engagement with others in society. Learning how to engage in recreational activities with peers without disabilities can greatly expand the opportunities available to persons with mental retardation (Schleien et al., 1995). Recreation leaders should provide social skills training in age-appropriate leisure situations. Programs should be designed to encourage socialization among participants. It has been shown that recreation activities based on cooperation between participants with and without disabilities are usually more effective than activities of a competitive or individualistic nature when social interaction is the goal (Schleien et al., 1997). An example of this would be for persons with and without mental retardation to work together on completing a puzzle.

Chapter Summary

This chapter examined the cognitive domain and addressed the following issues:

- Difficulty in assessing and evaluating the cognitive domain due to the lack of standardized definitions and measurements
- IQ testing as a popular but controversial method used to discriminate between individuals
- Cognitive functioning by using an information-processing model (Figure 2.1)
- Piaget's explanation of intellectual development and four phases in the progression of cognitive capabilities
- Prevalence, potential causes, and characteristics of mild and severe mental retardation
- Significant life span issues and available therapeutic recreation services for persons with mental retardation

Answers Exercise 2.1

1. Sandbox
2. Man overboard
3. I understand
4. Reading between the lines
5. Long underwear
6. Crossroads
7. Downtown
8. Tricycle
9. Split level
10. Three degrees below zero
11. Neon lights
12. Partly sunny
13. Highchair
14. Paradise
15. Touchdown
16. Six feet underground
17. Mind over matter
18. He's beside himself
19. Backward glance
20. Life after death
21. GI overseas
22. Space program
23. See-through blouse
24. Just between you and me

References

Adams, J. (1967). *Human memory.* New York, NY: McGraw-Hill.

American Association on Mental Retardation. (1992). *Mental retardation: Retardation, classification and systems of supports* (9th ed.). Washington, DC: Author.

Anderson, J. and Bower, G. (1973). *Human associative memory.* Washington, DC: Vith Winston.

Anderson, S. and Allen, L. (1985). Effects of a leisure education program on activity involvement and social interaction of mentally retarded persons. *Adapted Physical Activity Quarterly, 2*(2), 107–116.

Balla, D., Styfco, S., and Zigler, E. (1971). Use of the opposition concept and outer directedness in intellectually average, familiar retarded, and organically retarded children. *American Journal of Mental Deficiency, 75,* 663–680.

Baroff, G. (1986). *Mental retardation: Nature, cause and management* (2nd ed.). New York, NY: Hemisphere.

Baroff, G. (1991). *Developmental disabilities: Psychosocial aspects.* Austin, TX: Pro-Ed.

Bates, P. and Renzaglia, A. (1982). Language instruction with a profoundly retarded adolescent: The use of a table game in the acquisition of verbal labeling skills. *Education and Treatment of Children, 5*(1), 13–22.

Bedini, L., Bullock, C., and Driscoll, L. (1993). The effects of leisure education on the successful transition of students with mental retardation from school to adult life. *Therapeutic Recreation Journal, 27*(2), 70–82.

Beirne-Smith, M., Patton, J., and Ittenbach, R. (1994). *Mental retardation* (4th ed.). New York, NY: Macmillan.

Belmont, J. (1971). Medical-behavioral research in mental retardation. *International Review of Research in Mental Retardation, 5,* 1–81.

Berg, C. and Emanuel, I. (1987). Relationship of prenatal care to the prevention of mental retardation and other problems of pregnancy outcome. In *Developmental handicaps: Prevention and treatment* (pp. 45–70). (ERIC Document Reproduction Service No. 276 192).

Brown, R., Brown, P., and Bayer, M. (1994). A quality of life model: New challenges arising from a six-year study. In D. Goode (Ed.), *Quality of life for persons with disabilities: International perspectives and issues.* Cambridge, MA: Brookline Books.

Bruininks, R. (1974). Physical and motor development of retarded persons. *International Review of Research in Mental Retardation, 7,* 209–261.

Bucher, C., Shivers, J., and Bucher, R. (1984). Leisure education and counseling. *Recreation for today's society* (2nd ed.). Englewood Cliffs, NJ: Prentice-Hall.

Bullock, C. C. and Howe, C. Z. (1991). A model therapeutic recreation program for the reintegration of persons with disabilities into the community. *Therapeutic Recreation Journal, 27*(2), 70–82.

Cattell, J. (1963). Theory of crystallized intelligence: A critical experiment. *Journal of Educational Psychology, 54,* 1–22.

Chinn, K. and Joswiak, K. (1981). Leisure education and leisure counseling. *Therapeutic Recreation Journal, 15*(4), 4–7.

Coleman, D. (1993). Leisure-based social support: Leisure dispositions and health. *Journal of Leisure Research, 25*(4), 350–361.

Dattilo, J. (1987). Recreation and leisure literature for individuals with mental retardation: Implications for outdoor recreation. *Therapeutic Recreation Journal, 21*(1), 9–17.

Dattilo, J. (1994). *Inclusive leisure services: Responding to the rights of people with disabilities.* State College, PA: Venture Publishing, Inc.

Dattilo, J. (1996). Mental retardation. In D. Austin and M. Crawford (Eds.), *Therapeutic recreation: An introduction* (2nd ed., pp. 130–149). Boston, MA: Allyn & Bacon.

Dattilo, J. and Murphy, W. (1991). *Leisure education program planning: A systematic approach.* State College, PA: Venture Publishing, Inc.

Dattilo, J. and Rusch, F. (1985). Effects of choice on leisure participation for persons with severe handicaps. *Journal of Association for Persons with Severe Handicaps, 10,* 194–199.

Dattilo, J. and Schleien, S. (1991). The benefits of therapeutic recreation in developmental disabilities. In C. Coyle, W. B. Kinney, B. Riley, and J. Shank (Eds.), *Benefits of therapeutic recreation* (pp. 69–134). Philadelphia, PA: Temple University.

deCharms, R. (1968). *Enhancing motivation: Change in the classroom.* New York, NY: Irvington.

DeGraff, D. G., Jordan, D. J., and DeGraff, K. H. (1999). *Programming for parks, recreation, and leisure services: A servant leadership approach.* State College, PA: Venture Publishing, Inc.

de la Cruz, F. (1985). Fragile X syndrome. *American Journal of Mental Deficiency, 90,* 119–123.

Dorland's Medical Dictionary (23rd ed.). (1957). Philadelphia, PA: Saunders.

Dunn, L. (Ed.). (1973). *Exceptional children in schools: Special education in transition* (2nd ed.), New York, NY: Holt, Rinehart, and Winston.

Edgerton, R. and Bercovici, S. (1976). The cloak of competence: Years later. *American Journal of Mental Deficiency, 80,* 485–497.

Epstein, M., Polloway, E., Patton, J., and Foley, R. (1989). Mental retardation: Student characteristics and services. *Education and Training of the Mentally Retarded, 24,* 7–16.

Erikson, E. (1968). *Identity: Youth and crisis.* New York, NY: Norton.

Erlenmeyer-Kimling, L. and Jarvik, L. (1963). Genetics and intelligence: A review. *Science, 142,* 1477–1479.

Farrell, P. and Lundegren, H. M. (1991). *The process of recreation programming: Theory and technique* (3rd ed.). State College, PA: Venture Publishing, Inc.

Gabel, H., McDowell, J., and Cerreto, M. (1983). Family adaptation to the handicapped infant. In S. Garwood and R. Fewell (Eds.), *Educating handicapped infants.* Rockville, MD: Aspen.

Gagne, R. (1977). *The conditions of learning* (3rd ed.). New York, NY: Holt, Rinehart, and Winston.

Garber, H. (1988). *The Milwaukee project: Preventing mental retardation in children at risk.* Washington, DC: American Association on Mental Retardation.

Gollesz, V. (1994). Quality of life of people with disabilities in Hungary after leaving school. In D. Goode (Ed.), *Quality of life for persons with disabilities: International perspectives and issues.* Cambridge, MA: Brookline Books.

Green, F. and Schleien S. (1991). Understanding friendship and recreation: A theoretical sampling. *Therapeutic Recreation Journal, 25*(4), 29–40.

Greeno, J. and Bjork, R. (1973). Mathematical learning theory and the new "mental forestry." *Annual Review of Psychology, 24,* 81–116.

Grossman, H. (Ed.). (1983). *Classification in mental retardation.* Washington, DC: American Association on Mental Deficiency.

Gunzburg, H. (1968). *Social competence and mental handicap.* Baltimore, MD: Williams & Wilkins.

Heber, R. F. (1961). A manual on terminology and classification in mental retardation (Rev. ed.). *Monograph supplement to the American Journal of Mental Deficiency,* 62.

Heyne, L., Schleien, S., and McAvoy, L. (Eds.). (1993). *Making friends: Using recreation activities to promote friendship between children with and without disabilities.* Minneapolis, MN: Institute on Community Integration (UAP).

Hill, A. (1974). Idiot savants: A characterization of abilities. *Mental Retardation, 12,* 12–13.

Iso-Ahola, S. (1980). *The social psychology of recreation and leisure.* Dubuque, IA: Wm. C. Brown.

Iso-Ahola, S. E. (1994). Leisure lifestyle and health. In D. M. Compton and S. E. Iso-Ahola (Eds.), *Leisure and mental health* (pp. 42–60). Park City, UT: Family Development Resources, Inc.

Iso-Ahola, S. and Weissinger, E. (1984). Leisure and well-being: Is there a connection? *Parks & Recreation, 18,* 40–44.

Jensen, A. (1971). The IQs of MZ twins reared apart. *Behavior Genetics, 2,* 1–10.

Kagan, J. (1970). On class differences and early development. In V. Denenberg (Ed.), *Education of the infant and young child.* New York, NY: Academic Press.

Kausler, D. (1982). *Experimental psychology and human aging.* New York, NY: Wiley & Sons.

Kiernan, W., McGaughey, M., and Schalock, R. (1988). Employment environment and outcome for adults with developmental disabilities. *Mental Retardation, 26,* 279–288.

Kleiber, D. A., Brock, S. C., Lee, Y., Datillo, J., and Caldwell, L. (1995). The relevance of leisure in an illness experience: *Realities of a spinal cord injury. Journal of Leisure Research, 27*(3), 283–299.

Koch, R., Friedman, E., Azen, C., Wenz, E., Parton, P., Ledue, X., and Fishler, K. (1988). Inborn errors or metabolism and the prevention of mental retardation. In F. J. Menolascino and J. Starle (Eds.), *Preventive and curative intervention in mental retardation* (pp. 61–90). Baltimore, MD: Paul H. Brookes.

Kozol, J. (1991). *Savage inequalities: Children in America's schools.* New York, NY: Crown.

Kraus, R. (1990). *Recreation and leisure in modern society.* New York, NY: Harper Collins.

Kraus, R. (1997). *Recreation and leisure in modern society* (5th ed.). Menlo Park, CA: Addison Wesley Longman, Inc.

Kraus, R. and Shank, J. (1992). *Therapeutic recreation service, principles and practices* (4th ed.). Dubuque, IA: Wm. C. Brown.

Lachiewicz, A., Harrison, C., Spridigliozzi, G., Callahan, N., and Livermore, J. (1988). What is the fragile X syndrome? *North Carolina Medical Journal, 49,* 203–208.

Lindsay, P. and Norman, D. (1972). *Human information processing: An introduction to psychology.* New York, NY: Academic Press.

MacNeil, R. D. and Anderson, S. C. (1999). Leisure and persons with developmental disabilities: Empowering self-determination through inclusion. In P. Retish and S. Reiter (Eds.), *Adults with disabilities: International perspectives in the community.* Mahwah, NJ: Lawrence Erlbaum Associates.

Mahon, M. J. and Bullock, C. C. (1992). Teaching adolescents with mild retardation to make decisions in leisure through the use of self-control techniques. *Therapeutic Recreation Journal, 26*(3), 9–26.

McLaren, J. and Bryson, S. (1987). Review of recent epidemiological studies of mental retardation: Prevalence, associated disorders and etiology. *American Journal of Mental Retardation, 92,* 243–254.

Menolascino, F. and Egger, M. (1978). Medical dimensions of mental retardation. Lincoln, NE: University of Nebraska Press.

Moss, S. (1994). Quality of life and aging. In D. Goode (Ed.), *Quality of life for persons with disabilities: International Perspectives and issues.* Cambridge, MA: Brookline Books.

Musland, R., Sarason, S., and Gladwin, T. (1958). *Mental subnormality.* New York, NY: Basic Books.

National Therapeutic Recreation Society. (1994). *Standards of practice for therapeutic recreation services and annotated bibliography.* Arlington, VA: Author.

Nirje, B. (1969). The normalization principle and its human management implications. In R. Kugel and W. Wolfensberger (Eds.), *Changing patterns in residential services for the mentally retarded* (pp. 179–195). Washington, DC: President's Committee on Mental Retardation.

Novak, A. and Heal, L. (Eds.). (1980). *Integration of developmentally disabled individuals into the community.* Baltimore, MD: Paul H. Brookes.

Orelove, F. and Sobsey, R. (1987). *Multiple disabilities: A transdisciplinary approach.* Baltimore, MD: Paul H. Brookes.

Patterson, I. And Carpentar, G. (1994). Participation in leisure activities after the death of a spouse. *Leisure Sciences, 16,* 105–112.

Piaget, J. (1952). *The origins of intelligence in children* (2nd ed.). New York, NY: International and Universities Press.

Pollingue, A. B. and Cobb, H. B. (1986). Leisure education: A model facilitating community integration for moderately/severely mentally retarded adults. *Therapeutic Recreation Journal 20*(3), 54–62.

Polloway, E., Epstein, M., Patton, J., Culliman, D., and Luebke, J. (1986). Demographic, social, and behavioral characteristics of students with educable mental retardation. *Education and Training of the Mentally Retarded, 21,* 27–34.

Richardson, S. (1978). Careers of mentally retarded young persons: Services, jobs, and interpersonal relationships. *American Journal of Mental Deficiency, 82,* 349–358.

Rogers, R. and Simensen, R. (1987). Fragile X syndrome: A common etiology of mental retardation. *American Journal of Mental Deficiency, 91,* 445–449.

Rossman, J. R. (1995). *Recreation programming: Designing leisure experiences* (2nd ed.). Champaign, IL: Sagamore Publishing.

Rotter, J. (1954). *Social learning and clinical psychology.* Englewood Cliffs, NJ: Prentice-Hall.

Rynders, J. and Schleien, S. (1991). *Together successfully: Creating recreational and educational programs that integrate people with and without disabilities.* Arlington, TX: Association for Retarded Citizens of the United States.

Rynders, J., Spiker, D., and Horrobian, J. (1978). Underestimating the educability of Down's syndrome children: Examination of methodological problems in recent literature. *American Journal of Mental Deficiency, 82,* 440–448.

Schalock, R., Starle, J., Snell, M., Coutler, D., Polloway, E., Luckasson, R., Reiss, S., and Spitalnik, D. (1994). The changing conception of mental retardation: Implications for the field. *Mental Retardation, 32*(3), 181–193.

Schleien, S. (1991). Severe multiple handicaps. In D. Austin and M. Crawford (Eds.), *Therapeutic recreation: An introduction* (pp. 189–223). Englewood Cliffs, NJ: Prentice-Hall.

Schleien, S. (1993). Access and inclusion in community leisure services. *Parks & Recreation, 28*(4), 66–72.

Schleien, S., Kiernan, J., and Wehman, P. (1981). Evaluation of an age-appropriate leisure skills program for moderately retarded adults. *Education and Training of the Mentally Retarded, 16*(1), 13–19.

Schleien, S., Meyer, L., Heyne, L., and Brandt, B. (1995). *Lifelong leisure skills and lifestyles for persons with developmental disabilities.* Baltimore, MD: Paul H. Brookes.

Schleien, S., Ray, M., and Green, F. (1997). *Community recreation and people with disabilities: Strategies for inclusion* (2nd ed.). Baltimore, MD: Paul H. Brookes.

Schleien, S. and Wehman, P. (1986). Severely handicapped children: Social skills development through leisure skills programming. In G. Cartledge and J. Milburn (Eds.), *Teaching social skills to children: Innovative approaches* (2nd ed., pp. 219–245). Elmsford, NY: Pergamon Press.

Seligman, M. (1975). *Helplessness: On depression, development, and death.* San Francisco, CA: Freeman.

Shary, J. and Iso-Ahola, S. (1989). Effects of a control-relevant intervention on nursing home resident's perceived competence and self-esteem. *Therapeutic Recreation Journal, 23*(1), 7–16.

Siegenthaler, K. (1997, January). Health benefits of leisure. *Parks & Recreation,* 24–28.

Smith, R. W., Austin, D. R., and Kennedy, D. W. (1996). *Inclusive and special recreation* (3rd ed.). Madison, WI: Brown & Benchmark.

Suttie, J. M. and Ashman, A. F. (1989). *An acceptable standard of living and quality of life: Fact or fiction for aging persons with intellectual disability.* Paper presented to the 25th Annual Conference of the Australian Society for the Study of Intellectual Disability, Melbourne, Australia.

Tarjan, G., Wright, S., Eyman, R., and Keeran, D. (1973). Natural history of mental retardation: Some aspects of epidemiology. *American Journal of Mental Deficiency, 77,* 369–379.

Terman, L. (1916). *The measurement of intelligence.* Boston, MA: Houghton Mifflin.

Trader, B. R. and MacKinnon, J. (1998). Start with the arts to encourage confident and enthusiastic learners. *Parks and Recreation, 33*(5), 94–98.

U. S. Department of Education (1992). *To assure free appropriate public education of all handicapped children: Fourteenth annual report to Congress on the implementation of the Education of the Handicapped Act.* Washington, DC: U. S. Department of Education, Office of Special Education and Rehabilitative Services.

Van Andel, G. and Austin, D. (1984). Physical fitness and the mentally handicapped: A review of literature. *Adapted Physical Activities Quarterly, 3,* 207–220.

Verhoven, P., Schleien, S., and Bender, M. (1982). *Leisure education and the handicapped individual: An ecological perspective.* Washington, DC: Institute for Career and Leisure Development.

Voeltz, L., Wuerch, B., and Wilcox, B. (1982). Leisure and recreation: Preparation for independence, integration and self-fulfillment. In B. Wilcox and G. Bellamy (Eds.), *Design for high school programs for severely handicapped students* (pp. 175–209). Baltimore, MD: Paul H. Brookes.

Ward, M. (1988). The many facets of self-determination. *National Information Center for the Children and Youth with Disabilities: Transition Summary, 5,* 2–3.

Wechsler, D. (1958). *The measurement of appraisal of adult intelligence* (4th ed.). Baltimore, MD: Williams and Wilkins.

Wehman, P. (1979). Toward a recreation curriculum for developmentally disabled persons. In P. Wehman (Ed.), *Recreation programming for developmentally disabled persons* (pp. 1–13). Austin, TX: Pro-Ed.

Wehman, P. and Kregel, J. (Eds.). (1989). *Supported employment and transition: Focus on excellence.* New York, NY: Human Sciences Press.

Wehman, P. and Schleien, S. (1981). *Leisure programs for handicapped persons: Adaptations, techniques and curriculum.* Austin, TX: Pro-Ed.

West, M. and Parent, W. (1992). Consumer choice and empowerment in supported employment services: Issues and strategies. *Journal of the Association for Persons with Severe Handicaps, 17*(1), 47–52.

Westling, D. (1986). *Introduction to mental retardation.* Englewood Cliffs, NJ: Prentice-Hall.

Williams, R. and Dattilo, J. (1997). Effects of leisure education on self-determination, social interaction and positive affect of young adults with mental retardation. *Therapeutic Recreation Journal, 31*(4), 244–258.

Wolfensberger, W. (1972). *The principle of normalization in human services.* Toronto, Ontario: The Canadian Association for the Mentally Retarded.

York, J. (1994). A shared agenda for educational change. *Newsletter: The Association for Persons with Severe Handicaps, 20*(2), 10–11.

Zetlin, A. and Turner, J. (1985). Transition from adolescence to adulthood: Perspectives of mentally retarded individuals and their families. *American Journal of Mental Deficiency, 89,* 570–579.

Zigler, E. (1966). Research on personality structure in the retardate. In N. R. Ellis (Ed.), *International Review of Research in Mental Retardation, 1,* 77–108.

CHAPTER 3
AFFECTIVE DOMAIN

The word *affect* roughly equates to *emotion* or *mood*. The affective domain refers to those aspects of behavior related to feelings, emotions, attitudes, and personal-social skills. Terms such as personality, motivation, self-concept, and adaptation are commonly used in reference to this domain.

The diverse disorders associated with the affective domain fall under the broad label of mental illness. They include:

- Anxiety-based disorders (obsessive–compulsive behavior, hypochondria, phobias)
- Affective disorders (depression)
- Psychotic disorders (schizophrenia, paranoia)
- Personality disorders (antisocial and criminal behavior)
- Substance abuse and addictive disorders
- Behavior disturbances of childhood and adolescence (conduct disorder, attention deficit hyperactivity disorder)

These disorders share one thing in common: They manifest themselves in behavior away from the normal. This abnormal behavior becomes the focal point for both the diagnosis and treatment of disorders associated with the affective domain.

This chapter presents a broad overview of abnormal behavior. We begin by presenting an historical overview of abnormality, including past explanations for and treatment of individuals who displayed abnormal behavior. Next, we discuss early 20th-century efforts to differentiate and classify the multitude of behaviors labeled as abnormal. This will be followed by a section that highlights a variety of theoretical perspectives on the nature of abnormality. We then discuss some general casual factors associated with abnormal behavior. The chapter will conclude with a section on current thinking about the classification of mental disorders.

Abnormal Behavior: Competing Perspectives

The word abnormal literally means away from the norm. But what should be the "norm" in terms of human behavior? In the case of a physical abnormality, the norm implies structural and functional integrity of the body. In this case the boundary between normality and pathology is usually quite clear. On the psychological level, however, we have no normal model of human functioning to serve as a base for comparison. Thus, there can be considerable confusion and debate over the boundaries between normal and abnormal.

Any definition of abnormal must be somewhat arbitrary. Definitions generally represent one of two competing perspectives: a cultural basis or an individual and/or group adjustment basis.

According to the cultural perspective, abnormal behavior deviates from social expectations within a given culture. The individual's culture defines normal (and abnormal)—a behavior that is expected is considered to be within the norm. Public nudity, for instance, is considered acceptable behavior in some societies, but unacceptable in the United States. Individuals who may choose to practice it would most likely be viewed as abnormal by society at large.

The second perspective defines abnormal behavior based on individual and/or group adjustment. Some degree of social conformity is essential to group cohesion, but when this behavior endangers group/individual well-being it is considered maladaptive. This maladaptive view of abnormal behavior will be the underlying definition for this text.

Historical Views of Abnormal Behavior

Many of our current views (and misconceptions) about mental disorders have their roots in approaches tried long ago. We see an evolution from beliefs grounded in folklore and superstition to those based on scientific evidence and from a focus on supernatural and demonic causes to biologic and psychosocial causes. The course of this evolution has not been a steady one; it has been marked by brief periods of great advancement followed by long periods of destructive backward surges. Despite years of scientific investigation and efforts at public education about mental disturbances, we are still not free of the culturally conditioned constraints of our past. Many attitudes toward people who are different are still formed in part by fear and superstition.

Ancient Times: Demons and Spirits

The earliest known treatment of abnormal behavior was practiced by Stone Age cave dwellers some half million years ago. For certain forms of mental disturbances, such as convulsive attacks, the *shaman* (healer) commonly used a form of treatment known as trephination. *Trephination* consisted of chipping away a circular hole in the skull of the victim. The opening, called a trephine, presumably permitted the evil spirit causing the disorder to escape from the skull of the victim.

References to abnormal behavior in the early writings of the Chinese, Egyptians, and Greeks show that they generally attributed such behavior to possession by a demon or, in some cases by a god (Davison & Neale, 1986). While such an explanation seems illogical by current standards, at that time many incomprehensible occurrences (e.g., storms, earthquakes, sickness) were explained in terms of good and bad spirits. It was a very easy transition to extend this theory to peculiar and incomprehensible human behavior.

In some cases, if the behavior seemed to have a religious or mystical significance, it was thought that the individual was possessed by a good spirit and he or she was treated with admiration and respect. Most possessions, however, were considered to be the work of evil spirits. The goal was to make the body as unpleasant a host as possible, thus encouraging the bad spirits to leave.

A primary type of treatment for demonical possession was exorcism. Exorcism took many forms, from prayer, incantations, and noise making to the use of horrible-tasting concoctions to magical rites. Extreme cases employed physical abuse such as starvation, burning, and flogging. The popularity of books and motion pictures dealing with themes of possession and exorcism suggest that these primitive ideas retain appeal today.

Early Philosophical and Medical Explanations

The roots of modern understanding of mental disorders can be traced to the Golden Age of Greece. Hippocrates (460–377 B.C.), the father of modern medicine, denied the intervention of deities and demons in the development of disease, and insisted that mental disorders had natural causes and required treatment like other diseases. Hippocrates also recognized the brain as the central organ of intellectual activity and suggested that mental disturbances were due to brain pathology. Hippocrates also first recognized the importance of heredity and predisposition and their possible relationship to physical and mental disorders.

Hippocrates classified the varieties of mental disorders into three general categories—mania, melancholia, and phrentis (brain fever)—and provided detailed descriptions of the specific disorders included in each category. The methods of treatment advocated by Hippocrates included tranquility (stress reduction), exercise, and vegetable diets—all methods far in advance of the exorcistic measures commonly practiced at the time. Although he falsely believed in the existence of four bodily fluids or "humors" (blood, black bile, yellow bile, and phlegm) that when out of balance led to ill health, his emphasis on the importance of bodily balance to mental health may be seen as a precursor of today's focus on the prevention and treatment of mental illness.

Later Greek and Roman physicians continued with similar work. Cicero (106–43 B.C.), for example, believed that body ailments could be the result of emotional factors. Treatments prescribed for mental patients often included pleasant surroundings and therapeutic activities including parties, dances, musical concerts, and walks. Some Roman physicians used warm baths, massage, and other physical therapies to make their patients comfortable. Many contemporary writers in the field of therapeutic recreation have suggested that the profession can trace its roots to this period of time (Kraus & Shank, 1992; Carter, Van Andel & Robb, 1995).

The Middle Ages: Return to Demonology

The Middle Ages in Europe (about A.D. 500–1500) revived ancient superstition and demonology. Individuals with mental disorders often became targets of cruel forms of "treatment."

In the early stages of the medieval period, treatment of the mentally disturbed was left largely to the clergy. Monasteries frequently served as refuges and places of confinement. Persons with mental disorders likely were attended by clergy who emphasized prayer, the touching of holy relics, and visits to holy places as preferred forms of treatment for abnormal behavior.

However, with the passage of time ancient theological explanations for abnormal behavior became widespread and mild and gentle treatment was replaced by harsh and punitive action. It was generally believed that cruelty to people afflicted with mental disorders was punishment for the devil residing within them, and authorities felt justified in driving out the demons by increasingly unpleasant methods. Flogging, starvation, immersion in hot water, and other forms of torture intended to make the body an unpleasant residence for devils and demons. Undoubtedly many individuals who might have been restored to health by more humane measures were driven into a hopeless condition of derangement by such abusive treatment.

By the latter part of the 15th century a popular explanation for abnormal behavior was spiritual possession. Such individuals were believed to have made a pact with the devil that gave them certain supernatural powers. It was thought that they could cause disease, storms, floods, injuries, and crop destruction, as well as turn themselves into animals. In short, they were witches.

Concern over the number of possessed individuals (and the consequences of their presence), continued to grow throughout the period until finally a papal decree issued in 1484 called for aggressive measures to detect and destroy witches. To be convicted of witchcraft was a serious matter—the penalty for conviction was usually death. For many death was by burning, but only after torture and mutilation (Coleman, Butcher & Carson, 1984).

The 16th Century: Birth of the Asylum

The belief in demons and witches as the cause of abnormal behavior gradually disappeared throughout the 16th century and was replaced by scientific explanations. More importantly, human and therapeutic approaches to treating individuals afflicted by mental disorders slowly replaced the torture and cruelty that characterized treatment during the previous period.

Representative of the scientific skepticism that began to emerge in the 16th century was a book written by Oxford-educated Reginald Scot (1538–1599). *Discovery of Witchcraft*, published in 1584, convincingly denied the existence of demons, devils, and evil spirits as the cause of mental disorders. As Scot (in Castiglioni, 1946, p. 253) wrote:

> These women are but diseased wretches suffering from melancholy, and their words, actions, reasoning, and gestures show that sickness has affected their brains and impaired their powers of judgment.

You must know that the effects of sickness on men, and still more on women, are almost unbelievable. Some of these persons imagine, confess, and maintain that they are witches and are capable of performing extraordinary miracles through the arts of witchcraft; others, due to the same mental disorder, imagine strange and impossible things which they claim to have witnessed.

Although many refuted Scot's thesis, including King James I of England, persistent advocates of science continued their testimonies throughout the next two centuries. Eventually explanations of mental disorders based upon observation and reason replaced demonology. This culminated in the development of modern experimental and clinical psychological approaches.

From the 16th century on, an accepted treatment for persons with mental disorders was confinement in special institutions commonly referred to as *asylums*. These early asylums were primarily modifications of penal institutions, where inmates experienced extremely harsh and cruel conditions. It was not uncommon for patients to be shackled to the walls in their dark, unlighted cells for most of the day, then chained in a different position so that they might sleep on straw spread on the floor during the night. They were poorly fed and their cells were seldom cleaned (Selling, 1943). Once admitted, most inmates died in these asylums amid conditions of incredible filth and cruelty.

The 18th Century: Birth of Humane Treatment

A movement toward humanitarian treatment of patients received its first great impetus from the work of Philippe Pinel (1745–1826) in France. Pinel, placed in charge of the largest hospital for the insane in Paris, boldly acted upon his theory that mental patients, if treated with kindness and consideration, would not respond like vicious beasts or criminals. Pinel ordered chains to be removed, permitted patients to move about hospital grounds, and ordered his staff to treat residents with kindness. The effect was as Pinel anticipated: order and peace replaced the previous noise, filth, and abuse. Residents who had previously been considered hopeless began to respond to this change in treatment. Some even recovered to the point of being permitted to leave the hospital (Selling, 1943). Pinel eventually repeated his experiment at another hospital in France with the same results. His successor, Jean Esquirol (1772–1840), continued Pinel's approach and helped in the establishment of 10 new mental hospitals, which placed France in the forefront of humane treatment for the mentally disturbed.

At about the same time that Pinel was reforming care for the mentally ill in France, William Tuke established the York Retreat, a pleasant country home in England where mental patients lived and worked in a kindly Quaker atmosphere. As word of Pinel's work spread, Samuel Hitch, a prominent English medical psychologist, introduced trained nurses into the wards at the Gloucester Asylum and placed trained supervisors at the head of the nursing staffs. These innovations improved the care of mental patients and helped to change public attitudes toward this illness.

Pinel's and Tuke's experiments in humanitarian methods strongly influenced Benjamin Rush (1745–1813), the founder of American psychiatry. While associated with the Pennsylvania Hospital in 1783, Rush encouraged more humane treatment of the mentally disturbed. He later authored the first systematic treatise on psychiatry in America and became the first American to organize a course on psychiatry.

Another prominent American associated with arousing public awareness regarding the inhuman treatment accorded the mentally ill was Dorthea Dix (1802–1887). Based in part on her experiences teaching in a women's prison, Dix became an outspoken advocate for the mental hygiene movement, which focused on the physical well-being of the mental patients in hospitals. Her efforts raised many millions of dollars to build suitable hospitals in the United States and Canada. She established some 22 mental hospitals, an astonishing record considering the degree of superstition and ignorance that still prevailed with respect to mental illness (Grob, 1994).

By the close of the 18th century the use of humane approaches to the treatment of the mentally ill was widespread. One form of treatment, moral therapy, was increasingly used in many of the same mental hospitals that had once chained and tortured the patients under their care. This approach, which stemmed largely from the original ideas of Pinel, has been described by Rees (1957):

> The insane came to be regarded as normal people who had lost their reason as a result of having been exposed to severe psychological and social stresses. These stresses were called the moral causes of insanity, and moral treatment aimed at relieving the patient by friendly association, discussion of his difficulties, and the daily pursuit of purposeful activity; in other words, social therapy, individual therapy, and occupational therapy. (pp. 306–307)

The 20th Century: Changing Attitudes, Expanding Knowledge

By the end of the 19th century the mental hospital had become a familiar landmark in America. While the living conditions within these facilities had markedly improved over the course of 200 years, to the general public the institution remained a frightening place, with its occupants viewed as strange. Gradually public attitudes toward mentally ill individuals improved; these attitudes were strongly influenced by Clifford Beers In 1908, Beers, a Yale graduate and former patient in three institutions, published the book, *A Mind That Found Itself*. The book described Beers' experiences while a patient in mental hospitals. It received broad acclaim and launched Beers on a campaign dedicated to make the public better understand the need for reform in the care of individuals who were mentally ill (Grob, 1994).

At about the same time that the mental hygiene movement gained momentum, many scientific discoveries occurred that profoundly affected our understanding of abnormal behavior. For example, biomedical research discovered that one of the leading causes of insanity was syphilis and further study produced a cure for the disease. This marked perhaps the first time in history that a mental disorder was successfully treated by a medical science. It also marked a notable transformation from believing in demons as the cause of mental illness to a scientific understanding of how brain pathology can cause a specific disorder.

Along with advances in biological causation, research into psychological and sociocultural factors which impact human behavior also progressed. Wilhelm Sundt (1832–1920) established the first experimental psychology laboratory at the University of Leipzig in 1879. Wundt's experimental methods set the standards for countless later studies of abnormal behavior. M. McKeen Cattell (1860–1944) brought Wundt's experimental strategies to the United States and greatly contributed to our understanding of individual differences in mental processing. William Healy (1869–1963) became the first scientist to describe juvenile delinquency as a symptom of the phenomenon known as urbanization, adding sociocultural factors to the list of causative agents. Additionally, outlets for publication of empirical research emerged (e.g., *Journal of Abnormal Psychology*, first published in 1906) and opened many new avenues for communicating information. This expansion of knowledge developed a gradual acceptance of mental patients as afflicted individuals who need professional attention. Another consequence has been the growth in the scientific study of abnormal behavior (Grob, 1983).

We have come a long way from the days when abnormal behavior was explained by possession by demons. Understanding this developmental sequence helps us to understand the emergence of modern concepts related to mental disorders. We now discuss three broad interpretations currently used to explain the sources of deviant behavior: biological, psychosocial, and sociocultural viewpoints.

Sources of Deviant Behavior: Biological Viewpoint

Many professionals, especially those with medical backgrounds, believe that abnormal behavior is the product of aberrant biophysical processes occurring in the brains of affected persons. This *biological viewpoint*, holds that a mental disorder is similar to a medical disease except that the primary symptoms are behavioral rather than physiological. In its extreme form, this viewpoint discounts psychological factors and the psychosocial environment of the individual as causal factors in mental disorders, and instead views abnormality as a disease of the central nervous system.

As evidence acquired through experimental science began to replace demonology as a source of knowledge about mental illness, support for the biological viewpoint developed quickly. Many early scientific discoveries, such as the relationship between syphilis and brain pathology, supported the biological view that mental disorder is an illness based on the pathology of an organ—in this case the brain. The earliest disorders recognized to have biological roots were those associated with gross destruction of brain tissue.

As research and experimentation progressed, however, the biological viewpoint accommodated new knowledge. It is now understood that many conditions may temporarily disrupt the information-processing capabilities of the brain, consequently altering behavior, without inflicting permanent damage or death of the brain cells involved. Alcohol intoxication is a common example used to emphasize this point. The normal functioning of the brain is altered due to changes in the brain's chemistry, which can result in changes in behavior. Once the chemical balance is restored, however, normal behavior may again occur.

This is a basic tenet of the biological perspective today—that a biochemical imbalance in the brain can result in abnormal behavior. Several biophysical therapies that are practiced today reinforce this view, including the use of psychotropic drugs (e.g., antipsychotic, antidepressant, antianxiety) and electroconvulsive therapy.

Sources of Deviant Behavior: Psychosocial Viewpoint

There are many more psychosocial interpretations of abnormal behavior than biological ones, reflecting the greater complexity of humans as whole persons versus humans as simply biological organisms. This section briefly summarizes three psychosocial explanations of human behavior: psychoanalytic, behavioristic, and humanistic.

Psychoanalytic Perspective

The individual most closely identified with the psychoanalytic perspective is Sigmund Freud (1856–1939). Freud's revolutionary ideas about human behavior were based on the clinical study of individual patients who consulted him for treatment. Freud came to strongly believe that some mental disorders had a psychological basis (not a biological basis) and directed much of his attention toward attempting to explain how psychologically caused mental disturbances come about.

Central to Freud's theory was the important role played by unconscious processes in determining behavior. Freud discovered that in a hypnotic state patients often recalled details and memories about problems that tended to be repressed in a fully conscious state. Once this repressed information was brought to the surface, he found that patients were often able to discuss their problems more freely and consequently were often able to resolve them. He eventually produced the same results without the use of hypnosis. He called this new method *free association*. The principles involved in analyzing and interpreting what a patient says and does with the intent of helping him or her make a more adequate adjustment came to be known as *psychoanalysis*.

The psychoanalytic perspective assumes that an individual's behavior results from the interaction of three key subsystems within the personality: the id, ego, and superego. The *id* is the source of instinctual drives for pleasure and satisfaction. Completely selfish, the id concerns itself with immediate gratification of instinctual needs without reference to moral considerations. The *ego* mediates between the demands of the id and the realities of the external world. The ego meets id demands, but in such a way as to ensure the well-being and survival of the individual. The *superego* is concerned with right and wrong—our conscience. An outgrowth of learning the taboos and values of a society, the superego becomes an additional inner control system that copes with the uninhibited desires of the id.

Freud viewed the interplay among these subsystems as crucial in determining behavior. Often conflicts arise because the id, ego, and superego strive for different goals. These intrapsychic conflicts produce *anxiety*, an uncomfortable psychological state that forces the individual to undertake corrective action. Often the ego can cope with anxiety by rational measures; if these fail, however, the ego may resort to irrational protective measures such as denial or rationalization. These *ego defense mechanisms* alleviate painful anxiety by pushing painful ideas out of consciousness and giving the individual a distorted view of reality instead of dealing directly with the problem. This creates an undesirable schism between reality and the individual's perception of reality. Freud believed that the hurtful memories and forbidden desires driven from our consciousness are repressed and stored in the depths of our unconscious mind. Although we remain unaware of such unconscious material, it continues to seek expression and may be reflected in fantasies and dreams when ego controls are temporarily lowered. Until such unconscious material is brought to our awareness—via psychoanalysis, for example—it presumably leads to irrational and maladaptive behavior.

Although Freud's work has many critics, he greatly advanced the understanding of abnormal behavior. Through the research techniques he developed, he demonstrated the importance of early childhood experiences in later personality adjustment and maladjustment. Moreover, he demonstrated that certain abnormal mental phenomena occur as a result of overemploying normal ego defense mechanisms. This realization that the same psychological principles apply to both normal and abnormal behavior.

Behavioristic Perspective

Behavioristic psychologists believe that only the study of directly observable behavior and the conditions which stimulate and reinforce it should serve as a basis for formulating scientific principles of human behavior.

The central theme of *behaviorism* is the role of learning in human behavior. Although this perspective developed through research in the laboratory rather than through clinical practice with patients, its implications for explaining and treating abnormal behavior was soon evident.

Behaviorism traces its roots to the work of Russian physiologist Ivan Pavlov (1849–1936). Pavlov's experiments focused upon simple forms of learning known as *conditioning*. Pavlov demonstrated that a dog could be taught to salivate to a nonfood stimulus, such as the sound of a bell, after the stimulus had been regularly followed by the presentation of food. Pavlov's research established that behavior can be learned and that the environment provides source of much of this learning.

American psychologist John Watson (1878–1958) viewed Pavlov's work as an opportunity to study behavior through the observation of systematic changes brought about by rearranging stimulus conditions. This approach became known as behaviorism. As a consequence of his work, Watson changed the focus of psychology from the study of inner (psychoanalytic) to outer behavior.

Watson's approach placed heavy emphasis on the role of the social environment in conditioning personality development and behavior, both normal and abnormal. Watson believed conditioning shaped human behavior. He suggested that abnormal behaviors were the product of unfortunate earlier conditioning and could be modified through reconditioning.

While Watson studied stimulus conditions (i.e., what occurs before a behavior) and their relation to behavioral responses, Edward Thorndike (1874–1949) and B. F. Skinner (1904–1990) explored the fact that over time behavior tends to be influenced by the consequences it produces. Behavior that operates on the environment is instrumental in producing certain outcomes. Those outcomes, in turn, determine the likelihood that the behavior will be repeated. This type of learning came to be called *instrumental conditioning* or *operant conditioning*.

As previously stated, learning provides the central theme of the behavioristic approach. Since they believe that most human behavior is learned, behaviorists address the question of how learning occurs. The same principles that apply to learning appropriate behavior also apply to learning inappropriate and/or abnormal behavior. Behaviorists view maladaptive behavior as the result of (a) failing to learn necessary adaptive behaviors or competencies or (b) learning ineffective or maladaptive responses.

For the behaviorist therapy focuses on changing specific behaviors. This usually includes the elimination of undesirable behaviors and the learning of desirable ones. This process of applying learning principles to changing behavior is called behavior modification. Variations of behavior modification programs are widely practiced and have been demonstrated to successfully alter behavior in a variety of settings with a wide variety of individuals (Dattilo & Murphy, 1987).

Perhaps the greatest strength of behaviorism is its preciseness and objectivity. The therapist specifies what behavior is to be changed, states how it is to be changed, and evaluates its effectiveness objectively by the degree to which the stated goals have been achieved. On the other hand, the behavioristic perspective has been criticized for being concerned only with symptoms, for ignoring the problems of value and meaning that may be important for those seeking help, and for denying the possibility of individual choice and self-direction. Whatever its limitations, the behavioristic perspective continues to have a significant impact on the treatment of people with mental disorders.

Humanistic Perspective

The humanistic perspective focuses on people's conscious experiences and perceptions—freeing them from self-limiting attitudes and assumptions so that they may develop their human potential and live fuller lives. It emphasizes growth and self-actualization rather than the cure of a disorder. This perspective is also concerned with processes about which we have little scientific information, such as love, hope, creativity, and self-fulfillment.

The humanistic perspective has also been referred to as the evolved primate perspective, owing to its belief in the evolutionary uniqueness and status of the human species. Humanistic psychologists view human nature as fundamentally good and place strong emphasis on our inherent capacity for responsible self-direction. At the same time, humanistic psychologists disagree with the negative and pessimistic picture of human nature portrayed by psychoanalytic theory, which stresses the overwhelming power of irrational unconscious impulses, and the behavioristic theory, which stresses environmental conditions and conditioned responses to explain human behavior. In this sense, the humanistic perspective tends to be as much a statement of values—of how we ought to view the human condition—as it is an attempt to explain deviance and abnormality.

This perspective has been strongly influenced by psychologists such as Gordon Allport, Abraham Maslow, Carl Rogers, and Fritz Perls. It has been suggested that this view emerged in the 1950s and 1960s when many middle-class Americans realized their simultaneous material affluence and spiritual emptiness (Coleman et al., 1984).

While the humanistic perspective tends to be diverse, common underlying themes of humanistic psychology can be outlined.

Self as a Unifying Theme

Consciousness of self (self-concept) has always been a focus of the humanistic perspective. Humanistic psychologists emphasize the importance of individuality. Carl Rogers (1951) developed a systematic formulation of the self-concept. Rogers has stated his views in a series of propositions:

- Individuals exist in a private world of experience with I, me, or myself as the center
- Individuals strive toward the maintenance, enhancement, and actualization of the self
- Individuals react to situations in ways consistent with their self-concept and worldview
- Perceived threats to the self activate coping mechanisms intended to preserve one's sense of self
- Under normal conditions we behave in rational and constructive ways and choose pathways toward personal growth and self-actualization

Focus on Values and Personal Growth

Humanistic psychologists emphasize personal values and value choices in achieving a meaningful life. They emphasize the need to develop values based upon our own experiences and feelings. To develop personally meaningful values, we must have a clear sense of who we are and what we want to become— our self-identity.

According to the humanistic view, abnormal behavior blocks or distorts personal growth and natural tendencies toward physical and mental health. This can result from exaggerated use of ego defense mechanisms, unfavorable conditions, faulty learning, or excessive stress.

Positive View of Human Nature and Potential

In contrast to the psychoanalytic and behavioristic perspectives, the humanistic approach holds a much more positive view of human nature and potential. Despite the presence of violence and cruelty throughout history, humanistic psychologists believe that under favorable conditions we are rational creatures who seek to behave in a friendly, cooperative, and constructive manner. They regard selfishness, aggression, and cruelty as pathological behavior resulting from inaccurate information, frustration, or social and economic deprivation.

Criticism of the humanistic perspective usually focuses upon the fact that many of its claims and explanations are not readily subject to empirical investigation. It also tends to emphasize present and future with far less emphasis upon the past—especially past factors that according to other fields of psychopathology may have caused current problems. Nonetheless, the humanistic perspective introduced a new dimension to our thinking about abnormal behavior. Because it views abnormality as a failure to sufficiently develop our human potential, it has moved our thinking on abnormal behavior out of the realm of deviance. This broadened perspective allows for a much more positive view of human nature and the roots of mental disturbance.

Sources of Deviant Behavior: Sociocultural Viewpoint

By the early 20th century, sociology and anthropology had developed into independent scientific disciplines. Both fields contributed greatly to our understanding of the role played by sociocultural factors in human development and behavior. Human beings are influenced by their environment. Our personality reflects both the people and relationships to which we are exposed, as well as the larger society—its institutions, norms, values, and attitudes—of which we are a part. In this light, it became evident that a relationship exists between sociocultural conditions and mental disorders. Patterns of both mental and physical disorders in a given society may change over time as sociocultural conditions change.

The relationships between sociocultural factors such as poverty, discrimination, or illiteracy and maladaptive behavior during childhood or adulthood are complex. It is one thing to observe that an indi-

vidual with a psychological disorder has come from harsh environmental circumstances. It is quite difficult, however, to show empirically that these circumstances were both necessary and sufficient conditions for producing the disorder. Moreover, specific evidence supports the view that many psychological disturbances are universal. For example, schizophrenia can be found among nearly all cultures, from the most primitive to the most technologically advanced (World Health Organization, 1975).

Cultural influences, however, cannot be disregarded. While there may be universal illnesses, there evidence also suggests that cultural factors influence what disorder develops, the form it takes, and how the condition is treated (Murphy, 1978). With the recognition of sociocultural influences, the almost exclusive concern with the individual patient has broadened to include a concern with societal, communal, familial, and other group settings as contributors to mental disturbances. The sociocultural viewpoint has introduced programs designed to alleviate social conditions that foster maladaptive behavior and provided community facilities for the treatment of possible prevention of mental disorders.

Causal Factors in Abnormal Behavior

Now that we have described several theoretical viewpoints concerning abnormal behavior, we turn our attention to causal factors. In most cases, a typical behavior does not suddenly appear out-of-the-blue. Usually a pattern of factors that rendered an individual vulnerable in respect to the particular circumstances can be pieced together, although often it can only be done in retrospect. In this section we look at some origins of human vulnerabilities—weak spots that under certain circumstances could make us susceptible to behaving abnormally. We discuss these causal factors in three broad categories: biological, psychological, and sociocultural.

Biological Causal Factors

Biological factors influence all aspects of our behavior, including our intellectual capabilities, basic temperament, stress tolerance, and adaptive resources. A wide range of biological conditions—faulty genes, diseases, and injuries that interfere with normal development and functioning—are potential causes of abnormal behavior.

In this section we will focus on four categories of biological factors particularly relevant to an understanding of the development of maladaptive behavior: genetic defects, constitutional liabilities, brain dysfunction, and physical deprivations.

Genetic Defects

Perhaps the most basic of biological causal factors is our genetic endowment. Except for identical twins, no two human beings have ever begun life with the same genetic endowment. Since our biology influences our behavior, it is hardly surprising that certain vulnerabilities have their source at this level. Some inherited defects cause structural abnormalities that interfere directly with the normal development of the brain. Such defects are often associated with the chromosomal abnormalities. When abnormalities occur in the structure or number of chromosomes a wide range of malformations and disorders may occur. The most common disorder associated with chromosome abnormality is Down syndrome. Although there remains little direct evidence linking chromosomal irregularities and mental illness, research on Alzheimer's disease has shown that many of the characteristic symptoms (e.g., plaques and tangles found in brain cells) also frequently occur among individuals with Down syndrome. This might suggest a chromosomal link to Alzheimer's disease; however, such an association remains speculative at this point.

Another source of vulnerability related to our genetic endowment is the inheritance of faulty genes. *Genes* are the long molecules of deoxyribonucleic acid (DNA) that occur at various locations on the chromosome. Individual genes sometimes contain information that causes bodily processes to malfunction. Huntington's chorea and Tay-Sachs disease are examples of genetic disorders causing gross neurological impairment. Such disorders are relatively rare and seldom directly associated with abnormal behavior. It seems clear that genes can affect behavior only indirectly, through their influence on the physical and chemical properties of the body whose development they regulate. One notable exception is schizophrenia, wherein genetic endowment may indeed be a primary causative agent.

Constitutional Liabilities

In addition to genetic endowment, a second category of biological causal factors may be identified by the broad term constitutional liabilities. The term constitutional describes any characteristic that is either innate or acquired so early and in such strength that it is functionally similar to a genetically determined characteristic. Physical impairments are among the traits included in this category.

A look at everyday situations affirms that physical appearance does play an important role in personality development and social adjustment. Physical beauty is highly valued in our society. One need only to attend a social gathering, glance through popular magazines, attend a movie, watch television, or note the billions of dollars spent on beauty enhancing products to see the influence of appearance on people's behavior and their feelings about themselves.

Physically attractive persons have advantages in life not shared by the less attractive. Does it follow that those less attractive may be more vulnerable to maladaptive behavior? Although some early research has sought to establish a direct link between physical appearances and psychopathology (Glueck & Glueck, 1968; Napoleon, Chassin & Young, 1980) most experts believe that the link is not primarily biological, but rather a product of social learning.

Individuals with physical impairments, especially impairments which are visibly evident, clearly experience social stresses not faced by their nonimpaired peers (Wright, 1960). Common and undesirable reactions to physical impairments include feelings of inferiority, self-pity, and hostility. Another obstacle to good stress management that a person with a physical disability faces is the tendency to accept the role of being "handicapped," which society often seems to expect and encourage. As a consequence of such obstacles, the individual may develop psychological conditions which may be more disabling than the physical impairment (Wright, 1960).

Brain Dysfunction

A third category of biological causal agents includes brain dysfunction. Significant damage or loss of brain tissue places a person at risk for psychopathology. Brain damage decreases an individual's capacity to cope with stress in everyday life. As cognitive capacity diminishes, an individual will usually demonstrate declines in functional competence, which in turn contributes a significant source of stress. Among the major sources of brain dysfunction in modern society are diseases of older adulthood, including Alzheimer's disease and cardiovascular insufficiency. Approximately 25% of elderly persons may suffer from diseases of the brain at some point in their lives (Jenike, 1989).

Physical Deprivations

The final category of biological causal agents includes conditions associated with physical deprivation or disruption. Digestive, circulatory, and other bodily functions operate in such a way as to maintain the body's physiological equilibrium and integration. Prolonged or severe disruption of this equilibrium— either due to deprivation or to excess of our basic needs—can threaten our survival or at the very least leave us vulnerable to other stresses.

Chronic deprivation may result in lowered resistance to stress. Insufficient rest, inadequate diet, or attempts to maintain a full schedule under the handicap of a severe cold, fatigue, or emotional strain may deplete a person's adjustive resources and result in increased predisposition to personality disorganization. Studies of volunteers who have gone without sleep for periods of 72 to 98 hours show increasing disorganization as the sleep loss progresses, including disorientation of time and place and feelings of depersonalization (Berger, 1970). Physical and mental deprivations were also key strategies employed during the Korean War to render soldiers more amenable to brainwashing (Farber, Harlow & West, 1956).

Perhaps the most tragic deprivation of all is seen in young children who are malnourished. Severe malnutrition during infancy not only impairs physical development and lowers resistance to disease, but also stunts brain growth and results in markedly lowered intelligence (Amcoff, 1980). Malnutrition contributes to lowered resistance to stress and consequently higher vulnerability to mental disorders and abnormal behavior. Researchers have also documented an increased incidence of psychoses and other mental disturbances among adults who follow a "crash diet" to achieve rapid weight loss (Robinson & Winnik, 1983).

Severe hunger, thirst, and fatigue can be extremely painful. The precise influence of physical pain on behavior has never been fully delineated, although observations indicate that it can be great. Through the centuries torture and pain have been used to elicit confessions as well as for punishment. When consistent and severe, pain may gradually wear down the sufferer's adjustive resources and lead to overwhelming feelings of hopelessness and despair.

Psychosocial Factors

Humans have a highly developed sense of self. Terms such as self-esteem, self-concept, self-image, self-worth, and self-confidence reflect our awareness of our own uniqueness and our own behavior, especially in the presence of others. Our perceptions of ourselves are the products of learning. The various influences operating upon us, and the manner in which they contribute to the perspectives we develop, may with good fortune outfit us with resourcefulness and resilience in facing the challenges that inevitably come our way. Unfortunately, positive outcomes are not guaranteed. In this section we will consider four categories of psychosocial factors associated with abnormal behavior: self-actualization, early deprivation or trauma, inadequate parenting, and pathogenic family structures.

Self-actualization

Humans have a basic core of psychological strivings necessary to maintain a healthy state. Although wide individual differences in psychological motives exist, five appear to be vital to an individual's sense of maintenance and actualization. Disruption or blocking of any of these can make us more vulnerable to abnormal behavior.

Understanding, order, and predictability. Humans strive to understand and achieve a meaningful picture of their world. Unless we can envision order and predictability in our environment, we cannot work out an intellectual response to it. Rules, laws, and social standards reflect this need for order and predictability. When new information contradicts existing assumptions, we experience cognitive dissonance—an unpleasant state of tension that may remain until the discrepancy can be reconciled. The inability to reconcile sources of cognitive dissonance has been theorized to impair one's sense of health and well-being (Iso-Ahola & Weissinger, 1984).

Adequacy, competence, and security. Each of us needs to feel capable of dealing with life's problems. Confidence in our ability to deal with problems leads to feelings of competence and security. Security is reflected in our preference for jobs with tenure, insurance policies and savings accounts that protect us against unplanned contingencies, and society's emphasis upon law and order. Feelings of incompetence or insecurity may have widely differing effects on behavior, but pervasive and chronic feelings of insecurity typically lead to fearfulness, apprehension, or learned helplessness (Seligman, 1975).

Love, belonging, and approval. To love and to be loved are crucial to healthy personality development. Studies have confirmed that the most pervasive of all influences toward healthy development of children was the love and warmth imparted by caregivers (Main & Weston, 1981). The need for close ties to other people continues throughout life and becomes especially important in times of severe stress or crisis.

Self-esteem, worth, and identity. These relate to the psychological need to feel good about oneself and worthy of the respect of others. Self-esteem has its early foundation in parental affirmation of worth and in mastery of early developmental tasks. It depends heavily on the values and standards of others, especially individuals who we deem as significant in our lives. If we can measure up to those standards—in terms of physical appearance, educational achievement, or economic status—we can approve of ourselves and feel worthwhile. The relationship between positive self-evaluation and success is well-documented (Marecek & Mettee, 1972; Rogers, 1959), which leads to the conclusion that positive self-esteem is a dominant attribute of psychologically healthy people.

Personal growth and fulfillment. We strive not only to maintain ourselves, but also to express ourselves and to maximize our potentialities. These strivings for fulfillment take different forms with different people, depending on their abilities, values, and life situations. In general, however, as human beings we seem to strive for similar ideals:

- Developing and using our potentials
- Enriching the range and qualities of our experiences
- Establishing and maintaining meaningful relationships
- Becoming the "self" that we feel we should be

These strivings represent a basic core of psychological requirements that significantly impact our behavior.

Early Deprivation or Trauma

In addition to the pursuit of these strivings, a second category of psychosocial causal factors is related to early deprivation or trauma. In contrast to physical deprivation, the deprivation referred to here relates to an absence of adequate care from and interaction with parents or parental substitutes during the formative years. It can occur in intact families where parents are unwilling or unable to provide for a child's needs for nurturing. Its most severe manifestations are usually witnessed, however, among abandoned or orphaned children, who may either be institutionalized or placed in a succession of foster homes.

The consequences of parental deprivation have been addressed by a variety of theorists representing a host of psychosocial viewpoints. All viewpoints consider the effects of parental deprivation to be potentially very serious. Faulty development, including marked retardation of speech and language development, emotional apathy, and impoverished play activities have all been observed in children who experienced such deprivation (Coleman et al., 1984).

In one study of 38 adolescents who had been institutionalized before age 3, it was found that 16 to 18 years after discharge from the orphanage, 4 were diagnosed as psychotic, 21 as having a character disorder, 4 as mentally retarded, and 2 as neurotic (Beres & Obers, 1950). These findings received general confirmation in a more recent review of child abandonment by Burnstein (1981). In general, it would appear that *affectionless psychopathy*, characterized by the inability to form close interpersonal relationships and often by antisocial behavior, is a syndrome common among children deprived of adequate parental care.

Another dimension of parental deprivation is associated not with separation, but rather with parents who neglect or devote little attention to the child in the home. The possible effects of such deprivation has been well-documented. Children who have been victims of such treatment tend to be aggressive and impulsive (Lefkowitz, Huesmann, Walder & Eron, 1973; Patterson, 1979), often have serious difficulty giving and receiving affection (Pringle, 1965), and may have difficulty forming meaningful relationships with others (Yates, 1981).

A severe early traumatic experience in the life of a child may also produce psychological wounds that never heal completely. A near drowning experience or the divorce of one's parents may be sufficient to produce long-term consequences such as an excessive fear of water or fear of developing close relationships that may endure for years or a lifetime. The after effects of early traumatic experiences depend heavily on the support and reassurance given the child by parents or other significant persons. Nonetheless, a child exposed to repeated traumatic experiences or one who fails to receive support from caretakers is likely to show a disruption in normal personality development (Meyer, 1993).

Inadequate Parenting

A third category of psychosocial causal factors may be labeled inadequate parenting. Many behavioral tendencies of individuals are the product of early social interactions with others—chiefly parents or primary caretakers. While interpretations of these events may differ depending upon the psychosocial perspective utilized, all theorists accept the general principle that certain deviations in parenting can have profound effects on the child's subsequent ability to cope with life's challenges. The following list highlights several patterns of parental influence that appear with great regularity in the background of children who show emotional disturbances.

Overprotection and restrictiveness. Overprotective parents tend to smother a child's growth in their attempt to protect their offspring from even the slightest dangers in the environment. Abnormal behaviors associated with this parenting pattern include excessive fears and over anxiousness. Restrictiveness, the tendency of some parents to rigidly enforce rules and standards, stifles a child's sense of autonomy and freedom. While restrictiveness may foster well-controlled children, it can also nurture fear, dependency, submission, and repressed hostility.

Unrealistic demands. Some parents place excessive pressure on their children to live up to unrealistically high standards. These standards may relate to academic or athletic performance or may focus on moral issues, particularly sex, drugs, or alcohol. According to Coopersmith (1967), unrealistic expectations and demands—either too high, too low, or too rigid—can cause faulty development and maladjustment.

Overpermissiveness and indulgence. This form of parenting is marked by the uninhibited submission of parental control to the child. In so doing, parents cater to the child's slightest whims and fail to teach and reward desirable standards of behavior. Overly indulged children are characteristically selfish and demanding and often display antisocial and aggressive behavior (Sears, 1961).

Faulty discipline. Faulty discipline refers to parental practices in which consistently "the punishment does not fit the crime." It includes the lack of disciplinary measures, inconsistent disciplinary practices, and excessively severe or harsh forms of punishment. Faulty discipline tends to increase such undesirable behaviors as aggression, rebellion, and social deviancy.

Undesirable parental models. Because children tend to observe and imitate the behavior of their caretakers, parental behavior influences the way the youngster learns to think, feel, and act. Examples of undesirable models to which a child may be exposed include parents who make faulty assumptions about reality or

values, or who depend excessively on defense mechanisms in coping with daily problems. Exposure to such models can clearly increase the likelihood that children will also engage in such undesirable behaviors. Undesirable parental models are undoubtedly one important reason why mental disorders, delinquency, crime, and other forms of maladaptive behavior tend to run in families.

Pathogenic Family Structures

The final category of psychosocial causal factors to be considered is concerned with pathogenic family structures. In a pathogenic family structure the total familial context is abnormal. Considerable evidence (Lidz, Fleck & Cornelison, 1965; Roff & Knight, 1981) suggests a strong causal relationship between pathogenic family structures and the eventual diagnosis of severe mental disturbances among children raised in such environments. The following are a few examples of such family structures.

Discordant families. In a discordant family one or both of the parents is not gaining satisfaction from the relationship and may express his or her feelings of frustration in hostile ways. Seriously discordant relationships are likely to be frustrating, hurtful, and generally pathogenic in the effects on all members of the family. Children who grow up in discordant families are likely to find it difficult to establish and maintain intimate relationships.

Disturbed families. A disturbed family is characterized by one or both parents behaving in grossly eccentric or abnormal ways which keeps the home environment in a constant state of emotional turmoil. Not only does the situation produce faulty parental models, but often as parents attempt to maintain their own equilibrium the children may be denied the love and guidance that they need. Moreover, children in these situations almost inevitably become enmeshed in the emotional conflicts of the parents.

Disrupted families. A disrupted family is incomplete, whether as a result of the death of one parent or by separation or divorce. The death of a parent or divorce can have traumatic effects on a child. Feelings of insecurity and rejection are common reactions to such events. Unquestionably, disruptions within the family involve very real stresses for children. This may help explain why delinquency and other maladaptive behaviors occur more frequently among children and adolescents from disrupted homes than among those from intact ones (Coleman et al., 1984).

Antisocial families. Families that overtly or covertly engage in behaviors that violate the values of the wider community are referred to as antisocial families. Such antisocial values and behaviors usually disrupt relationships within the family, as well as provide undesirable models for children.

Sociocultural Factors

The sociocultural viewpoint on abnormality grew out of observations of varying value and behavior patterns among different cultural groups and societal institutions. These observations brought an increased appreciation of the power of social and cultural forces in shaping behavior and personality. In every society there may be many social and cultural influences that increase the vulnerability to the development of abnormal behavior.

One example of the sociocultural environment influencing personality development and behavior is the learning of gender roles. Many societies associate physical prowess with masculinity and reinforce it by exposing males to physically challenging experiences such as competitive sports at very young ages. Femininity, in contrast, is often associated with nurturing activities such as doll play or babysitting and the avoidance of physically demanding involvement. In such societies both the *sissy* (a label traditionally applied to males who seek to avoid physically demanding activities) and the *tomboy* (a label traditionally applied to females involved in physically demanding activities) will probably experience social backlash for their failure to conform to role expectations. The price one has to pay for nonconformity to accept gender roles is often high, frequently producing emotional and psychological scars that increase one's vulnerability to maladaptive behavior.

On a broader level, a variety of social experiences and situations can significantly influence the development of abnormal behavior. For instance, an inverse correlation seems to exist between socioeconomic standing and the prevalence of abnormal behavior—the lower the socioeconomic level, the higher the incidence of maladaptive behavior (U. S. Department of Health and Human Services, 1999; Eron & Peterson, 1982). Many persons in society have been subjected to attacks on their self-esteem and to demoralizing stereotypes due to prejudice and discrimination. Elevated rates of abnormal behavior have been associated with factors such as economic and employment problems (Dooley & Catalano, 1980). Recession and inflation coupled with high unemployment lead to chronic anxiety for

many people, and these conditions are typically accompanied by increases in certain types of maladaptive behavior, such as depression, suicide, and crime (Brenner, 1973). Periods of pervasive social change—much like what Toffler labeled as future shock in his 1970 book by the same title—can produce profound confusion, uncertainty, and a sense of helplessness among some individuals. These reactions are well-established predisposing conditions for abnormal reactions to stressful events (Frank, 1978).

Classification of Mental Disorders

Our understanding of mental disturbances has steadily progressed throughout the past several centuries. During this time there has been a general movement away from superstition and demonic explanations for abnormal behaviors. Consistent with such a movement has been an increasing need to develop accurate, consistent, and specific information about mental illness. This section reviews the *Diagnostic and Statistical Manual of Mental Disorders* 4th edition (*DSM-IV*), published by the American Psychiatric Association (APA, 1994) The *DSM-IV* is the most widely used organizational scheme for mental disorders in the United States.

The delineation of various categories of maladaptive behavior is a necessary first step toward introducing some order into discussions regarding the nature, causes, and treatment of such behavior. Additionally, diagnostic classification helps to keep accurate statistical counts of the incidence of various disorders, an important objective in terms of meeting medical insurance company needs.

The *Diagnostic and Statistical Manual of Mental Disorders I* was published by the American Psychiatric Association in 1952. Subsequently, three more editions were published: *DSM-II* in 1968, *DSM-III* in 1980, and *DSM-IV* in 1994. Each successive edition has sought to improve its clinical usefulness for professionals who diagnose and treat patients. The *DSM* system seeks to specify the exact symptoms that must be observed for a given diagnostic label to be applied. The intent is to remove as many subjective elements from the diagnostic process as possible. In addition, it is important to recognize that the *DSM* does *not* attempt to classify people—what actually is being classified are disorders that people have.

DSM-IV (APA, 1994) evaluates an individual's behavior according to five dimensions or axes. Each axis refers to a different domain of information that may help to plan treatment and predict outcomes. The first four axes are detailed in **Table 3.1**.

The first three axes assess an individual's present condition. Axis I is for reporting all the various disorders in the classification except for the personality disorders and mental retardation (which are reported on Axis II).

Axis II is for reporting personality disorders and mental retardation and for noting prominent maladaptive personality features and defense mechanisms. Personality disorders and mental retardation are listed on a separate axis to ensure that consideration will be given to the presence of these conditions which might otherwise be overlooked when attention is directed to the usually more pronounced Axis I disorders.

Axis III identifies currently existing general medical conditions that may be relevant to the understanding or management of an individual's mental disorder.

More than one diagnosis may be recorded on Axes I and III and, in exceptional cases, on Axis II. A person may have multiple psychiatric symptoms or medical conditions (Axes I and III, respectively) and, much more rarely, may manifest more than one personality disorder (Axis II).

The last two axes provide assessments of broader aspects of the individual's situation. This might include stressors that have contributed to the current disorder (Axis IV) and an overview of how well the individual has been coping in recent months (Axis V).

Axis IV is used for reporting psychosocial and environmental problems that may affect the diagnosis, treatment, and prognosis of mental disorders (Axes I and II). A psychosocial or environmental problem may be a negative life event (e.g., the death of a spouse) or a problem related to an inadequacy of social support or personal resources. In addition to contributing to the initiation or exacerbation of a mental disorder, psychosocial problems may also develop as a consequence of a person's psychopathology.

Axis V is for reporting the clinician's judgment of the individual's overall level of functioning. This information helps in developing a plan of treatment and measuring the impact of intervention. The reporting of overall functioning on Axis V is done using the Global Assessment of Functioning (GAF) Scale (see **Table 3.2**, page 52).

Perhaps the main advantage to using a diagnostic classification system such as the one developed in *DSM-IV* (APA, 1994) is that it allows for a comprehensive and systematic evaluation of mental disorders and related problems. In addition, the *DSM-IV* system facilitates the process of documentation. The documentation format recommended by the American Psychiatric Association is the Multiaxial Evaluation Report Form.

The form has five sections that correspond to the five axes found in the *DSM-IV*. For Axis I and II, the evaluator specifies the diagnosed disorder by the *DSM-IV* numerical code and name. When more than one disorder has been diagnosed each would be listed. In situations where the diagnosed disorder corresponds to only one Axis, the second Axis is left blank. If a general medical condition is present, this is identified next using the *DSM-IV* code number and name. Psychosocial and environmental problems are addressed in the next section, using both a checklist to specify the presence of a primary set of problems as well as a narrative to provide a more detailed description. The score on the GAF Scale is the last item of information on this instrument.

The Multiaxial Evaluation Report Form (see **Table 3.3**, page 53) is a straightforward method for documenting relevant information about individuals with mental disorders. It may be used both as an initial assessment of an individual's status as well as an evaluation form to measure client progress. While the Therapeutic Recreation Specialist is seldom asked to complete the Multiaxial Evaluation Report Form, they should become familiar with it, as it provides the baseline information needed to develop an individualized therapeutic recreation program.

Mental Illness in Contemporary Society

Despite the extraordinary progress in terms of our understanding and treatment of people with mental disorders in the past century, mental illness remains one of the most serious public health challenges faced by our society. The seriousness of the problem was recently underscored by the publication of a comprehensive report, *Mental Health: A Report of the Surgeon General* (U. S. Department of Health and Human Services, 1999). This groundbreaking document confirmed that mental health problems continue to take a tremendous social, emotional, and economic toll on nations all over the world.

According to the surgeon general's report, devastating mental disorders such as schizophrenia, depression, bipolar disorder, Alzheimer's disease, behavioral disorders, and a range of other illnesses affect nearly

Axis I
Clinical disorders
Other conditions that may be a focus of clinical attention

    Disorders usually first diagnosed in infancy, childhood, or adolescence (excluding mental retardation, which is diagnosed on Axis II)

    Delirium, dementia, amnestic, and other cognitive disorders

    Mental disorders due to a general medical condition

    Substance-related disorders

    Schizophrenia and other psychotic disorders

    Mood disorders

    Anxiety disorders

    Somatoform disorders

    Factitious disorders

    Dissociative disorders

    Sexual and gender identity disorders

    Eating disorders

    Sleep disorders

    Impulse control disorders not elsewhere classified

    Adjustment disorders

    Other conditions that may be a focus of clinical attention

Axis II
Personality disorders
Mental retardation

    Paranoid personality disorder

    Schizoid personality disorder

    Schizotypal personality disorder

    Antisocial personality disorder

    Borderline personality disorder

    Histrionic personality disorder

    Narcissistic personality disorder

    Avoidant personality disorder

    Dependent personality disorder

    Obsessive-compulsive personality disorder

    Personality disorder not otherwise specified

    Mental retardation

Axis III
General medical conditions
(with ICD-9-CM codes)

    Infectious and parasitic diseases (001–139)

    Neoplasms (140–239)

    Endocrine, nutritional, and metabolic diseases and immunity disorders (240–279)

    Diseases of the blood and blood-forming organs (280–289)

    Diseases of the nervous system and sense organs (320–389)

    Diseases of the circulatory system (390–459)

    Diseases of the respiratory system (460–519)

    Diseases of the digestive system (520–579)

    Diseases of the genitourinary system (580–629)

    Complications of pregnancy, childbirth, and the puerperium (630–676)

    Diseases of the skin and subcutaneous tissue (680–709)

    Diseases of the musculoskeletal system and connective tissue (710–739)

    Congenital anomalies (760–779)

    Certain conditions originating in the perinatal period (780–799)

    Injury and poisoning (800–999)

Axis IV
Psychosocial and environmental problems

    Problems with primary support

    Problems related to the social environment

    Educational problems

    Occupational problems

    Housing problems

    Economic problems

    Problems with access to healthcare services

    Problems related to interaction with the legal system and crime

    Other psychosocial and environmental problems

Table 3.1 Axes of the DSM-IV (APA, 1994, pp. 26–30)

Global Assessment of Functioning (GAF) Scale

100–91	Superior functioning in a wide range of activities, life's problems never seem to get out of hand, is sought out by others because of his or her many positive qualities. No symptoms.
90–81	Absent or minimal symptoms (e.g., mild anxiety before an exam), good functioning in all areas, interested in and involved in a wide range of activities, socially effective, generally satisfied with life, no more than everyday problems or concerns (e.g., an occasional argument with family members).
80–71	If symptoms are present, they are transient and expectable reactions to psychosocial stressors (e.g., difficulty concentrating after a family argument), no more than slight impairment in social, occupational, or school functioning (e.g., temporarily falling behind in schoolwork).
70–61	Some mild symptoms (e.g., depressed mood and mild insomnia) OR some difficulty in social, occupational, or school functioning (e.g., occasional truancy, theft within the household), but generally functioning pretty well, has some meaningful relationships.
60–51	Moderate symptoms (e.g., flat affect and circumstantial speech, occasional panic attacks) OR moderate difficulty in social, occupational, or school functioning (e.g., few friends conflicts with peers or coworkers).
50–41	Serious symptoms (e.g., suicidal ideation, severe obsessive rituals, frequent shoplifting) OR any serious impairment in social, occupational, or school functioning (e.g., no friends, unable to keep a job).
40–31	Some impairment in reality testing or communication (e.g., speech is at times illogical, obscure, or irrelevant) OR major impairment in several areas, such as work or school, family relations, judgment, thinking, or mood (e.g., depressed man avoids friends, neglects family, and is unable to go to work; child frequently beats up younger children, is defiant at home, and is failing at school).
30–21	Behavior is considerably influenced by delusions or hallucinations OR serious impairment in communication or judgment (e.g., sometimes incoherent, acts grossly inappropriate, suicidal preoccupation) OR inability to function in almost all areas (e.g., stays in bed all day, no job, home, or friends).
20–11	Some danger of hurting self or others (e.g., suicide attempts without clear expectation of death, frequent violent, manic excitement) OR occasionally fails to maintain minimal personal hygeine (e.g., smears feces) OR gross impairment in communication (e.g., largely incoherent or mute).
10–1	Persistent danger of severely hurting self or others (e.g., recurrent violence) OR persistent inability to maintain minimal personal hygeine OR serious suicidal act with clear expectation of death.
0	Inadequate information

Table 3.2 Global Assessment of Functioning (GAF) Scale (APA, 1994, p. 32)

Multiaxial Evaluation Report Form

The following form is offered as one possibility for reporting multiaxial evaluations. In some settings, this form may be used exactly as is. In other settings, the form may be adapted to satisfy special needs.

Axis I
Clinical disorders
Other conditions that may be a focus of clinical attention
Diagnostic code   DSM-IV name

— — —.— —   _____
— — —.— —   _____
— — —.— —   _____

Axis II
Personality disorders
Mental retardation
Diagnostic code   DSM-IV name

— — —.— —   _____
— — —.— —   _____
— — —.— —   _____

Axis III
General medical conditions
ICD-9-CM code   ICD-9-CM name

— — —.— —   _____
— — —.— —   _____
— — —.— —   _____

Axis IV
Psychosocial and environmental problems
☐ Problems with primary support group *Specify* _____
☐ Problems related to the social environment *Specify* _____
☐ Educational problems *Specify* _____
☐ Occupational problems *Specify* _____
☐ Housing problems *Specify* _____
☐ Economic problems *Specify* _____
☐ Problems with access to healthcare services *Specify* _____
☐ Problems related to interaction with the legal system and crime *Specify* _____
☐ Other psychosocial and environmental problems *Specify* _____

Axis V
Global assessment of functioning scale
Score _____   Time frame _____

Table 3.3 Multiaxial Evaluation Report Form (APA, 1994, p. 34)

one in five Americans in any given year. Approximately 15% of adults who have a diagnosed mental disorder in one year also experience substance-related disorder, which complicates the primary problem. In addition, while most mental disorders can be successfully treated, the report concludes that nearly two thirds of all people with diagnosable mental disorders do not seek help (U. S. Department of Health and Human Services, 1999).

The burden of mental illness on health and productivity in the United States and throughout the world is just now beginning to be fully appreciated. Using a *disability-adjusted life year* (a measure that expresses the number of healthy years lost to premature death and years lived with a disability of specified severity and duration), it has been estimated that mental illness ranks as the second leading burdening disease in economically advanced nations. In the United States mental disorders collectively account for more than 15% of the overall burden of disease, ranking just behind cardiovascular conditions. (Murray & Lopez, 1996).

These data underscore the importance and urgency of treating and preventing mental disorders and of promoting mental health in our society. Untreated mental disorders lead to lost productivity, unsuccessful relationships, and significant distress and dysfunction. It may prevent an individual from fulfilling social norms and social expectations at home, work, or in his or her community. Mental disorders in adults can have a significant and continuing effect on children in their care. For about one in five Americans, mental illness presents a significant barrier to living a full, rich, and satisfying life. But just as importantly, we have begun to recognize that mental illness not only takes a toll on the person who is ill, it also takes a toll on the broader society in which the individual lives.

Chapter Summary

This chapter examined the affective domain and addressed the following issues:

- Nature of deviance and the response of different societies toward people who behaved in abnormal manners
- Historical explanations for abnormal behavior and past treatment of persons with mental illness
- Role of biological, psychological, and sociocultural factors in the causation of mental illness
- Identifiable biological, psychological, and sociocultural factors associated with deviant behavior
- Explanation and classification of mental disorders, including a review of the *DSM* system

References

Amcoff, S. (1980). The impact of malnutrition on the learning situation. In H. M. Sinclair and G. R. Howat (Eds.), *World nutrition and nutrition education*. New York, NY: Oxford University Press.

American Psychiatric Association. (1952). *Diagnostic and statistical manual of mental disorders*. Washington, DC: Author.

American Psychiatric Association. (1968). *Diagnostic and statistical manual of mental disorders* (2nd ed.). Washington, DC: Author.

American Psychiatric Association. (1980). *Diagnostic and statistical manual of mental disorders* (3rd ed.). Washington, DC: Author.

American Psychiatric Association. (1994). *Diagnostic and statistical manual of mental disorders* (4th ed.). Washington, DC: Author.

Beres, D. and Obers, S. J. (1950). The effects of extreme deprivation in infancy on psychic structure in adolescence. In R. S. Eissler (Ed.), *The psychoanalytic study of the child* (Vol. 5). New York, NY: International University Press.

Berger, R. J. (1970). Morpheus descending. *Psychology Today, 4*(1), 33–36.

Brenner, M. H. (1973). *Mental illness and the economy*. Cambridge, MA: Harvard University Press.

Burnstein, M. H. (1981). Child abandonment: Historical, sociological, and psychological perspectives. *Human Development, 11*, 213–221.

Carter, M., Van Andel, G., and Robb, G. (1995). *Therapeutic recreation: A practical approach*. Prospect Heights, IL: Waveland Press.

Castiglioni, A. (1946). *Adventures of the mind*. New York, NY: Knopf.

Coleman, J. C., Butcher, J. M., and Carson, R. C. (1984). *Abnormal psychology in modern life* (7th ed.). Glenville, IL: Scot, Foresman and Company.

Coopersmith, S. (1967). *The antecedents of self-esteem*. San Francisco, CA: Freeman.

Dattilo, J. and Murphy, W. (1987). *Behavior modification in therapeutic recreation*. State College, PA: Venture Publishing, Inc.

Davison, G. and Neale, J. (1986). *Abnormal psychology: An experimental clinical approach* (4th ed.). New York, NY: John Wiley & Sons.

Dooley, D. and Catalino, R. (1980). Economic changes as a cause of behavior disorder. *Psychological Bulletin, 87*, 45–468.

Eron, L. D. and Peterson, R. A. (1982). Abnormal behavior: Social approaches. In M. R. Rosenzweig and L. W. Porter (Eds.), *Annual Review of Psychology, 33*, 231–265.

Farber, J. E., Harlow, H. F., and West, L. J. (1956). Brainwashing, conditioning, and DDD (disability, dependency, and dread). *Sociometry, 19*, 271–85.

Frank, J. D. (1978). *Persuasion and healing* (2nd ed.). Baltimore, MD: Johns Hopkins University Press.

Glueck, S. and Glueck, E. (1968). *Nondelinquents in perspective*. Cambridge, MA: Harvard University Press.

Grob, G. N. (1983). *Mental illness and American society*, 1875–1940. Princeton, NJ: Princeton University Press.

Grob, G. N. (1994). *The mad among us: The history of the care of America's mentally ill*. New York, NY: Free Press.

Iso-Ahola, S. E. and Weissinger, E. (1984). Leisure and well-being: Is there a connection? *Parks & Recreation, 19*(6), 40–44.

Jenike, M. A. (1989). *Geriatric psychiatry and psychopharmacology*. St. Louis, MO: Mosby.

Kraus, R. and Shank, J. (1992). *Therapeutic recreation services: Principles and practices*. Dubuque, IA: Wm. C. Brown.

Lefkowitz, M. M., Huesmann, L. R., Walder, L. O., and Eron, L. D. (1973). Developing and predicting aggression. *Science News, 103*(3), 40.

Litz, T., Fleck, S., and Cornelison, A. R. (1965). *Schizophrenia and the family*. New York, NY: International University Press.

Main, M. and Weston, D. R. (1981). The quality of a toddler's relationship to mother and to father: Related to conflict behavior and the readiness to establish new relationships. *Child Development, 52*, 932–940.

Marecek, J. and Mettee, D. R. (1972). Avoidance of continued success as a function of self-esteem, level of esteem certainty and responsibility for success. *Journal of Personality and Social Psychology, 22*, 98–107.

Meyer, R. G. (1993). *The clinician's handbook* (3rd ed.). Boston, MA: Allyn & Bacon.

Murphy, H. B. (1978). Cultural influences on incidence, course and treatment response. In L. C. Wynne, R. L.

Cromwell, and S. Matthysse (Eds.), *The nature of schizophrenia: New approaches to research and treatment* (pp. 586–594). New York, NY: Wiley.

Murray, C. J. and Lopez, A. D. (Eds.). (1996). *The global burden of disease. A comprehensive assessment of mortality and disability from disease, injuries, and risk factors in 1990 and projected to 2020.* Cambridge, MA: Harvard School of Public Health.

Napoleon, N., Chassin, L., and Young, R. D. (1980). A replication and extension of "physical attractiveness and mental illness." *Journal of Abnormal Psychology, 89,* 250–253.

Patterson, G. R. (1979). Treatment for children with conduct problems: A review of outcome studies. In S. Feshbach and A. Fraczek (Eds.), *Aggression and behavior change: Biological and social processes.* New York, NY: Praeger.

Pringle, M. L. K. (1965). *Deprivation and education.* New York, NY: Humanities Press.

Rees, T. P. (1957). Back to moral treatment and community care. *Journal of Mental Science, 103,* 303–313.

Robinson, S. and Winnick, H. Z. (1983). Severe psychotic disturbances following crash diet weight loss. *Archives of General Psychiatry, 29*(4), 559–562.

Roff, J. D. and Knight, R. (1981). Family characteristics, childhood symptoms, and adult outcome in schizophrenia. *Journal of Abnormal Psychology, 90,* 510–520.

Rogers, C. R. (1951). *Client-centered therapy.* Boston, MA: Houghton Mifflin.

Rogers, C. R. (1959). Toward a theory of creativity. In H. H. Anderson (Ed.), *Creativity and its cultivation* (2nd ed.). New York, NY: Harper & Row.

Sears, R. R. (1961). Relation of early socialization experiences to aggression in middle childhood. *Journal of Abnormal Social Psychology, 63,* 466–492.

Seligman, M. E. P. (1975). *Helplessness: On depression, development and death.* San Francisco, CA: W. H. Freeman and Co.

Selling, L. S. (1943). *Man against madness.* New York, NY: Garden City Books.

Toffler, A. (1970). *Future shock.* New York, NY: Random House.

U. S. Department of Health and Human Services. (1999). *Mental health: A report of the surgeon general.* Washington, DC: Author.

World Health Organization. (1975). *Schizophrenia: A multinational study.* Geneva, Switzerland: Author.

Wright, B. (1960). Physical disability: A psychological approach. New York, NY: Harper & Brothers.

Yates, A. (1981). Narcissistic traits in certain abused children. American Journal of Orthopsychiatry, 51, 55–62.

CHAPTER 4
ANXIETY-RELATED DISORDERS

The affective domain deals with some of the most personal levels of human functioning. Disturbances in the brain (the source of affective functioning), whether derived from biological, psychosocial, or sociocultural roots, produce mental illness.

Mental illness is identified in terms of behavioral manifestations. This means that in most cases the diagnosis of some form of mental illness is made on the basis of symptoms or behaviors displayed by the individual. All the disorders discussed in this chapter manifest themselves in relation to persistent feelings of danger or apprehension. These feelings of anxiety are so strong they produce self-injurious or socially inappropriate behaviors. Thus, these abnormal behaviors are the product of perceived stress in one or more aspects of the individual's environment.

This chapter covers three broad categories of emotional disorders: anxiety disorders, somatoform disorders, and dissociative disorders. Each of these categories will be subdivided into representative specific disorders. After presenting general descriptive information about each disorder, we will discuss associated features, prevalence, and potential treatments. At the end of the chapter we will present possible implications for therapeutic recreation practice.

Anxiety Disorders

Anxiety is characterized by subjective feelings of threat, dread, or apprehension, or by a sense of impending disaster associated with varying degrees of arousal and uneasiness. Like physical pain, anxiety leads to changes in behavior, thus affecting learning and adaptation. Severe anxiety serves as a primary initiator of maladaptive functioning and psychological disturbance. However, although maladaptive, individuals who suffer from anxiety disorders seldom display gross distortions of reality or experience hallucinations or the delusions often associated with other forms of mental illness.

Anxiety may be described as having two components: psychological and somatic. The psychological component varies from individual to individual and is strongly influenced by the personality and coping mechanisms. Somatic or bodily manifestations can usually be succinctly described by the individual and vary in their severity. We discuss five categories of anxiety disorders: panic disorder, phobias, obsessive-compulsive disorder, posttraumatic stress disorder, and generalized anxiety disorder.

Panic Disorder

Panic disorder is a syndrome characterized by the recurrence of sudden, unexpected panic attacks. In panic disorder an abrupt and inexplicable attack of a host of jarring symptoms overwhelm the individual, including:

- Labored breathing
- Heart palpitations
- Chest pain
- Feelings of choking and smothering
- Dizziness, sweating, and trembling
- Intense apprehension, terror, and feelings of doom
- Feelings of being outside of one's body (depersonalization)
- Fear of losing control or going crazy

The panic attacks occur frequently—weekly or more often. The attacks typically last for about 15 minutes, although they may last for hours (Hoehn-Saric & McLeod, 1988). Sometimes the panic attacks are linked to specific situations, such as using public transportation, but they may also occur spontaneously without a situational trigger. Diagnostic criteria specifies that the attacks are followed by at least one month of persistent concern about having additional attacks or worry about the implications or consequences of the attacks (APA, 1994).

The frequency and severity of panic attacks can vary widely. Some individuals experience panic attacks over many years that fluctuate in frequency and intensity but never completely stop. Others have discrete periods of attacks separated by long panic-free intervals. Most often, persons seeking treatment experienced a fluctuating course of attacks over several years. The disorder is recurrent (i.e., its symptoms occur repeatedly) and episodic (i.e., each occurrence is a separate incidence). In at least 50% of cases the course is chronic (i.e., continuing over time) (Keller & Baker, 1992).

The onset of panic disorder is variable—the average age of onset is 24 and about 40% of patients have an onset after age 30 (Matuzas, Jack, Andriukaitis, Olson & Hernandez, 1993). Studies estimate a lifetime prevalence of panic disorder to be between 1.5% and 3.5% (APA, 1994). The syndrome is also frequently associated with other psychiatric conditions, including generalized anxiety disorder, major depressive disorder, and substance-related disorder, as well as a high risk of suicide (Fawcett, 1992).

The *Diagnostic and Statistical Manual of Mental Disorders IV* (*DSM-IV*) identifies panic disorder as a separate and distinct disorder; however, it is better understood within the context of two subclassifications: panic attack and agoraphobia (APA, 1994).

A *panic attack* is described as a discrete period of intense fear or discomfort. The attack has a sudden onset and builds to a peak rapidly (usually in 10 minutes or less). Frequently the attack is accompanied by a sense of imminent danger or impending doom and an urge to flee one's present situation.

DSM-IV recognizes three characteristic types of panic attacks (APA, 1994):

1. Unexpected panic attacks that seem to occur spontaneously and are not identified with a situational trigger
2. Situationally bound panic attacks that almost invariably occur upon exposure to or anticipation of a situational trigger
3. Situationally predisposed panic attacks that are likely to occur upon exposure to a situational trigger, but do not always occur upon exposure

Agoraphobia (from the Greek *agora*—place of assembly, marketplace) is a cluster of fears centering around public places and being unable to escape or find help should the individual suddenly become incapacitated. Fears of shopping, encountering crowds, or traveling are often part of agoraphobia. Agoraphobic fears also typically involve situations that include being alone and away from places of comfort (e.g., one's home). The anxiety may lead to pervasive avoidance of the source of discomfort, leading to an impaired ability to carry out basic activities of daily life. Undoubtedly agoraphobia is a very distressing condition; consider how limiting it must be to be afraid of leaving one's house.

The condition often begins with recurrent panic attacks. It often includes symptoms such as dizziness, tension, loss of bladder control, compulsions, depression, and a fear of "going mad." It is one of the most common phobias treated in clinical settings; however, many of the more severe cases may be untreated as sufferers are unable to leave their home to seek therapy. Most agoraphobics (75% to 90%) are women who begin to experience symptoms after the onset of puberty (Davidson & Neale, 1986).

The *DSM-IV* (APA, 1994) classification system distinguishes between two forms of panic disorder:

1. Panic disorder without agoraphobia—recurrent and unexpected panic attacks with the absence of agoraphobia
2. Panic disorder with agoraphobia—anxiety about being in public places or situations from which escape may be difficult or embarrassing. Due to these fears, the person either restricts travel, needs a companion when away from home, or endures these situations despite intense anxiety.

Treatment for Panic Disorder

Since the hallmark of panic disorder is periodic episodes of intense anxiety and psychological discomfort, treatment attempts to develop a sense of mastery over anxiety and a controlled relaxation response. Relaxation training using techniques like progressive muscle relaxation, meditation, and yoga has proven helpful for many individuals suffering from panic disorder. Meyer (1993) suggests that conducting relaxation training in a group setting is beneficial because it can lead to the awareness that others share this problem, it encourages discussion of anxieties associated with the syndrome, and it increases the likelihood of entering group therapy.

The development of an educational program designed to inform individuals about panic disorder—to provide information about its characteristics, its prevalence, factors that can exacerbate or ameliorate symptoms, and the effectiveness of available treatments—can be very helpful as well. Such a program can provide reassurance that the symptoms are part of an identifiable syndrome shared by many others, and that effective treatment is available. Matuzas and his colleagues claim that an education program alone "can bring about remarkable improvement and, occasionally, a complete remission" (1993, p. 162).

Pharmacological intervention is also an important part of a treatment program for panic disorder. From a physical perspective, antidepressant drugs appreciably reduce the frequency and intensity of panic attacks for many individuals (Matuzas & Jack, 1991). Perhaps just as importantly, these agents may provide psychological relief in the sense that it gives individuals confidence that control over their symptoms is available (Foa & Kozak, 1986).

Phobias

A *phobia* is a disrupting, fear-mediated avoidance that is out of proportion to the danger actually posed by a particular object or situation. For example, when a fear of spiders (provided there is not objective danger) leads to a level of distress sufficient to disrupt common life activities, the label phobia is likely to be applied.

A plethora of complex terms have been formulated as names for such unwarranted avoidance patterns. In each case the suffix *phobia* (from the Greek god *Phobos*, who frightened his enemies) is preceded by a Greek word for the feared object of situation. Among the more familiar terms are claustrophobia (fear of closed places), acrophobia (fear of heights), and agoraphobia (fear of public places).

The *DSM-IV* (APA, 1994) describes three major phobias: agoraphobia without history of panic disorder, specific phobia, and social phobia.

Agoraphobia without History of Panic Disorder

This diagnosis may be attributed to individuals who display the characteristics associated with agoraphobia, but who have never met the criteria for panic disorder. In this disorder, anxiety associated with being in places or situations from which escape may be difficult or embarrassing is present, but actual panic attacks do not occur. Individuals with agoraphobia usually worry about experiencing a variety of symptoms (e.g., dizziness, loss of bladder or bowel control, difficulty breathing) while away from home. Sometimes they have experienced these symptoms in the past and they dread reexperiencing them should they leave home. The age of onset is usually between 20 and 40 and the disorder occurs far more frequently in women. Youthful experiences such as the refusal to go to school or parental overprotectiveness are sometimes viewed as early signs of the disorder (Matuzas et al., 1993).

Specific Phobia

Specific phobia, formerly referred to as simple phobia, is what most people typically associate with the term: fear of heights, animals, flying, and the like. Exposure to the phobic stimulus almost invariably provokes an anxiety response. The avoidance and distress caused by the feared situation often interfere with the person's normal routines and daily functioning, thus increasing his or her anxiety.

The *DSM IV* (APA, 1994) recognizes four subtypes of specific phobias:

1. Animal Type—fear is generated by animals or insects
2. Natural Environment Type—fear cued by objects in the natural environment such as storms, heights, or water
3. Blood-Injection-Injury Type—fear cued by seeing blood or an injury, receiving an injection, or other invasive medical procedures
4. Situational Type—fear generated by a specific situation such as bridges, tunnels, flying, driving, or enclosed places

As with other forms of phobia, the person recognizes that his or her fear is irrational and out of proportion to the threat caused by the actual object or situation. Even when there is an element of active danger in the situation or object, such as the fear of heights, the individual's reaction is disproportionate to the level of risk encountered. Specific phobia is usually a relatively chronic disorder, frequently starting in childhood, and more commonly diagnosed in females than males. In community samples, a one-year prevalence rate of about 9% has been reported. Lifetime prevalence rates range from 10% to 11.3% (APA, 1994).

Social Phobia

A *social phobia* is a persistent, irrational fear generally linked to the presence of other people. Social phobics are characterized by anxiety about possible scrutiny of their behaviors by others, usually accompanied by anticipatory anxiety or panic and/or acting in a manner that will be considered shameful by others (Walker, Norton & Ross, 1991). The individual tries to avoid a particular situation in which he or she might be scrutinized and reveal signs of nervousness or behave in an embarrassing way. Social phobias often center on such behaviors as speaking in public (the most common form of this disorder), using public lavatories, eating in public, or blushing uncontrollably. Individuals with social phobia may take extreme measures to avoid these situations, or they may endure them with extreme anxiety. While the fear of speaking in public or anxiety over other social situations is not uncommon, they do not constitute social phobia unless exposure to the feared situation almost invariably provokes anxiety which may take the form of a panic attack (APA, 1994). As with other phobias, the individual with a social phobia recognizes that his or her fear is excessive or unreasonable.

This disorder, although not uncommon, rarely incapacitates (Meyer, 1993). Social phobics seek help much less frequently than do agoraphobics (Davison & Neale, 1986). This disorder usually begins in late childhood or early adolescence and men seek treatment slightly more often than do women (Matuzas et al., 1993). Lifetime prevalence rates are reported at between 3% and 13% (APA, 1994).

Treatment for Phobias

Behavior therapy is useful for most individuals who experience phobias. In addition to reducing avoidance, it may prevent a recurrence of symptoms and increase self-confidence. A key component in most behavioral therapy interventions is *relaxation training*. Relaxation can be taught using techniques such as meditation, progressive muscle relaxation, or biofeedback.

A principle behavioral treatment for phobias is *systematic desensitization*. Using this technique, the phobic individual imagines a sense of increasingly frightening scenes while in a relaxed state. Gradually, starting with the situations causing the least fear, phobics are asked to face the feared situations in fantasy or in reality. While they are doing this, therapists instruct them to use previously learned relaxation responses. Once initiated, the therapist attempts to work with the patient through progressively more fearful situations. Systematic desensitization seems to be an effective treatment, especially for the social phobias (Hecker & Thorpe, 1992).

Fearful individuals may also be treated using the behavioral technique called *modeling*. This technique usually involves exposing the phobic person to a model (either in person or on film) who deals with anxiety-provoking situations in a fearless way. The individual being treated is then asked to imitate the behavior of the model. Modeling is employed using a *graded-task approach* (i.e., one step at a time) or *flooding* (exposing phobic individuals to fearful situations all at once and for prolonged periods). Role-playing that develops specific skills may help some individuals and may be used to give social phobics a sense of control that allows them to go on if an anticipated and feared mistake does occur.

Pharmacological treatments (drug therapy) may be combined with other techniques in the treatment of phobias. Drug treatment is not curative, but the use of pharmacological agents such as antidepressants have proven helpful in reducing the frequency and intensity of panic attacks and some of the accompanying anxious

mood experienced by people suffering from phobias (Matuzas et al., 1993).

Oftentimes the use of support groups can help alleviate the sense of isolation experienced by individuals with phobias. A group may also enhance the person's social networks and can be a source of information, understanding, and encouragement.

Obsessive–Compulsive Disorder

Obsessive–compulsive disorder (OCD) is a classification of anxiety disorder characterized by the presence of obsessions or compulsions. These obsessions or compulsions form the predominant clinical manifestation of the illness.

Obsessions are persistent thoughts, impulses, or images that recurrently and urgently intrude into the conscious awareness and are perceived as intrusive and senseless. The person with OCD attempts to ignore or suppress such thoughts and images, but his or her efforts are unsuccessful. Failure to ignore or neutralize these obsessions contributes to the sense of distress. The most common obsessions are repetitive thoughts of contamination, violence, doubts about religion, one's duties, and self-doubts (Meyer, 1993).

Compulsions are impulses to action resulting in repetitive and intentional behaviors (e.g., hand washing) performed in a ritualistic fashion in response to obsession or according to rules that the individual feels must be applied rigidly. These behaviors seem to be undertaken as countermeasures to prevent or reduce the distress caused by the initial obsessive thought or idea. Compulsions help to allay the feelings of anxiety and dread that accompany obsessions.

While most people probably experience intrusive, senseless thoughts, urges, and impulses at some time in their lives, and have engaged in some meaningless rituals, for individuals who suffer from OCD these thoughts and rituals are sufficiently severe to cause marked distress and interfere with daily functioning.

Several features characterize OCD. First, the obsessive thoughts are ego-alien—they are not experienced as part of one's normal psychological being. They are undesired, unacceptable, and involuntary. Second, people with OCD understand the obsessions are products of their own mind and not imposed from without. No matter how vivid and compelling the ideas, the person with OCD recognizes them as absurd, irrational, and unreasonable. Third, the compulsion to perform an act is coupled with a strong need to resist it and a sense of mounting tension relieved only by yielding to the compulsion. However, the performance of the compulsive act, while it may relieve tension, provides no sense of pleasure to the person. Finally, efforts to hide symptoms from others are common due to fears of shame, embarrassment, or being stigmatized (Israni, Janicak & Davis, 1993).

The manifestation of obsessions and compulsions are varied and complex. They may occur alone or together, they may be experienced as thoughts or impulses, and they may range from simple acts to highly complicated patterns of thinking and ritualized behavior. Obsessions may take the form of intrusive thoughts (e.g., preoccupation with past deeds or a sense of guilt over some disastrous event), images (often involving violent or sexual themes), impulses (e.g., the urge to shout obscenities or jump in front of a moving car), or rituals (e.g., repeated showering, or the use of highly elaborate routines to complete common activities). Any deviation in the routine causes anxiety and compels the individual to repeat the action over and over (Israni et al., 1993).

A frequent consequence of OCD is the negative effect it can have on the individual's relations with other people, especially family members. A person with the irresistible need to wash his or her hands every few minutes or count every tile in a floor is likely to cause concern and even resentment in a spouse, children, friends, or coworkers. The undesirable effects on others can have additional consequences, engendering feelings of anxiety and depression in the obsessive-compulsive person and setting the stage for even further deterioration of personal relationships.

The usual age for onset of OCD is late adolescence or early adulthood. It often follows some stressful event such as pregnancy, childbirth, family conflict, or difficulties at work. This syndrome occurs proportionately more often in middle- or upper-class individuals. Individuals with OCD are brighter on average than individuals with other anxiety disorders, perhaps because obsessions are intellectual coping strategies for anxiety (Kozak, Foa & McCarthy, 1988).

Obsessive–compulsive disorder has traditionally been thought to be relatively rare, at least as compared to other anxiety disorders. Recent estimates, however, indicate about 2.5% of the general population have a history of obsessive-compulsive symptoms, with about 1.6% displaying the symptoms at any given time (Israni et al., 1993). The previous underestimation may be due to the embarrassment experienced by some individuals who may have the syndrome but who are reluctant to seek treatment.

Treatment of Obsessive–Compulsive Disorder

The most common form of behavioral treatment for OCD is exposure plus response prevention. In this technique the patient is brought in direct contact with the feared object or obsessional cue. The exposure can be made using *participant modeling* (the therapist first makes contact with the feared object and then requests the patient to follow suit) or *flooding* (the patient is encouraged directly into the anxiety-provoking situation). The exposure followed by *response prevention*, in which the patient is persuaded not to carry out the compulsive act. This may mean removal of sources of compulsive behavior (e.g., taking soap and towels away from a sink for an individual who compulsively washes his or her hands in response to touching a doorknob). This combined approach to treatment reduces the capacity of obsessions to provoke anxiety and blocks the reinforcing compulsive action (Meyer, 1993).

Another technique that has been used successfully with OCD patients is *thought stopping*. This procedure asks the person with OCD to bring the obsessional thought into conscious awareness. On a cue (e.g., a signal from the therapist), the patient shouts, "Stop!" The patient eventually generalizes the experience and independently shouts, "Stop!" (or completes some other intrusion, such as snapping an elastic band on the wrist), each time the obsessional thought occurs. Thought stopping may be supplemented with *cognitive reframing*—visualizing a pleasant scene immediately after saying stop. As progress occurs, group therapy may be used to help encourage self-awareness and self-disclosure (Israni et al., 1993; Meyer, 1993).

Pharmacological treatment of OCD is usually used only when behavioral techniques do not produce desired results or when complicating psychological conditions (e.g., depression) exist.

Posttraumatic Stress Disorder

The anxiety disorders discussed so far in this chapter share an important characteristic: They cannot be adequately explained by environmental circumstances alone. In contrast, people diagnosed as having *posttraumatic stress disorder* (PTSD) have in their lives a major, salient, and powerful happening. As described in *DSM-IV* (APA, 1994, p. 424):

The person has experienced, witnessed, or been confronted with an event or events that involve actual or threatened death or serious injury, or a threat to the physical integrity of oneself or others. The person's response (to the event) involved intense fear, helplessness, or horror.

In posttraumatic stress disorder, a traumatic event, such as rape, combat, or a natural disaster, leads to difficulties with concentration and memory, an inability to relax, impulsiveness, a tendency to be easily startled, disturbed sleep, anxiety, depression, and a psychic numbing. Previously enjoyed experiences lose their interest. Individuals become detached from others and from events of daily life. In the case of shared trauma that injured or took the lives of companions, a sense of intense guilt for having survived often results.

The traumatic event is persistently reexperienced in a variety of manners. Flashbacks, vivid and intrusive recollections of the painful event, and recurring nightmares or frightening dreams are common. The individual usually experiences intense psychological distress (e.g., anxiety, disorganization, fear) and physiologic reactivity (e.g., nausea, breaking into a cold sweat) upon exposure to environmental cues or reminders that symbolize or resemble the traumatic event (APA, 1994).

Traumatic events commonly evoke emotional responses and behaviors aimed at reducing stress. Normal responses to trauma may include anxiety, depression, and physical irritability. Themes related to the event may produce distressing thoughts or may intrude upon dreams. However, with the normal response these symptoms cause only momentary disturbances in functioning and usually diminish in a few weeks. The diagnosis of PTSD is characterized by severe symptoms which do not resolve within a few weeks, which may cause impairment in functioning in an array of activities of daily life, and which may lead to maladaptive responses including withdrawal, substance abuse, and depressive reactions.

Community-based studies reveal lifetime prevalence for PTSD at between 1% and 4%; however, among at-risk individuals (e.g., combat veterans, victims of criminal violence), prevalence rates are generally much higher (APA, 1994).

Treatment of Posttraumatic Stress Disorder

Evidence supports the use of therapeutic exposure and cognitive reframing as the most widely used treatment

for PTSD (Hecker & Thorpe, 1992). Techniques such as systematic desensitization or flooding often supplement exposure. The use of support groups also appears to be helpful in the amelioration of stress-related disorders. These groups provide an opportunity for victims to express their feelings about what they have experienced and to receive reassurance that their reactions are normal and transient. At present, there are no pharmacological treatments specific to PTSD, although mild tranquilizers are sometimes used to provide temporary relief from symptoms.

Interest in providing treatment to victims of combat-induced stress expanded rapidly after World War II. Based upon this work the principle of immediacy has been established as a key goal in crisis intervention. Because it has been found that emotional problems following a disaster escalate over time if not given early attention (Matuzas et al., 1993), immediacy emphasizes early awareness, detection, treatment, and return to typical life situations for victims of traumatically induced stress. We often see this principle employed as mental health professionals are quickly mobilized to aid individuals who have been exposed to a severely traumatic event (e.g., shootings in schools, hurricanes, airplane crashes).

Generalized Anxiety Disorder

Central features of *generalized anxiety disorder* (GAD) include excessive anxiety, worry, and apprehension that occur on most days for an extended period of time. The individual is chronically and persistently anxious in many life situations. In contrast to *situational anxiety disorder*, which produces anxiety when an individual is confronted with a specific situation (e.g., encountering a snake), there does not seem to be a specific focus to this sense of apprehension. Instead, the individual's anxiety is general and involves any number of different events. While the disorder is chronic in nature, patients may experience acute episodes punctuated by disabling periods of anxiety.

A variety of somatic symptoms are associated with GAD. General feelings of restlessness or being on edge, difficulty in concentrating, irritability, muscle tension, and sleep disturbances are among the symptoms established in the *DSM-IV* (APA, 1994). Other common complaints include sweating, flushing, pounding heart, upset stomach, diarrhea, cold, clammy hands, dry mouth, and a lump in the throat. Rapee (1991) claims that the essential feature of GAD is "chronic autonomic hyperactivity" similar to the general physiological-stress syndrome originally described by Hans Selye (1956). Restlessness, fidgeting, trembling, inability to relax, and being easily startled mark this syndrome.

As for the state of mind, the person is generally apprehensive, often imagining and worrying about impending disasters. Individuals are frequently impatient, irritable, and easily distracted. While often easily discouraged, indecisive, and mildly depressed, most individuals usually manage to struggle through their days. If treatment is sought, it is often preceded by periods of significant distress that causes impairment in social, occupational, or other areas of daily functioning (Sharma, Andriulcaitis & Davis, 1993).

The prevalence of anxiety disorders in the general population is conservatively estimated to be from 2% to 4.7% (Sharma et al., 1993). Many experts feel that this figure is probably low due to poor recognition of anxiety syndromes. Among psychiatric patients, a primary diagnosis of anxiety disorder is an estimated 5% to 15% (Sharma et al., 1993). Anxiety disorders are twice as common in women as in men (APA, 1994).

Treatment of Generalized Anxiety Disorder

The initial treatment for GAD usually attempts to reduce the chronic state of autonomic arousal, often by using a combination of therapies. Biofeedback has also proven helpful in the treatment of autonomic tension (Schwartz, 1987). *Biofeedback* employs a measuring device to reward patients for a relaxation response by providing them with immediate feedback on functions such as pulse rate, skin temperature, and eye movement. Concomitantly, teaching the client a controlled relaxation response (e.g., meditation, yoga) has successfully been used with GAD patients (Wolpe, 1987). Pharmacological treatment in the form of tranquilizers is also often used during initial stages of treatment to help relieve symptoms of autonomic arousal.

As treatment progresses the emphasis shifts toward attacking underlying causes of the pervasive anxiety. Often this entails efforts to help the individual acquire skills that might engender a sense of competence or self-efficacy (Bandura, 1977). The skills may be taught by verbal instructions, modeling, or operant shaping. As a client begins to gain more control over the anxiety, a technique such as client-centered therapy (Rogers, 1951) may become the primary treatment mode.

Somatoform Disorders

Somatoform disorders are characterized by the presence of bodily symptoms that suggest a physical defect or dysfunction, but for which no physiological basis can be found. The symptoms of somatoform disorders are not believed to be under conscious control; thus despite the inability to identify physiological reasons for the dysfunction the victims are not malingering. Somatoform disorders occur more frequently in women (Kellner, 1986).

The *DSM-IV* (APA, 1994) identifies four major subcategories of somatoform disorders: somatization disorder, conversion disorder, somatoform pain disorder, and hypochondriasis. There is also a catchall category, somatoform disorder not otherwise specified, in which individuals are placed if they fit the general criteria for somatoform disorders but not the specific criteria of the other four major categories.

Somatization Disorder

Somatization disorder is a chronic syndrome marked by multiple somatic complaints beginning before the age of 20. This disorder, formerly known as Briquettes' syndrome, is commonly associated with complaints about pain (e.g., head, abdomen, back, joint, or extremities), gastrointestinal symptoms (e.g., nausea, diarrhea, bloating), sexual symptoms (e.g., sexual indifference, irregular menses, excessive menstrual bleeding, or vomiting throughout pregnancy), and pseudoneurological symptoms (e.g., blindness or double vision, loss of touch or pain sensation, impaired coordination, hallucinations, paralysis or localized weakness, seizures, amnesia). These symptoms and/or complaints are recurrent, but despite medical attention no apparent physical cause can be identified.

Persons with this disorder make frequent visits to physicians. They often describe their symptoms in a vague but exaggerated manner. Patients are given to histrionics, presenting their complaints in overly dramatic fashion or as part of a long and complicated medical history. Because of their preoccupation with symptoms and their history of suffering, and because exhaustive testing fails to uncover pathological or organic sources for their symptoms, physicians often come to believe that such people are faking their condition. Hence, medical personnel are inclined to put them in the category of "crank" and avoid spending time with them (Meyer, 1993).

Somatization disorder typically begins in late adolescence and is diagnosed predominantly in women. Its prevalence may be as high as 1% of the female population. Evidence suggests that it runs in families and is more common in female relatives of patients with the disorder (Lewis & Flaherty, 1993).

Conversion Disorder

Conversion disorder is similar to somatization disorder in many respects. In the conversion disorder, however, a specific symptom or set of symptoms is the focal point of the individual's concerns. The symptom (or symptoms) typically mimics neurological abnormalities that impair sensorimotor functioning. Classic conversion symptoms include partial or complete paralysis of arms or legs, seizures and coordination problems, sensations of pricking or tingling or creeping on the skin, difficulty in vocalizing, and partial or complete blindness. Individuals diagnosed with conversion disorder often manifest an attitude referred to as *la belle indifference*, which refers to the lack of concern about the apparent serious implications of the disorder. They appear to be aware at some level that their symptoms do not predict the further dire consequences normally associated with them.

For many years conversion disorder was associated with the condition known as hysteria. *Hysteria* refers to a psychological condition characterized by extreme excitability often in response to environmental cues. An individual who acts hysterically behaves in an abnormal manner in response to some event or situation. In like fashion, conversion disorder is considered to be a psychological response to perceived sources of stress. The term conversion originally was derived from Sigmund Freud, who believed that energy or a repressed instinct is diverted into sensory-motor channels and blocks functioning. Thus, anxiety and psychological conflict convert into physical symptoms.

Conversion symptoms usually develop in adolescence or early adulthood. Some experts believe that a dependent or histrionic personality predisposes individuals to the development of conversion symptoms (Meyer, 1993), but little definitive information exists. Prevalence rates are not established, but the disorder appears to be less prevalent now than it was in the first part of the century (Lewis & Flaherty, 1993). While females are more likely than males to be diagnosed with conversion disorder today, during both world wars a large number of males developed conversion-like difficulties in combat (Ziegler, Imboden & Meyer, 1960).

Somatoform Pain Disorder

Somatoform pain disorder is a conversion disorder that specifically involves pain not due to physical cause. The individual with this disorder frequently describes pain symptoms that do not follow known anatomic patterns, and extensive diagnostic work cannot reveal evidence of organic pathology. As with other forms of conversion disorder, persons with this syndrome tend to be highly suggestible. They often "doctor shop" and seek repeated evaluations in search of an organic cause of their pain. They commonly develop a history of extensive medical treatment and take significant dosages of pain medicine. Rejecting psychological explanations for their symptoms and avoiding psychiatric care are common. Moreover, they are likely to adopt the role of invalid in response to rewards from those around them (Lewis & Flaherty, 1993).

The *DSM-IV* (APA, 1994) recognizes two subcategories of pain disorder: pain disorder associated with psychological factors, and pain disorder associated with both psychological factors and a general medical condition.

While the *DSM-IV* (APA, 1994) claims that somatoform pain disorder may be relatively common, little is known about actual prevalence rates. Because individuals who experience this disorder typically reject psychological explanations, they are often treated by medical personnel. Their symptoms may also mask other undiagnosed disorders such as depression or posttraumatic stress disorder (Benedikt & Kolb, 1986). Somatoform pain disorder may occur at any age.

Hypochondriasis

A *hypochondriac* is preoccupied with fears of having a serious disease. As evidence of their ill health, hypochondriacs consistently and unreasonably interpret normal or relatively unimportant bodily and physical changes as indicative of serious physical disorder. They are constantly alert to new symptoms that they interpret as further evidence of their disorder. Their preoccupation with illness persists despite medical reassurances of health. Hypochondriasis resembles somatization disorder in many respects, except that the hypochondriac is preoccupied with the fear of having a specific and serious physical disease, rather than with the symptoms themselves. Hypochondriacs do not fear becoming sick—they are certain they already are sick.

Complaints expressed by hypochondriacs are often vague and dramatic, and they wax and wane with difficulties in the person's life. Meyer has suggested that this disorder reflects a distorted coping strategy employed by the patient in an attempt to avoid a feeling of loss of control and in that sense it parallels the panic disorder described previously (1993, p. 132). The symptoms described by the hypochondriac serve to help avoid tasks or demands that they feel are being placed upon them.

A number of common factors have been observed in the development of hypochondriasis (Kellner, 1986). Two of the primary factors identified by Kellner include:

1. Personal history marked by substantial exposure to an atmosphere of illness. This could include a family member who was diagnosed with a serious illness, or a significant individual who was also hypochondrial.

2. A strong dependency relationship with a family member who expressed normal love and affection during periods when the hypochondriac has been ill.

The prevalence of hypochondriasis is difficult to assess, but the disorder is considered relatively common in medical practice. A diagnosis of hypochondriasis is made in about 1% of psychiatric patients. The disorder affects both sexes equally and may appear at any age. It is seen most frequently in the age range of 30 to 40 for men and 40 to 50 for women (Lewis & Flaherty, 1993). It is believed that there are many "closet hypochondriacs"—individuals who may not constantly visit physicians, yet who are heavily involved in health fads and who closely monitor their bodily functions (Meister, 1980).

Treatment of Somatoform Disorders

The primary focus of treatment for somatoform disorders is the development of a trusting relationship between the patient and the caregiver, wherein the patient can begin to accept other explanations for his or her "symptoms" and "illnesses." In this regard the use of psychotherapeutic approaches such as client-centered therapy (Rogers, 1951), which promote empathetic understanding on the part of the caregiver, seems very appropriate. The therapist must assure the patient that he or she understands that his or her experience of suffering is real, even if an organic source cannot be identified. Such reassurance helps the patient to understand that his or her condition is not being dealt with lightly, and it also allows him or her a "face-saving" way of dropping the somatoform system.

Along with supportive psychotherapy, specific techniques such as reality therapy (Glasser, 1980) can be appropriate. *Reality therapy* is a systematic approach to treatment that focuses on present behavior. The therapist guides the client to enable them to see themselves accurately, face reality, and to fulfill their own needs without harming themselves or others. This approach encourages the client to take personal responsibility for his or her own behavior. According to advocates for reality therapy, personal responsibility is equated with mental health.

Cognitive and behavioral therapy techniques such as *distraction* and *imaging* may also be appropriate. These approaches emphasize efforts to direct clients' attention to pleasant, nonstressful experiences rather than perceived symptoms of bodily pain or discomfort.

Creating an altered state of consciousness by means of *hypnosis* has also proven effective in treating some individuals with somatoform pain disorder (Lewis & Flaherty, 1993) and conversion disorder (Meyer, 1992). Hypnotic induction procedures bring about a heightened state of selective attention in which the client "tunes out" irrelevant stimuli. One hypnotic phenomena used widely in therapy is *posthypnotic suggestion*. Suggestions are made by the therapist during the hypnotic state for behavior to be carried out later in the waking state, with the subject remaining unaware of the source of the behavior. For example, the subject may be told that he or she will no longer experience pain associated with a somatoform disorder upon coming out of the hypnotic state. Such an approach can produce short-term relief for some individuals with somatoform disorders.

In situations where it is believed that somatoform-like behaviors are reinforced by family members, family therapy may be helpful. *Family therapy* provides an opportunity for therapists to observe the responses of family members to the clients' symptoms and to deal directly with interpersonal and social issues that may be complicating recovery. According to Brown (1991), family therapy may be particularly beneficial in the treatment of hypochondriasis.

Dissociative Disorders

Dissociative disorders are characterized by a sudden disruption of the normal functions of consciousness. This disturbance is almost always temporary, and usually involves loss of memory or a sudden sense of loss of identity. Important personal events cannot be recalled, or customary identity is temporarily lost. The individual may even wander far from his or her usual surroundings. The *DSM-IV* (APA, 1994) distinguishes among five major dissociative disorders: dissociative amnesia, dissociative fugue, dissociative identity disorder (multiple personality disorder), depersonalization disorder, and dissociative disorder not otherwise specified. We will briefly highlight the first four of these conditions.

Dissociative Amnesia

Dissociative amnesia is characterized by the sudden inability to recall important personal information. It can be information about a specific topic or memories of the immediate or distant past. *Localized amnesia* involves events occurring during a specific period of time following a traumatic event (e.g., after an automobile accident). Somewhat less common, *selective amnesia*, involves the inability to recollect only some of the events during a certain period of time. *Generalized amnesia*, failure to recall all events in one's life, and *continuous amnesia*, failure to recall events subsequent to a specific time up to and including the present, may also occur as a form of this disorder. Unlike forms of amnesia caused by organic conditions (e.g., trauma to the brain), in dissociative amnesia both the onset and termination of memory loss is rapid and complete recovery is common (Weiler & Jacobson, 1993).

Diagnostic criteria set by *DSM-IV* (APA, 1994) require evidence of one or more episodes of inability to recall important personal information that had been previously stored in memory. The memory failure is too significant to be explained by ordinary forgetfulness, and it is not explained by blackouts such as may occur with heavy alcohol or drug use. The amnesia usually is associated with a particularly traumatic or stressful event such as an unexpected loss.

This disorder is most commonly observed in adult and adolescent females undergoing significant stress or in young men during wartime. It is rarely diagnosed in older adult populations. The prevalence rate is believed to be about 7% in the general population (Weiler & Jacobson, 1993), but a far smaller percentage is actually seen in clinical practice.

Dissociative Fugue

The predominant feature of *dissociative fugue* is sudden, unplanned travel away from home or customary workplace along with an assumption of a new identity and confusion about one's previous identity. Individuals in the fugue state may appear perplexed and disoriented. Although they are seldom able to recall the behaviors carried out

while in a fugue state, recovery is usually complete (Meyer, 1993). The fugue usually lasts only hours to days, and after recovery there is no recollection of what occurred during the fugue.

The syndrome often occurs as a reaction to a severe psychosocial stressor, such as the unexpected death of a spouse or the sudden loss of a job. It is sometimes facilitated by alcohol or drug abuse. The age of onset varies, but is primarily between 20 and 40. The prevalence rate for dissociative fugue in the general population is only about 0.2% (Weiler & Jacobson, 1993).

Dissociative Identity Disorder (Multiple Personality Disorder)

Multiple personality disorder (MPD) is characterized by the presence of two or more distinct identities or personalities in the same individual. At least two of these identities or personalities alternately take control of the person's behavior. The dominant personality at any particular time determines the individual's behavior.

Each individual personality is complex and integrated, with its own behavior patterns and set of social relationships. The different personalities are often starkly contrasting (e.g., Dr. Jekyll and Mr. Hyde) and transition from one personality to another is usually sudden. Personalities may claim to be of a different race, age, or sex than the host. One personality may be aware of the other personalities or may report hearing voices of other personalities or even engaging in activities with the others.

Persons with MPD usually come into treatment because they notice some peculiarities in their world: general confusion about interactions with other people or loss of memories. A different personality may then be discovered through therapy.

The disorder is most commonly observed in young adult and adolescent females. The prevalence rate for MPD is about 3% of the general population (Weiler & Jacobson, 1993). Growing evidence suggests that a predisposing factor in MPD is a history of severe abuse as a child, especially incest, rape, bestiality, or pornography. Many victims allege abuse as a result of various cults, especially those associated with satanic activities (Weiler & Jacobson, 1993). Victims develop "new" personalities in a subconscious attempt to protect their "true" personalities from the abuse. These new personalities are thought to be a way of coping with extremely disturbing events and sometimes with the individual's own unacceptable reactions to them (Davison & Neale, 1986).

Depersonalization Disorder

The predominant feature of *depersonalization disorder* is the persistent and recurring sensation of feeling detached from one's own mental processes or physical body. In a depersonalization episode individuals rather suddenly lose the sense of self. Their limbs may seem drastically changed in size, or they may have the impression that they are outside of the bodies, viewing themselves from a distance. Sometimes they feel mechanical—as if they are moving through a dream in a world that has lost its reality.

Depersonalization disorder does not resemble other dissociative reactions since consciousness is never truly segmented from reality and significant memory loss is not a factor. Because there is no better place for depersonalization disorder in the *DSM-IV* (APA. 1994) and because it includes dissociation from the usual sense of reality, it is listed with the dissociative disorders.

Many people experience moments of depersonalized detachment at times. While most people are not really bothered by such experiences, others feel as if they are "going crazy" or "losing their minds." When depersonalization experiences cause significant distress or impairment in important areas of daily functioning, the clinical diagnosis of depersonalization disorder may be appropriate.

This disorder focuses on an experience of changing identity, a situation particularly common during the adolescent years. Not surprisingly, adolescents are most frequently diagnosed with the disorder. The prevalence rate for this condition in the general population is 2.4% (Weiler & Jacobson, 1993). Males and females experience the condition at similar rates.

Treatment of Dissociative Disorders

Dissociative disorders have long been associated with Sigmund Freud's concept of repression. With dissociative amnesia, dissociative fugue, and MPD, people have forgotten earlier experiences of their lives. Since these people may be unaware even of having forgotten something, the hypothesis that they have repressed portions of their lives is compelling. Consequently, psychoanalytic treatment is more commonly used with these psychiatric disorders than most others. Hypnosis, in particular, has been successfully used to gain access to subconscious material or in the case of MPD, to help get in touch with dissociated subpersonalities (Meyer, 1992).

Psychotherapy, such as client-centered therapy (Rogers, 1951), may also help to interpret and to deal with possible conflicts that contribute to a person's condition. Since the goal of treatment is to help the individual recover lost memories and integrate the stressful event into one's consciousness, a supportive environment and an empathetic therapist may provide enough of a sense of safety and potential for reassurance that he or she seeks. Since both dissociative amnesia and dissociative fugue are often a response to an identifiable stressor, the techniques previously discussed in the treatment of posttraumatic stress disorder are also applicable.

Although repressed memories seem not to be a primary issue in depersonalization disorder, psychotherapy using a client-centered approach would seem to be an appropriate strategy to help deal with issues of detachment and separation. In one of the few documented cases of treating persons diagnosed with depersonalization, Yablonsky (1976) supported the use of psychodrama, which allows the individual to act out his or her fantasies about his or her own reality.

Implications for Therapeutic Recreation

The possible roles which therapeutic recreation (TR) may play with respect to anxiety, somatoform and dissociative disorders will be discussed using the three levels of service delivery defined by Peterson and Gunn (1984): participation, leisure education, and therapy.

Participation

The recreation participation component provides clients with the opportunity to experience freely chosen activities and to utilize recreational resources available in their home communities. The theoretical rationale for recreation participation is the same for individuals who experience anxiety, somatoform, or dissociative disorders as it is for all people: to experience enjoyable, personally meaningful use of their free time. When discussing the influence of leisure upon health, Iso-Ahola wrote: "leisure becomes a tool by which health is pursued and obtained; that is, leisure provides time and environment in which health behaviors are practiced . . . a lifestyle that promotes and is conducive to health" (1994, p. 43). Health as defined by Iso-Ahola (1994) is a multidimensional concept that includes physical, psychological, emotional, and spiritual components.

Recreation participation has the potential to improve one's perceived quality of life.

Because most individuals diagnosed with one of the disorders described in this chapter will be treated on an outpatient basis, efforts to promote their involvement in community-based recreational activities should be encouraged. Therapeutic recreation professionals can play a critical role in facilitating this process. Additionally, because persons who experience anxiety, somatoform, or dissociative disorders seldom require special accommodations to participate in community-based recreational opportunities, efforts to include them are usually far less complicated than what may be required for other populations with special needs.

Leisure Education

The leisure education component serves to address leisure-related skills, attitudes, and knowledge. Leisure education programs intend to empower consumers to exercise personal choice in terms of their leisure involvement. While an unquestionably valuable component of a TR program, in reality, most leisure education programs are associated with clinically based TR programs working with clients in preparation for reintegration into the community. Thus, given that the psychiatric disorders discussed in this chapter seldom involve institutionalization, literature specifically linking leisure education and anxiety, somatoform, and dissociative disorders was not identified by the authors.

Therapy

The treatment component involves direct intervention utilizing TR services to "help the individual free himself from the constraints that are limiting his personal growth and healthy choices of behavior" (Kinney & Kinney, 1996, p. 65). In terms of the disorders reviewed in this chapter, the most basic problem shared by each is the inability to cope with perceived stress in one's environment. Recognizing this fact, the potential benefits of TR intervention would seem intuitively obvious. Several authors (Coleman & Iso-Ahola, 1993; Finnicum & Zeiger, 1998; Iso-Ahola & Weissinger, 1984) have discussed leisure's mediating effects upon stressful events in life. In each case, it has been suggested that leisure may impact health by providing a buffering effect, which helps an individual absorb or protect oneself against sources of stress in his or her daily life.

While it may be true that leisure promotes psychological health by helping people cope with stress, individuals diagnosed with an anxiety, somatoform, or dissociative disorder obviously experience stress in markedly different ways than people who are psychologically healthy. While studies linking recreation intervention specifically to the treatment of anxiety, somatoform, or dissociative disorders are very rare, inferences may be drawn from several related areas of research.

Aerobic exercise programs have been identified as producing beneficial effects on the psychological well-being of individuals with psychiatric disorders, including anxiety disorders (Martinsen, 1987; McCann & Holmes, 1984). Other investigators have examined the effects of anaerobic exercises, particularly weightlifting, on the same populations (Auchus & Kaslow, 1994; Pelham, Campagna, Rituo & Birnie, 1993). Each of these studies reported improvement in both the physical and psychological states of their subjects. Auchus and Kaslow (1994), who developed a weightlifting program for five female clients, stated that the effects of the program included increased strength and muscle size, as well as an enhanced sense of mastery, control, and self-esteem. This study also reported an improvement in the perceived psychological well-being in all five of the subjects studied.

In similar fashion, both Hales and Travis (1987) and Schwartz (1989) have suggested that supervised exercise programs should be investigated as a major therapy (either alone or in combination with other modalities) for panic disorders and other anxiety syndromes. According to Schwartz (1989), a carefully monitored exercise program can help the anxiety-prone individual become familiar and comfortable with the physical sensations of adrenergic arousal (i.e., arousal associated with the stimulation of the adrenal glands), which then may be generalized to other everyday situations which are associated with crippling terror. In addition to the possible reduction of anticipatory anxiety, the exercise programs will also enhance physical fitness and improve health and longevity (Schwartz, 1989, p. 1358).

Physical exercise and therapeutic recreation may have similar enjoyable effects in terms of anxiety relief. Allowing anxiety-prone participants to select their own types of activities should produce a greater feeling of control. The TR specialist working with individuals diagnosed with anxiety-related problems would take advantage of activities that possess characteristics known to be more effective in reducing stress. These include activities that promote abdominal breathing, (e.g., aerobic activities such as swimming or cycling), noncompetitive, process-oriented activities (e.g., cooking or gardening), and self-paced, repetitive and rhythmical activities (e.g., juggling or dancing) (Hall, 1994).

Since several of the disorders identified in this chapter involve fears associated with being in public places or with strangers, TR professionals might employ activities which promote social skills training with such clients. The intent of such training would be to promote self-confidence and to reduce anxiety for individuals who may experience panic attacks while in the presence of unfamiliar people or places. Skalko's (1991) review of social skill training for persons with chronic mental illness is a worthwhile resource for TR specialists working with anxiety-related disorders.

Therapeutic recreation would also seem to hold promise for persons who experience phobias. Earlier we discussed common behavioral treatments for phobias, including systematic desensitization, modeling, and role-playing. Owing to the stress-reducing nature of recreation activities, the use of TR services in conjunction with such behavioral techniques seems particularly appropriate.

Finally, as our earlier review of anxiety, somatoform, and dissociative disorders indicated, people with these conditions have an unusually strong need to feel "in control." In contrast to other forms of therapy where control over the course and direction of intervention is dictated by the therapist, TR services provide opportunities for clients to engage in activities in which a sense of mastery and success may be inferred (Iso-Ahola, MacNeil & Szymanski 1981). According to Dattilo and Kleiber (1993), "for people receiving TR services, a sense of control is particularly important in establishing self-determination" (p. 60). This sense of self-determination may be the vital pathway between overcoming anxiety and fear and achieving a desired state of psychological health.

Chapter Summary

This chapter examined anxiety-related disorders and addressed the following issues:

- Overview of three broad categories of physiological disturbances: anxiety disorders, somatoform disorders, and dissociative disorders
- Characteristics of specific anxiety disorders, including panic disorder, phobias, obsessive-compulsive disorder, posttraumatic stress disorder, and generalized anxiety disorder
- Behavioral, humanistic, and pharmacological interventions for treating anxiety disorders
- Characteristics and treatments of specific somatoform disorders, including somatization disorder, conversion disorder, somatoform pain disorder, and hypchondrias
- Characteristics and treatments of specific dissociative disorders, including dissociative amnesia, dissociative fugue, dissociative identity disorder (multiple personality disorder), and depersonalization disorder
- Implications of anxiety disorders, somatoform disorders, and dissociative disorders for therapeutic recreation

References

American Psychiatric Association. (1994). *Diagnostic and statistical manual of mental disorders* (4th ed.). Washington, DC: Author.

Auchus, M. and Kaslow, N. (1994). Weightlifting therapy: A preliminary report. *Psychosocial Rehabilitation Journal, 18*(2), 99–108.

Austin, D. and Crawford, M. (Eds.). (1996). *Therapeutic recreation: An introduction* (2nd ed.). Boston, MA: Allyn & Bacon.

Bandura, A. (1977). Self-efficacy: Toward a unifying theory of behavioral change. *Psychological Review, 84*, 191–215.

Benedikt, R. and Kolb, L. (1986). Preliminary findings on chronic pain and posttraumatic stress disorder. *American Journal of Psychiatry, 143*, 908–910.

Brown, F. (Ed.). (1991). *Reweaving the family tapestry.* New York, NY: W. W. Norton.

Coleman, D. and Iso-Ahola, S. (1993). Leisure and health: The role of social support and self-determination. *Journal of Leisure Research, 25*, 111–128.

Dattilo, J. and Kleiber, D. (1993). Psychological perspectives for therapeutic recreation research: The psychology of enjoyment. In M. Malkin and C. Howe (Eds.), *Research in therapeutic recreation: Concepts and methods.* State College, PA: Venture Publishing, Inc.

Davidson, G. and Neale, J. (1986). *Abnormal psychology: An experimental clinical approach* (4th ed.). New York, NY: John Wiley & Sons.

Fawcett, J. (1992). Suicide risk factors in depressive disorders and in panic disorder. *Journal of Clinical Psychiatry, 53*(Supplement), 9–13.

Finnicum, P. and Zieger, J. (1998). Managing stress through outdoor recreation. *Parks & Recreation, 33*(8), 46–51.

Foa, E. and Kozak, M. (1986). Emotional processing of fear: Exposure to corrective information. *Psychological Bulletin, 99*, 20–35.

Glasser, W. (1980). Two cases in reality therapy. In G. Belin (Ed.), *Contemporary psychotherapies.* Chicago, IL: Rand McNally.

Hales, R. and Travis, T. (1987). Exercise as a treatment option for anxiety and depressive disorders. *Medicine, 152*, 299–302.

Hall, E. (1994). Exercise and depression: Beyond physical fitness. In D. Compton and S. Iso-Ahola (Eds.), *Leisure and mental health* (pp. 307–319). Park City, UT: Family Development Resources, Inc.

Hecker, J. and Thorpe, G. (1992). *Agoraphobia and panic.* Boston, MA: Allyn & Bacon.

Hoehn-Saric, R. and McLeod, D. (1988). Panic and generalized anxiety disorder. In C. Last and M. Hersen (Eds.), *Handbook of anxiety disorders.* Elmsford, NY: Pergamon.

Iso-Ahola, S. E. (1994). Leisure lifestyle and health. In D. Compton and S. E. Iso-Ahola (Eds.), *Leisure and mental health* (pp. 42–60). Pine City, UT: Family Development Resources, Inc.

Iso-Ahola, S., MacNeil, R., and Szymanski, D. (1980). Social psychological foundations of therapeutic recreation: An attributional analysis. In S. Iso-Ahola (Ed.), *Social psychological perspectives on leisure and recreation* (pp. 390–413). Springfield, IL: Charles C. Thomas.

Iso-Ahola, S. and Weissinger, E. (1984). Leisure and well-being: Is there a connection? *Parks and Recreation, 19*(6), 40–44.

Israni, T., Janicak, P., and Davis, J. (1993). Obsessive-compulsive disorder. In J. Flaherty, J. Davis, and P. Janicak (Eds.), *Psychiatry: Diagnosis and therapy* (2nd ed., pp. 145–155). Norwalk, CT: Appleton & Lange.

Keller, M. and Baker, L. (1992). The clinical course of panic disorder and depression. *Journal of Clinical Psychiatry, 53*(Supplement), 5–8.

Kellner, R. (1986). *Somatization and hypochondriasis.* London, UK: Praeger.

Kinney, J. and Kinney, T. (1996). Psychiatry and mental health. In D. Austin and M. Crawford (Eds.), *Therapeutic recreation: An introduction* (2nd ed., pp. 57–77). Boston, MA: Allyn & Bacon.

Kozak, M., Foa, E., and McCarthy, P. (1988). Obsessive-compulsive disorder. In C. Last and M. Hersen (Eds.), *Handbook of anxiety disorders.* Elmsford, NY: Pergamon.

Lewis, J. and Flaherty, J. (1993). Somatoform disorders. In J. Flaherty, J. Davis, and P. Janicak (Eds.), *Psychiatry: Diagnosis and therapy* (2nd ed., pp. 188–195). Norwalk, CT: Appleton & Lange.

Martinsen, E. (1987). The role of aerobic exercise in the treatment of depression. *Stress Medicine, 3*, 93–100.

Matuzas, W. and Jack, E. (1991). The drug treatment of panic disorder. *Psychiatric Medicine, 9*, 215.

Matuzas, W., Jack, E., Andriukaitis, S., Olson, S., and Hernandez, G. (1993). Panic disorder, phobias, and posttraumatic stress disorder. In J. Flaherty, J. Davis, and P. Janicak (Eds.), *Psychiatry: Diagnosis and therapy* (2nd ed., pp. 156–173). Norwalk, CT: Appleton & Lange.

McCann, I. and Holmes, D. (1984). Influence of aerobic exercise in depression. *Journal of Personality and Social Psychology, 46*(5), 1142–1147.

Meister, R. (1980). *Hypochondria*. New York, NY: Taplinger.

Meyer, R. (1992). *Practical clinical hypnosis*. Lexington, MA: Lexington Books.

Meyer, R. G. (1993). *The Clinician's Handbook*. Boston, MA: Allyn & Bacon.

Pelham, T., Campagna, P., Rituo, P., and Birnie, W. (1993). The effects of exercise on clients in a psychiatric rehabilitation program. *Psychosocial Rehabilitation Journal, 16*(4), 75–84.

Peterson, C. and Gunn, S. (1994). *Therapeutic recreation program design*. Englewood Cliffs, NJ: Prentice-Hall.

Rapee, R. (1991). Generalized anxiety disorder: A review of clinical features and theoretical concepts. *Clinical Psychology Review, 11*, 419–440.

Rogers, C. (1951). *Client-centered therapy*. Boston, MA: Houghton Mifflin.

Schwartz, C. (1989). Exercise and anxiety disorders. *American Journal of Psychiatry, 146*(10), 1358–1359.

Schwartz, M. (1987). *Biofeedback*. New York, NY: Guilford.

Selye, H. (1956). *The stress of life*. New York, NY: McGraw-Hill.

Sharma, R., Andriulcaitis, S., and Davis, J. (1993). Anxiety states. In J. Flaherty, J. Davis and P. Janicak (Eds.), *Psychiatry: Diagnosis and therapy* (2nd ed., pp. 133–144). Norwalk, CT: Appleton & Lange.

Skalko, T. (1991). Social skills training for persons with chronic mental illness. *The Journal of Physical Education, Recreation & Dance, 62*(4), 31–34.

Walker, J., Norton, G., and Ross, C. (Eds.). (1991). *Panic disorder and agoraphobia*. Pacific Grove, CA: Brooks/Cole.

Weiler, M. and Jacobson, D. (1993). Special psychiatric syndromes. In J. Flaherty, J. Davis, and P. Janicak (Eds.), *Psychiatry: Diagnosis and therapy* (2nd ed., pp. 284–297). Norwalk, CT: Appleton & Lange.

Wolpe, J. (1987). Carbon dioxide inhalation treatments of neurotic anxiety. *The Journal of Nervous and Mental Disease, 175*, 129–133.

Yablonsky, L. (1976). *Psychodrama: Resolving emotional problems through role-playing*. New York, NY: Basic Books.

Ziegler, F., Imboden, J., and Meyer, E. (1960). Contemporary conversion reactions: A clinical study. *American Journal of Psychiatry, 116*, 901–910.

CHAPTER 5 AFFECTIVE DISORDERS

Psychiatrists define *mood* as a sustained emotion that colors a person's view of the world. Moods affect our entire being, including how we think and feel, both emotionally and physically. They have a pervasive influence on physical energy and psychological motivation. Disruption in mood can have a far-ranging impact, affecting such things as sleep, appetite, concentration, self-esteem, and social life.

The word *affect* literally means to move or stir the emotions. *Affective disorders* are disturbances in moods that can produce intense suffering and discomfort. Affective disorders are among the most common of mental disturbances, and certainly one of the oldest diagnosed conditions. *Melancholia* (from the Greek *melan*, black and *choler*, bile) and *mania* (from the Greek *mainesthac*, to be mad) were two of the three types of mental disorders recognized by Hippocrates. The physician Aretaeus of Cappadocia had suggested a relationship between melancholia and the apparently opposite emotional state of mania (Davison & Neale, 1986). By the late 19th century, German psychiatrist Emil Kraopelin identified *manic–depressive illness* to be the disturbance of all patients showing *affective excess*—moods or emotions in excess of what may be expected in a given situation (Davison & Neale, 1986).

The *Diagnostic and Statistical Manual of Mental Disorders* (*DSM-IV*) identifies four types of mood disorders (American Psychiatric Association, 1994): major depressive disorder, dysthymic disorder, bipolar disorder, and cyclothymic disorder. This chapter discusses each of the four main types of disorders. We distinguish between the disorders in terms of characteristics and epidemiology, we present several theories that have been advanced to explain the cause of affective disorders, and we provide an overview of treatment options for these disorders. The chapter will conclude with a discussion of the implications for therapeutic recreation.

Classifications of Mood Disorders

Major Depressive Disorder

Our lives are filled with shifting mood states. We all have days when things seem to go well, when our routines seem to go as planned, and we may receive an unanticipated surprise or praise that pleases us. Our mood on these days is undoubtedly good. On the other hand, we all also experience days when we seem to experience one interruption after another, when even the simplest tasks seem difficult to complete or when the actions of our friends and family seem particularly irritating to us. On these days we are likely to be in a bad mood. Some people, however, are affected by a disturbance that alters these expected mood states for extended periods of time. No matter how well things seem to be going for them, they cannot seem to overcome their general sense of despair and sadness. These people may suffer from *major depressive disorder* (MDD).

Before describing MDD, it is important to clarify what distinguishes this disorder from other conditions in which depression is a central symptom. Often depressed states are associated with other psychological problems or medical conditions. Stressful events, such as the death of a loved one, the end of a relationship, or the loss of a job can sometimes trigger depression. Being diagnosed with a serious illness or medical condition can be directly associated with symptoms of depression, or a depressed mood may be the side effect of certain drugs prescribed to combat a medical condition. Agoraphobics may become dependent because of their inability to venture out of their homes. Alcoholics may be depressed by their inability to control their drinking and by the social and employment problems that their drinking has provoked. In these and many other instances depression is best viewed as secondary to another condition. With MDD, however, depression is the primary problem.

The diagnosis of major depressive disorder follows the occurrence of a major depressive episode. As described by the *DSM-IV,* this episode is distinguished by a change in functioning characterized by the presence of a generally depressed mood and the loss of interest or pleasure in life events and which lasts for at least a two-week period of time (APA, 1994). The episode is characterized by a wide variety of symptoms, including the following (Klein & Wender, 1993):

- Sad or depressed mood experienced most of the day, nearly every day

- Feelings of restlessness, anxiousness, and irritability

- Overwhelming feelings of hopelessness or helplessness (feeling "trapped")

- Loss of motivation to change one's situation

- Feelings of worthlessness

- Self-blame out of proportion to reality

- Loss of interest and pleasure in their normal activities

- Withdrawal from other people and previously enjoyable hobbies or recreational activities

- Marked decline in sex drive

- Changes in appetite and weight (losing weight without conscious dieting or rapid gain in weight)

- Difficulties in sleeping (insomnia) or oversleeping (hypersomnia)

- Decreased energy levels and feeling lethargic

- Decreased attention span, inability to concentrate, and difficulty completing tasks or making decisions

- Impaired ability to function at work or to complete intellectual tasks around the home

- Excessive feelings of guilt and self-blaming

- Recurrent thoughts of death or suicide

A single individual seldom displays all of the characteristic aspects of depression described here. The diagnosis of MDD is typically made if at least five of the symptoms have been present during the same two-week period, and particularly if they coexist with a mood of profound sadness that is out of proportion to a person's life situation. If there is a single major depressive episode, the formal *DSM-IV* (APA, 1994) diagnosis is *major depressive disorder, single episode*. The occurrence of more than one is diagnosed *major depressive disorder, recurrent*. Both require an absence of any manic episodes (i.e., mood characterized by joyful elation and hyperactivity).

Major depression can begin at any age. The mean age of onset is the mid to late twenties (Gaviria & Flaherty, 1993). While people between the ages of 25 and 44 are particularly vulnerable, anyone, of any age or either sex, can become depressed. This illness strikes an estimated 17 million American adults each year. The prevalence of major depression in the population of the United States is 3% to 5%. The lifetime risk is 3% to 12% for men and 20% to 26% for women (Gaviria & Flaherty, 1993).

Certain individuals have a higher risk of becoming depressed. One major factor associated with increased risk is having a history of depressive episodes. About 50% of people who have had one major depressive episode will have another at some point in their lives, and more than 70% of those who had two episodes will have a recurrence. Approximately 20% to 35% of those who suffer chronic depression have difficulty maintaining normal routines of daily life (APA, 1994). The risk is also higher for individuals having a first-degree relative with a diagnosis of major depression, bipolar disorder, or alcoholism. The occurrence of frequent major life changes, such as the death of a loved one or the loss of a job, can also increase one's vulnerability. Moreover, as statistics presented previously indicated, women appear to have a greater risk of developing depression at some point in their lives than men. Some of the risk factors affecting women include childbirth (e.g., postpartum depression), economic deprivation, low self-esteem, and sexual and physical abuse (McGrath, Keita, Strickland & Russon, 1990).

Many experts think depression is the illness that underlies the majority of suicides in the United States. Suicide is the eighth leading cause of death in America, and the third leading cause of death among people aged 15 to 24. Every day about 15 individuals ages 15 to 24 take their own lives. It is believed that one of the best strategies for preventing suicide is the early recognition and treatment of depression (APA, 1994).

In addition to increasing the risk of suicide, depression takes an economic toll on society. It was recently estimated that the yearly cost of depression to the U. S. economy was in excess of $43.7 billion. Most of this cost was in terms of lost economic productivity, although about $12.4 billion were spent on doctors, hospitals, and medications (Cooper, 1996).

Dysthymia

Dysthymia shares many of the same features as major depressive disorder, but is generally regarded as a milder form of the illness. Despite this fact, it still causes long-term suffering for its victims.

The person with dysthymic disorder is chronically depressed. A person with dysthymia may have good days in which these symptoms are not present, but such days do not occur for more than two months in a row during a two-year period (APA, 1994). Besides feeling blue and losing pleasure in usual activities, the person displays other signs of depression, such as poor appetite or overeating; insomnia or sleeping too much; feeling inadequate, ineffective, and drained of energy; being unable to concentrate or to think clearly; or avoiding the company of others.

Dysthymic disorder often has an early onset (childhood, adolescence, or early adulthood) as well as a chronic course. By the time they are adults, many affected people feel that they have been depressed for as long as they can remember. In addition, many people with dysthymia will also experience a major depressive episode. When this happens the person is said to have *double depression* (dysthymic disorder plus MDD), a much more serious medical condition.

The lifetime prevalence of dysthymia is approximately 4.5% to 10.5%, with women slightly more affected than men (Gaviria & Flaherty, 1993). Dysthymia affects about 3% of the population at any give time (APA, 1994). Some evidence supports the claim that the loss of a parent early in life increases the risk of being diagnosed with dysthymic disorder (Gaviria & Flaherty, 1993).

Bipolar Disorder (Manic-Depressive Illness)

Bipolar disorder, also known as *manic–depressive illness,* involves episodes of serious mania accompanied by one or more major depressive disorders. Individuals with this disorder may experience episodic periods of depression, but they also experience times in which they suddenly abound with joyful elation and become hyperactive, overconfident, and full of impractical, grandiose ideas. This elated mood state is referred to as a manic episode.

A *manic episode* is defined by a distinct period during which there is abnormally and persistently elevated, expansive, or irritable mood. This abnormal mood lasts for at least a week and is accompanied by some of the following symptoms (U. S. Department of Health and Human Services, 1995):

- Increased energy, activity, restlessness, racing thoughts, and rapid talking
- Excessive "high" or euphoric feelings
- Extreme irritability and distractibility
- Decreased need for sleep (often feeling rested after only a few hours)
- Unrealistic beliefs in one's abilities and powers
- Uncharacteristically poor judgment, including reckless behavior
- Sustained period of behavior which is noticeably different from usual
- Increased sexual drive, sexual indiscretions, or promiscuity

- Abuse of drugs, particularly cocaine, alcohol, and sleeping medications
- Provocative, intrusive, or aggressive behavior
- Denial that anything is wrong

The individual experiencing a manic episode is loud and incessant, full of puns, jokes, plays on words, rhyming, or interjections about objects or people that have attracted their attention. Their speech may be very difficult to interpret. The individual shifts rapidly from one topic to another. The person's need for activity may cause him or her to be annoyingly sociable and intrusive, constantly busy, and usually to the pitfalls of his or her endeavors. Any attempt to curb his or her behavior can bring quick anger and even rage. Mania usually comes on suddenly, over a period of a day or two. Untreated, episodes may last from a few days to several months.

While some individuals experience manic episodes without experiencing bouts of depression, the diagnosis of bipolar disorder involves mood swings that alternate between the two extremes; the person has episodes of mania that alternate with depression. Sometimes there may be milder episodes of the high mood, a condition known as *hypomania.* There can also be *mixed episodes*, in which both mania and major depression are present at the same time.

Compared to major depression, bipolar disorder is relatively rare. The lifetime risk of developing a bipolar disorder is estimated at about 1%. Bipolar disorder strikes men and women at about the same rate with the age of onset frequently in late adolescence or the early twenties. The rate of bipolar illness in first-degree relatives of bipolar patients is higher than might be expected in the general population. Close relatives of people with bipolar disorder are 10 to 20 times as likely as other people to develop a mood disorder (Gaviria & Flaherty, 1993).

Bipolar disorder is a recurrent disorder. Over 90% of people who have one manic episode will eventually have another. Roughly 60% to 70% of manic episodes occur immediately after a major depressive episode. Individuals who experience the disorder usually develop a characteristic pattern of manic and depressive episodes. Some people go directly from mania to depression and back again, while others return to their usual selves between episodes. The periods of mania, which can last from days to months, are usually briefer than those of depression (APA, 1996).

The timing and severity of episodes and the relative health of the individuals between episodes may be influenced by a variety of psychosocial factors, including personality style, presence or absence of a social support system, and stressful life events. Childbirth is an example of a stressor that may cause physiological and psychological changes that may produce a first or recurrent episode of mania (Gaviria & Flaherty, 1993).

Cyclothymic Disorder

Cyclothymia is a milder version of bipolar disorder. It involves less extreme alternating high and low moods. Cyclothymia includes episodes of hypomania and periods of less severe depressive symptoms. Although these symptoms are relatively mild, they may last for extended time periods and can still cause long-term disruption in an individual's life.

Cyclothymia always includes hypomanic episodes that last for at least four days. During these episodes the person will exhibit symptoms such as unrealistically high self-esteem, talkative behavior and racing thoughts, decreased need for sleep, distractibility, or continued reckless behavior. Despite the presence of these symptoms, the individual is able to continue daily routines. Depressive symptoms, which may be troubling to the individual, but are usually not severe, numerous, or long-lasting enough to meet the criteria for major depression, usually follow.

Up to 1% of the population will develop cyclothmyia at some point in their lives. Like bipolar disorder, this condition usually has its onset in adolescence or early adult life, and occurs about equally in men and women. There is a 15% to 50% risk that the person with cyclothymia will subsequently develop a bipolar disorder. Moreover, evidence suggests that both major depressive disorder and bipolar disorder appear to be more common among first-degree biological relatives of persons with cyclothymic disorder than among the general population (APA, 1994).

Theories of Causation

Sadness is a normal emotional state among human beings; everyone experiences sadness. Depression, which may be considered to be an extreme and prolonged state of sadness, is an abnormal condition. Efforts to differentiate between normal sadness and abnormal depression are extremely difficult. In this section we will briefly highlight several different theories which have been advanced to explain what might cause one individual to be labeled as *normal* with respect to the emotion of sadness, and a second to be

labeled as *abnormal* (or depressed). We will first consider several psychological theories of depression, after which we will examine two physiological theories.

Psychological Theories

Freud's *psychoanalytic theory* of depression identifies self-centeredness as the characteristic that differentiates depression from normal sadness. Freud associated depression with the tendency to be excessively dependent on other people for the maintenance of one's self-esteem. Predictably, Freud saw the potential for depression being created early in childhood during the oral period when the child's needs are either insufficiently or over-sufficiently gratified. Freud theorized that the person may remain psychologically "stuck" in this stage of development with its characteristic dependence upon others for the validation of one's self-esteem. As a consequence, the person may unconsciously interpret personal loss as the rejection or withdrawal of the affection that is needed to sustain the sense of self-worth. This theorizing is the basis for the widespread psychoanalytic view of depression as anger turned against oneself (Davison & Neale, 1986).

Cognitive theorists, such as Aaron Beck and Martin Seligman, suggest that our thoughts and our beliefs can cause abnormal emotional states like depression. The central thesis of Beck's theory (1967) is that depressed individuals feel as they do because they commit characteristic errors in logic. Beck reported that depressed patients tend to distort whatever happens to them in the direction of self-blame or the hopelessness of life. He refers to this as a "negative cognitive mindset." In childhood or adolescence depressed individuals have learned a negative cognitive mindset which is dominated by feelings of personal failings, misfortune, and overwhelming difficulties ahead. This negative mindset, once acquired, is activated whenever new situations they encounter resemble in some way the conditions under which the negative mindset was learned. Consequently, people diagnosed with depressive disorders tend to draw illogical conclusions about their experiences and come to evaluate negatively not only themselves, but their immediate world as well as their future (Beck, 1967).

Martin Seligman's *learned helplessness theory* suggests that although anxiety is the initial response to a stressful situation, it may be replaced by depression if the person comes to believe that control is unattainable. Initially Seligman's view explained the behavior of animals who received painful electric shock in experimental situations. Seligman observed that when confronted with uncontrollable aversive stimulation, his animals acquired a *sense of helplessness*—they seemed to give up efforts to avoid the electric shock and passively accepted the painful stimulation. Seligman demonstrated that once learned, this sense of helplessness affected their performance in other stressful situations. The animals seemed to lose their ability and motivation to learn to respond in an effective way to painful stimulation (Seligman, 1974).

Experiments with human beings have yielded results similar to those of experiments done with animals. For example, Hiroto and Seligman (1975) found that people who have been subjected to inescapable noise, or who have been confronted by unsolvable problems, fail later to escape noise and solve simple problems. Other studies demonstrated that in a laboratory setting, exposure to uncontrollable situations could elicit behavior similar to that observed in depressed individuals from nondepressed subjects (Klein & Seligman, 1976).

Abramson, Seligman, and Teasdale (1978) proposed a revised version of the learned helplessness model. The essence of the revised theory lies in the concept of *attribution*. The attributional revision of helplessness theory postulates that the way the person attributes failure will determine its subsequent effects. Attributing failures to internal characteristics or personal inadequacies is more likely to diminish self-esteem. People then become depressed when they believe either that desired outcomes are unattainable or that negative outcomes are unavoidable. The depression-prone individual shows a "depressive attributional style," a tendency to attribute bad outcomes to personal, stable faults of character. When persons with this style face stressful or unhappy experiences they become depressed and their self-esteem shatters (Peterson & Seligman, 1984). Thus, hurtful situations instill a sense of helplessness that can evolve into depression.

These same theories are usually applied to explain the depressive phase bipolar disorder. Individuals diagnosed with major depression and those with bipolar disorder suffer from low self-esteem. In contrast to the depressed state, in which this deficit in self-esteem manifests in terms of depressive-like behavior, the manic phase has been explained as a psychological defense mechanism employed by the individual against the debilitating effects caused by low self-image. In other words, an episode of manic behavior may be used to subconsciously defend oneself from feelings of inadequacy or uncontrollability (Davison & Neale, 1986).

Physiological Theories

Physiological processes have considerable effects on moods. As our earlier discussion of affective disorders indicated, the frequency of both depressive and bipolar disorders in first-degree relatives is considerably higher than those for the general population. While this does not prove genetic causation, the overwhelming evidence from family and twin studies suggests that both unipolar depression and bipolar disorder have heritable components (Davison & Neale, 1986).

What might be a physiological link to affective disorder? A leading set of theories has been proposed relating depression to neurotransmitters. *Neurotransmitters* are chemicals located on synaptic tips of axons in the human nervous system. For a nerve impulse to pass from one neuron to another, it must have a way of bridging the synaptic space that exists between neurons. Neurotransmitters serve as this bridge. Their release in response to a nerve impulse allows neurons to communicate with one another. One physiological theory of depression suggests that the disorder is caused by low levels of the neurotransmitter *norepinephrine;* a second points to low levels of *serotonin.* The norepinephrine theory also postulates that an excess of this neurotransmitter causes mania (Schildkraut, 1965).

Evidence for both of these theories has resulted from studying the actions of various drugs upon the central nervous system and the treatment of depression. Studies conducted as early as the 1950s found that two particular groups of drugs, the *tricyclics* and the *monoamine oxidase inhibitors,* seemed to be effective in relieving symptoms of depression. Studies further revealed that they also increase the levels of both norepinephrine and serotonin in the brains of animals (Davison & Neale, 1986).

These early experiments spawned further exploration into the possible biochemical link to affective disorders. While a physiological cause has not yet been proven, evidence strongly points to an inherited predisposition for bipolar disorder and relates the phenomenon of depression and mania to abnormalities in neurotransmitters in the brain. Support for these theories has led to the almost standard use of pharmacological agents to treat symptoms of depression and mania.

Treatment of Affective Disorders

Affective disorders are chronic pernicious illnesses associated with episodes of long duration, relapse, and recurrence, and psychosocial and physical impairment. The annual cost of depression in the United States is estimated to be in excess of $43 billion. A depressed employee will cost an employer about $6,000 annually; 72% of these costs relate to absenteeism and lost productivity (National Depressive and Manic-Depressive Association, 1997).

Fortunately, affective disorders are among the most treatable of the mental illnesses. Between 80% and 90% of all depressed people respond to treatment and nearly all who receive treatment experience at least some relief from their symptoms (APA , 1996). Current therapies used in the treatment of affective disorders may be classified in two broad areas: somatic therapies and psychological therapies.

Somatic Therapies

Somatic therapy uses agents that directly treat the physical body (e.g., drugs). Since ancient times, humans have used drugs to alleviate depression. Since the 1950s, tremendous strides have been made in understanding the effects of various medications upon affective disorders. Although new drugs are constantly being developed, the two traditional major subcategories of *antidepressants* used in recent times are the tricyclics and the monoamine oxidase (MAO) inhibitors.

Tricyclics include a variety of different drugs assumed to interfere with the re-uptake of certain neurotransmitters (e.g., norepinephrine and serotonin) by the nerve cell after it has fired (i.e., synapsed with another nerve cell). It is believed that when levels of these neurotransmitters fall, depression may result. Tricyclics are most often prescribed for people with depression characterized by fatigue, feelings of hopelessness, helplessness, excessive guilt, inability to feel pleasure, and loss of appetite. Common side effects associated with tricyclics include dry mouth, constipation, dizziness, and blurred vision.

MAO inhibitors prevent a certain enzyme (monoamine oxidase) from degrading monoamine (an organic compound) within the central nervous system. As with the tricyclics, MAO inhibitors act by facilitating the release of norepinephrine and serotonin within nerve cells. MAO inhibitors are often prescribed for

people with depression characterized by increased appetite, excessive sleepiness, anxiety, phobia, and obsessive–compulsive symptoms. Because the MAO inhibitors have more significant side effects, the tricyclics have been favored in recent years (Lickey & Gordon, 1991).

The tricyclics and MAO inhibitors require substantial trial-and-error adjustment of dosages to find the most effective level for the individual receiving treatment, and both require several days to several weeks before any positive effects occur. However, available evidence suggests that these agents are effective in combating depression and reducing the risk of relapse for the majority of persons who suffer from depression (Prien et al., 1984; Meyer, 1993).

The most popularly prescribed antidepressant, *fluoxetine* (Prozac), is neither a tricyclic nor an MAO inhibitor. Prozac acts as a very selective uptake inhibitor of the neurotransmitter serotonin. Scientists think a deficiency in serotonin may cause the sleep problems, irritability, and anxiety associated with depression. By helping to maintain sufficient levels of serotonin in the nervous system, Prozac may inhibit these symptoms. Owing to simplicity of prescription and limited side effects Prozac has become a popular drug for treating elderly patients with depression (APA, 1996; Meyer, 1993).

Lithium carbonate, a simple mineral salt, was first tried for the treatment of affective disorders in the 1940s, but was halted due to adverse side effects. Since then, however, refinements have made lithium therapy a highly effective treatment for mania. Identification of how lithium works to inhibit manic episodes remains unclear, but it appears to reverse the manic factor in approximately 75% of the cases treated (Lickey & Gordon, 1991). Lithium therapy is used to treat bipolar disorders in individuals of all ages.

Perhaps the most dramatic and controversial form of somatic therapy is *electroconvulsive therapy* (ECT). ECT deliberately induces a seizure and momentary unconsciousness by passing an electrical stimulus through the depressed individual's brain. In the procedure the patient is given a short-acting anesthetic, then an injection of a strong muscle relaxant before the current is applied. The convulsive spasms of the body muscles are barely perceptible to onlookers, and the patient awakens a few minutes later remembering nothing about the treatment. Clients typically receive 6 to 12 ECT treatments administered every other day or until the patient improves or it becomes evident that further treatment will be ineffective (APA, 1996).

Although ECT has been performed for decades, scientists still do not know precisely how it works to combat depression. Major theories that attempt to explain its effect include the following:

- Neurotransmitter theory—ECT works like antidepressant medication, changing the way the brain receives important mood-related chemicals
- Anticonvulsant theory—Shock-induced seizures teach the brain to resist seizures which dampens abnormally active brain circuits, stabilizing mood
- Neuroendocrine theory—Seizures cause the brain to release chemicals that regulate mood
- Brain damage theory—Shock damages the brain, causing memory loss and disorientation that creates a temporary illusion that problems are gone

While controversy remains about how ECT may work, many scientists are convinced that it can be an effective treatment for severe depression. Janicak, Comaty, and Dowd claim that "60 to 70% of seriously depressed patients will improve with standard antidepressants, whereas 80% or more will show improvement with ECT" (1993, p. 61).

Nonetheless, inducing a seizure remains a drastic procedure. Why would anyone subject himself or herself to such a treatment? The simple answer is that for many people suffering from severe depression ECT relieves their symptoms (Valenstein, 1986). ECT seems to be particularly effective for treating patients who cannot take medications due to heart conditions, old age, or severe malnourishment, or patients who do not respond to antidepressant medication. Given the real possibility of suicide among depressed people, the use of ECT (after other treatments have failed) is regarded by many as responsible and defensible.

Psychological Therapies

A variety of *psychological therapies* (psychotherapies) are also used with persons who suffer from affective disorders. Psychotherapies (talk therapies) involve verbal interaction between a trained professional and the patient. The therapist applies techniques based on established psychological principles to help the client gain insights about himself or herself and his or her situation. It is believed that with the acquisition of such insights the individual may become capable of changing his or her maladaptive feelings, thoughts, or behaviors.

Can psychotherapy produce therapeutic results among depressed individuals? Scientific evidence now supports that for some categories of patients and under certain circumstances, some types of cognitive behavior therapy and interpersonal therapy can be as effective as medications for producing relief from symptoms for depressed patients (Deakin, 1996).

Psychoanalytic or *psychodynamic treatment* views depression as the result of past conflicts which patients have pushed into their unconscious. This form of psychotherapy considers depression as anger turned inward, and attempts to help the patient achieve insight into his or her repressed conflict. It often encourages the release of hostility supposedly working inward. The therapist attempts to guide the patient to confront sources of guilt and then help the patient realize that such guilt is unfounded. Through this process of self-realization the patient can reduce feelings of inadequacy and loss, which are the source of the depression.

Cognitive behavior therapies are based upon the theory that people's emotions are controlled by their views and opinions of the world. Depression results when patients consistently berate themselves, expect to fail, make inaccurate assessments of what others think of them, and have a negative and hopeless attitude toward the world and the future. The therapist helps the client alleviate the negative thought patterns and beliefs by applying various techniques of verbal reinforcement and behavioral prescriptions. Two popular models of this form of psychotherapy are Aaron Beck's cognitive therapy (1976) and Albert Ellis' rational–emotive therapy (1984). Implicit in both approaches is the need for clients to learn to validate any self-made conclusions more objectively, a behavior notably absent in people who experience depression.

In Beck's *cognitive therapy* the therapist tries to persuade the depressed person to change his or her opinions of events and of the self. When the patient makes self-accusatory statements, for example, the therapist would attempt to offer examples contrary to these generalizations, and would suggest competencies that the client is overlooking or discounting. The therapist also attempts to help the client monitor his or her thought patterns to help identify negative attitudes or assumptions that contribute to depression. Beck also emphasized behavioral components, including activities which will provide clients with successful experiences and allow them to think well of themselves (Beck, 1976).

Ellis's *rational–emotive therapy* is founded upon the premise that sustained emotional reactions are caused by internal sentences that people repeat to themselves. The aim of therapy is to eliminate the "wrongheaded" sentences of disturbed people through a rational examination of them. Ellis believes that people constantly interpret what is happening around them and that sometimes these interpretations can cause emotional turmoil. A therapist's attention, according to Ellis, should be focused on these internal interpretations rather than on historical causes or overt behavior (Ellis, 1984).

Implications for Therapeutic Recreation

Participation

A considerable amount of research has focused on the relationship between depression and variables assumed to be associated with leisure involvement. For example, findings have revealed that individuals with depression have fewer social skills (Antonuccio, Ward & Tearnan, 1989; Lewinsohn, 1974), low social support (Coyne, 1976; Lewinsohn & Talkington, 1979) and low self-esteem (Billins & Moos, 1982).

Lewinsohn and Graf (1973) found that persons with depression not only engaged in a smaller number of different activities than nondepressed individuals, but also they repeated those activities less frequently. Lewinsohn (1974) also demonstrated that persons with depression scored significantly lower than nondepressed persons on scales measuring obtained pleasure from activity involvement. Wassman and Iso-Ahola (1985) also explained the possible linkage between leisure and depression. They found evidence that among a group of subjects diagnosed with clinical depression, higher frequencies of participation in recreation activities were associated with lower levels of depression.

The specific reasons for leisure's mediating effect upon depression have not yet been established, but several different explanations have been postulated. Iso-Ahola and Weissinger (1984, 1990) have explored the relationship between leisure and boredom, a psychological state common to individuals diagnosed with depression. They suggest that boredom is a psychological state associated with a lack of knowledge about potential leisure choices. To overcome a state of boredom one must be aware that his or her need for intrinsic rewards (e.g., feelings of self-determination) can be satisfied.

Maughn and Ellis (1991) and Ellis, Maughan-Pritchett, and Ruddell (1993) examined the impact of efficacy information provided during recreation participation upon efficacy judgments of adolescents diagnosed with major depression. The researchers found that measures of perceived freedom in leisure and self-reported skill in video games both improved for subjects provided with efficacy information during their involvement in recreational activities. Patrick (1994)

suggested that leisure involvement may help treat *anhedonia,* a condition marked by diminished interest or ability to experience pleasure, which is very common among individuals diagnosed with depression.

Although the specific effects leisure may have on depression are not yet proven, involvement in recreational activities can help these individuals to have feelings of pleasure and happiness, to feel better about themselves, to see some hope for the future, and to increase energy and interest levels. Participation in leisure experiences may help induce a positive mood (Iso-Ahola, 1994), thus helping to combat the sense of helplessness and hopelessness which often characterizes the psychological state of people with affective disorders.

In terms of therapeutic recreation programming, the use of structured activities that promote a sense of perceived control (Wassman & Iso-Ahola, 1985) may help lower levels of depression. Active involvement in enjoyable leisure experiences helps an individual cope with depressive symptoms. Successful participation in recreational activities is important for community reintegration following hospital treatment for depression.

Leisure Education

Leisure education seeks to clarify leisure values and to foster changes in attitudes that develop motivation and skills to participate in leisure experiences. Leisure education may encourage individuals with affective disorders to participate in activities that promote positive feelings and contribute to community involvement.

Although research designed to study the effects of leisure education programs on this population is limited, a few investigations merit attention. In a study designed to investigate the cognitive patterns of suicidal women, Malkin developed a rationale for the use of therapeutic recreation services as an intervention strategy for this population. Malkin concluded, "perhaps the most productive area of focus for women with depression and suicidal tendencies may be the Leisure Awareness Component of the Leisure Education Content Model (Peterson & Gunn, 1984)" (1991, p. 46). The author claimed that the value of this component lies in its ability to help individuals become aware of leisure and its potential benefits. The self-awareness aspect of this model includes an emphasis upon strengths, as well as limitations, which is very important for the self-deprecating tendencies of suicidal, depressed individuals.

Hickman (1994) conducted a study to examine the effects of leisure counseling programs on leisure independence, depression, and depression-related variables of adult women. Data revealed that leisure counseling can be an effective approach for counseling among depressed clients. The use of a combination of pleasant activities and social skills training had a significant effect on measure of perceived freedom in leisure, depression, and self-esteem for this sample. The investigator proclaimed that leisure counseling programs "could be used to alleviate depression among women in our society" (Hickman, 1994, p. 211).

A third study, conducted by Mahon, Bullock, Luken, and Martens (1996), investigated the efficacy of the reintegration through recreation (RTR) leisure education program upon the mastery of skills required for participation in recreation and community living among a sample of adults diagnosed with severe and persistent mental illness. This research specifically sought to determine the social validity (as a determiner of "value") of the RTR program. Three sets of individuals—the consumers, family members of consumers, and service providers—were surveyed. The results suggested that all three groups considered the program to be socially valid. This finding clearly supported the importance of leisure education as an intervention strategy for persons with severe and persistent mental illness.

Therapy

Several researchers have explored the possible benefits of *structured recreation activities* on the treatment of depression. Wassman and Iso-Ahola (1985) studied the relationship between recreation involvement and levels of depression among 14 patients diagnosed as having bipolar or major depression. Data strongly supported their hypothesis that levels of depression would increase as recreation participation decreased. This finding proved to be particularly true with respect to the use of structured recreation programs. The researchers postulated that the development of positive rapport between therapists and patients and the therapists' ability to enhance patients' feelings of accomplishment, control, and freedom contributed to lowered depression levels in the patients. They further speculated that structured recreation programs designed to meet the patients' needs and interests may offer necessary motivation to overcome symptoms of lower levels of energy and loss of interest in activities and events (Wassman & Iso-Ahola, 1985).

Patrick (1994) also advocated the role of structured recreation as a means of reducing various symptoms that inhibit recovery among individuals diagnosed with depression. In particular, he suggested that therapeutic recreation specialists are well-trained to help depressed patients overcome symptoms of boredom, resistance to involvement, and temporal dysfunction characterized by distorted expectations for the future. Patrick (1994) hypothesized that structured recreation programs have a restorative role to play in the treatment of depression, and that therapeutic outcomes, such as the rekindling of interest, the experience of pleasure, and the overcoming of a sense of hopelessness can be products of recreation intervention.

One form of recreational activity which has been well-documented in terms of its impact on psychological and mental states is *physical exercise* (Hall, 1994). Studies have shown that aerobic activity can reduce depression and can increase vigor and clearmindedness (Blumenthal, Williams, Needels & Wallace, 1982). Folkins and Sime (1981) reviewed eight separate investigations which all reported significant improvement in mood states as a result of exercise. Brown (1988) found that jogging five days a week was associated with significant reductions in depression scores.

If physical exercise has preventative qualities as suggested here, does it follow that it can be used in the treatment of depression? Evidence garnered from several different investigations supports this connection. Aerobic exercises were found to be as effective as different forms of psychotherapy in a study reported by Klein et al. (1985). Brown (1988) found that jogging five days a week for a 10-week period was associated with significant reductions in depression scores. Greist, Klein, Eischens, and Faris (1978) reported similar findings. Work completed by Dunn and Dishman (1991) and Martinsen (1990) demonstrated that physical exercise can have an antidepressive effect on patients with mild to moderate forms of depression. The available studies on the impact of anaerobic exercise on depressed patients (Doyne et al., 1987; Dunn & Dishman, 1991; Martinsen, Hoffort & Solberg, 1989), show similar patterns of improvement.

Other forms of physical activity have also shown promise in mediating depressed mood states. Chakravorty, Tunnell, and Ellis (1995) documented a decline in depression scores as a result of participation in ropes course sessions among hospitalized adults. Stewart, McMullen, and Rubin (1994) demonstrated that movement therapy activities could have a positive effect upon the moods of individuals diagnosed with major depression. Additionally, O'Kelly, Piper, Kerver, and

Fowler (1996) demonstrated the value of exercise groups as part of an insight-oriented, psychodynamic treatment program for outpatients with mood disorders.

The use of *aquatic therapy* to reduce depression and enhance mood has support in research literature. Weiss and Jamieson (1989) reported a significant drop in symptoms of depression among subjectively depressed women as a result of an aquatic therapy class. Stein and Motta (1992) summarized the findings of their investigation by concluding that for individuals with disabilities who are unable to withstand land-based weight training, water exercise may be a valuable option for enhancing self-esteem and decreasing depression. In addition, findings from a pair of studies conducted by Berger and Owen (1992) and Berger, Owen, and Man (1993) lend support to the belief that swimming positively influences mood. Nonetheless, it must be remembered that these benefits attributed to aquatic programs were produced using subjects who were not diagnosed with clinical depression; consequently, more research is needed to establish the efficacy of these programs for disabled individuals.

Pets have long been suspected of helping to reduce stress levels in humans. Not surprisingly, the use of animals as therapy for mental illness has been theorized to be an important part of activity-oriented treatment programs. McCandless, McCready, and Knight (1985) developed an excellent review of the potential benefits of animal therapy and a model therapeutic recreation program using animals to treat psychiatric patients.

Another intervention that has produced positive effects among severely depressed and suicidal women is *cognitive restructuring*. Malkin's (1991) study of 35 adult female inpatients diagnosed with depression, produced findings which supported the use of cognitive therapy techniques in the application of leisure counseling and leisure education programs for this population. According to Malkin, some cognitive therapy techniques specifically applicable to therapeutic recreation include graded task assignments activity schedules, and mastery and pleasure therapy (1991, p. 45).

Chapter Summary

This chapter examined affective disorders and addressed the following issues:

- Four types of mood disorders: major depressive disorder (MDD), dysthymic disorder, bipolar disorder (manic-depressive illness), and cyclothymic disorder
- Psychological and physiological theories of causation of affective disorders
- Somatic and psychological treatments of affective disorders
- Implications of mood disorders for therapeutic recreation services

References

Abramson, L., Seligman, M., and Teasdale, J. (1978). Learned helplessness in humans: Critique and reformulation. *Journal of Abnormal Psychology, 87,* 49–74.

American Psychiatric Association. (1994). *Diagnostic and statistical manual of mental disorders* (4th ed.). Washington: DC: Author.

American Psychiatric Association. (1996). *APA Online. Public Information: Depression.* Available online: http://www.psych.org/public_info

Antonuccio, D. O., Ward, C. H., and Tearnan, B. H. (1989). The behavioral treatment of unipolar depression in adult outpatients. In M. Hersen and P. M. Miller (Eds.), *Progress in behavior modification* (Vol. 24, pp. 152–191). New York, NY: Academic Press.

Beck, A. (1967). *Depression: Clinical, experimental, and theoretical aspects.* New York, NY: Harper and Row.

Beck, A. (1976). *Cognitive therapy and emotional disorders.* New York, NY: International Universities Press.

Berger, B. and Owen, D. (1992). Mood alteration with yoga and swimming: Aerobic exercise may not be necessary. *Perceptual and Motor Skills, 75,* 1331–1343.

Berger, B., Owen, D., and Man, F. (1993). A brief review of literature and examination of acute mood benefits of exercise in Czechoslovakian and United States Swimmers. *International Journal of Sport Psychology, 24,* 130–150.

Billings, A. G. and Moos, R. H. (1982). Psychological theory and research on depression: An integrative framework and review. *Clinical Psychology Review, 2,* 213–237.

Blumenthal, J. A., Williams, R. S., Needels, T. L., and Wallace, A. G. (1982). Psychological changes accompanying aerobic exercise in health middle-aged adults. *Psychosomatic Medicine, 44,* 529–536.

Brown, D. R. (1988). Exercise, fitness, and mental health. In C. Bouchard, R. J. Shephard, T. Stephens, J. R. Sutton, and B. D. McPherson (Eds.), *Exercise, fitness and health* (pp. 607–626). Champaign, IL: Human Kinetics.

Chakravorty, D., Tunnell, E., and Ellis, G. (1995). Ropes course participation and postactivity processing on transient depressed mood of hospitalized adult psychiatric patients. *Therapeutic Recreation Journal, 29*(2), 104–113.

Cooper, J. (1996, June 1). The deep dark tunnel of depression. *The Medical Reporter.*

Coyne, J. C. (1976). Depression and the responses of others. *Journal of Abnormal Psychology, 85,* 186–193.

Davison, G. and Neale, J. (1986). *Abnormal psychology: An experimental clinical approach.* New York, NY: John Wiley & Sons.

Deakin, J. (Ed.). (1996). *The biology of depression.* Washington, DC: American Psychiatric Press.

Doyne, E., Ossip-Klein, D., Bowman, E., Osborn, K., McDougall-Wilson, I., and Neimeyer, R. (1987). Running versus weightlifting in the treatment of depression. *Journal of Consulting and Clinical Psychology, 55,* 748–754.

Dunn, A. and Dishman, R. (1991). Exercise and the neurobiology of depression. In J. Holloszy (Ed.), *Exercise and sport science reviews* (Vol. 19, pp. 41–98). Baltimore, MD: Williams and Wilkins.

Ellis, A. (1984). Rational-emotive therapy. In R. J. Corsini (Ed.), *Current psychotherapy* (3rd ed.). Itasca, IL: Peacock Press.

Ellis, G. D., Maughan-Pritchett, M., and Ruddell, E. (1993). Effects of attribution based verbal persuasion and imagery on self-efficacy of adolescents diagnosed with major depression. *Therapeutic Recreation Journal, 27*(2), 83–92.

Folkins, C. H. and Sime, W. E. (1981). Physical fitness training and mental health. *American Psychologist, 36,* 373–389.

Gaviria, M. and Flaherty, J. (1993). Depression. In J. Flaherty, J. Davis, and P. Janicak (Eds.), *Psychiatry: Diagnosis & therapy* (2nd ed., pp. 46–75). Norwalk, CT: Appleton & Lange.

Griest, J., Klein, M., Eischens, R., and Faris, J. (1978). Running out of depression. *The Physician and Sports Medicine, 6*(12), 49–51.

Hall, E. G. (1994). Exercise and depression: Beyond physical fitness. In D. Compton and S. E. Iso-Ahola (Eds.), *Leisure and mental health* (pp. 307–319). Pine City, UT: Family Development Resources, Inc.

Hickman, C. M. (1994). Leisure counseling and depressed women. In D. Compton and S. E. Iso-Ahola (Eds.), *Leisure and mental health* (pp. 204–214). Pine City, UT: Family Development Resources, Inc.

Hiroto, D. and Seligman, M. (1975). Generality of learned helplessness in man. *Journal of Personality and Social Psychology, 31,* 311–327.

Iso-Ahola, S. E. (1994). Leisure lifestyle and health. In D. Compton and S. E. Iso-Ahola (Eds.). *Leisure and mental health* (pp. 42–60). Pine City, UT: Family Development Resources, Inc.

Iso-Ahola, S. E. and Weissinger, E. (1984). Leisure and well-being: Is there a connection? *Parks & Recreation, 18*(6), 40–44.

Iso-Ahola, S. E. and Weissinger, E. (1990). Perception of boredom in leisure: Conceptualizations, reliability and validity of the Leisure Boredom Scale. *Journal of Leisure Research, 22,* 1–7.

Janicak, P. G., Comaty, J., and Dowd, S. (1993). Electroconvulsive therapy for depression. In J. Flaherty, J. Davis, and P. Janicak (Eds.), *Psychiatry: Diagnosis & therapy* (2nd ed., pp. 61–68). Norwalk, CT: Appleton & Lange.

Klein D. and Seligman, M. (1976). Reversal of performance deficits in learned helplessness and depression. *Journal of Abnormal Psychology, 85,* 11–26.

Klein, D. and Wender, P. (1993). *Understanding depression: A complete guide to its diagnosis and treatment.* New York, NY: Oxford University Press.

Klein, M., Griest, J., Gurman, A., Neimeyer, R., Lesser, D., Bushnell, N., and Smith, R. (1985). A comparative outcome study of group psychotherapy vs. exercise treatment for depression. *International Journal of Mental Health, 13,* 148–177.

Lewinsohn, P. M. (1974). A behavioral approach to depression. In R. M. Friedman and M. M. Katz (Eds.), *The psychology of depression: Contemporary theory and research* (pp. 157–185). New York, NY: Wiley.

Lewinsohn, P. M. and Graf, J. (1973). Pleasant activities and depression. *Journal of Counseling and Clinical Psychology, 41,* 261–268.

Lewinsohn, P. M. and Talkington, J. (1979). Studies on the measurement of unpleasant events and relations with depression. *Applied Psychological Measurement, 3,* 83–101.

Lickey, M. and Gordon, B. (1991). *Medicine and mental illness.* New York, NY: W. H. Freeman.

Mahon, M. J., Bullock, C. C., Luken, K., and Martens, C. (1996). Leisure education for persons with severe and persistent mental illness: Is it a socially valid process? *Therapeutic Recreation Journal, 30*(3), 197–212.

Malkin, M. (1991). Cognitive evaluations of suicidal women: Implications for therapeutic recreation intervention. *Therapeutic Recreation Journal 25*(1), 34–49.

Martinsen, E., Hoffort, A., and Solberg, O. (1989). Comparing aerobic and nonaerobic forms of exercise in the treatment of clinical depression: A randomized trial. *Comprehensive Psychiatry, 30,* 324–331.

Martinsen, E. W. (1990). Benefits of exercise for the treatment of depression. *Sports Medicine, 9,* 380–389.

Maughan, M. and Ellis, G. D. (1991). Effect of efficacy information during recreation participation on efficacy judgements of depressed adolescents. *Therapeutic Recreation Journal, 25*(1), 50–59.

McCandless, P., McCready, K., and Knight, L. (1985). A model animal therapy program for mental health settings. *Therapeutic Recreation Journal* (2), 55–63.

McGrath, E., Keita, G., Strickland, B., and Russon, N. (1990). *Women and depression: Risk factor and treatment issues.* Washington, DC: American Psychological Association.

Meyer, R. G. (1993). *The clinician's handbook.* Boston, MA: Allyn & Bacon.

National Depressive and Manic-Depressive Association (1997, Jan. 22/29). Undertreatment of depression. *Journal of American Medical Association, 277,* 4.

O'Kelly, J., Piper, W., Kerber, R., and Fowler, J. (1996). Exercise groups in an insight-oriented, evening treatment program. *International Journal of Group Psychotherapy, 48*(10), 85–94.

Patrick, G. D. (1994). A role for leisure in the treatment of depression. In D. Compton and S. E. Iso-Ahola (Eds.). *Leisure and mental health* (pp. 175–190). Pine City, UT: Family Development Resources, Inc.

Peterson, C. and Seligman, M. (1984). Casual explanations as a risk factor for depression: Theory and evidence. *Psychological Review, 91,* 347–374.

Prien, R., Kupfer, D., Mansky, P., Small, J., Tuason, V., Voss, C., and Johnson W. (1984). *Archives of General Psychiatry, 41,* 1096–1104.

Schildkraut, J. (1965). The catecholamine hypothesis of affective disorders. *American Journal of Psychiatry, 122,* 509–522.

Seligman, M. (1974). Depression and learned helplessness. In R. J. Friedman and M. M. Katz (Eds.), *The psychology of depression: Contemporary theory and research.* Washington, DC: Winton-Wiley.

Stein, P. and Motta, R. (1992). Effects of aerobic and nonaerobic exercise on depression and self-concept. *Perceptual and Motor Skills, 74,* 79–89.

Stewart, N., McMullern, L., and Rubin, L. (1994). Movement therapy with depressed inpatients: A randomized multiple single case design. *Archives of Psychiatric Nursing, 8*(1), 22–29.

U. S. Department of Health and Human Services. (1995). *Bipolar disorder.* (NIH Publication #95–3679).

Valenstein, E. (1986). *Great and desperate cures: The rise and decline of psychosurgery and other radical treatments for mental illness.* New York, NY: Basic Books.

Wassman, K. B. and Iso-Ahola, S. E. (1985). The relationship between recreation participation and depression in psychiatric patients. *Therapeutic Recreation Journal, 29*(3), 63–70.

Weiss, C. and Jamieson, N. (1989). Women, subjective depression and water exercise. *Health Care for Women International, 10,* 75–88.

CHAPTER 6
SCHIZOPHRENIA

Schizophrenia is a complex, potentially devastating condition—the most disabling of the major mental illnesses. Andreasen (1999) called it "one of our most important public health problems" (p. 2). It typically strikes young people just as they are maturing into adulthood. Once it strikes, morbidity is high (60% of patients are receiving disability benefits within the first year after onset), as is mortality (the suicide rate is 10%). An estimated 1% of the world's population experiences this disorder. Despite its prevalence, schizophrenia is often misunderstood, and people with the disorder are stigmatized by both the medical profession and the public (Andreasen, 1999).

Schizophrenia is always associated with severe psychotic symptoms. *Psychotic* means out of touch with reality, or the inability to separate real from unreal experiences. Some people have only one such psychotic episode, others have many episodes during a lifetime but lead relatively normal lives during the interim periods. The individual with chronic schizophrenia often does not fully recover normal functioning and typically requires long-term treatment to control symptoms. Some chronic schizophrenic patients may never be able to function without assistance.

This chapter provides a basic overview of this puzzling disease. We first briefly discuss how the concept of schizophrenia has evolved over time. Next, we discuss essential features of the disorder and symptoms that differentiate this illness from other forms of mental disturbance. The discussion intends to differentiate between several of the common forms of the illness. We highlight prevalence and causes of schizophrenia, the course of the disease, and subtypes of schizophrenia. Different treatments associated with the disorder are also included. The chapter concludes with a discussion of the possible implications of schizophrenia for the field of therapeutic recreation.

Evolution of Schizophrenia

Two European psychiatrists, Emil Kraepelin and Eugen Bleuler, originally formulated the concept of schizophrenia. In 1898 Kraepelin presented his concept of dementia praecox, the early term for schizophrenia. *Dementia praecox* reflects Kraepelin's view of the two major aspects of the disorder: an early onset (praecox) and a progressive intellectual deterioration (dementia). The symptoms that Kraepelin described included hallucinations, delusions, attention difficulties, stereotyped behavior, and emotional dysfunction. Kraepelin's work, however, did not move beyond a description of the disease (Davison & Neale, 1986).

In contrast, Eugen Bleuler attempted to define the roots of the disorder. Unlike Kraeplin, Bleuler did not believe that the disorder necessarily had an early onset or that it inevitably progressed toward dementia. In 1908 Bleuler proposed the term *schizophrenia* to capture what he viewed as the essential nature of the condition. Psychoanalytic theory had a major influence upon Bleuler's view of schizophrenia. Bleuler believed that the various symptoms associated with the disorder were caused by underlying psychological processes—the same rationale applied by Freud to explain various other forms of mental disturbances. In addition, Bleuler also thought that Freudian concepts could account for the specific content of symptoms such as delusions and hallucinations. While Kraepelin's writings fostered an early description of the course of schizophrenia, Bleuler's work led to a broader concept of the disorder and a more pronounced theoretical emphasis (Davison & Neale, 1986).

Bleuler's emphasis upon a broader concept of schizophrenia received wide support by American psychiatrists. Adolf Meyer, for instance, adopted a flexible view of the disorder, which did not rely on specific symptoms or progressive deterioration for a definition. He viewed schizophrenia as an accumulation of faulty habits that had been building for a long period of time. Meyer labeled these habits as *substitutive reactions*. Meyer believed that these reactions had replaced ones appropriate to daily life and had become established as the person settled into a path of least resistance (Davison & Neale, 1986).

The American conception of schizophrenia was also broadened by researchers who identified additional subtypes of the disease. The *Diagnostic and Statistical Manual of Mental Disorders* (*DSM-IV*) (American Psychiatric Association, 1994) recognizes five subtypes, including paranoid type, disorganized type, catatonic type, undifferentiated type, and residual type.

Another important step in creating a broad concept of schizophrenia was the development of the *process–reactive dimension* in the 1960s and 1970s. Once Bleuler observed that the onset of the disease was not always at a young age and that deterioration was not certain, investigators began to identify other differences between those whose onset was later and who some-times recovered and those whose onset was earlier and who usually deteriorated further. Some schizophrenics had experienced a gradual (often beginning in their young years) but insidious onset of characteristic symptoms of the disorder. Others, usually those identi-fied later in life, had a rapid onset of more severe symptoms. The term *process* indicated some sort of basic physiological malfunction in the brain believed to be associated with the insidiously developmental form of the disorder. The term *reactive* indicated the type that appeared rather suddenly. While process schizophrenia, which is associated with a long history of adjustment problems, may be equated with Kraepelia's original description of dementia praecox, the inclusion of the reactive form in the definition of the disorder helped to extend the American concept (Davison & Neale, 1986).

Our understanding of schizophrenia was broadened further by a prevailing interest in the treatment of the disorder. Kraepelin viewed progressive intellectual deterioration as an inevitable consequence of the disease. In contrast, both Bleuler and Meyer rejected the notion of inevitability and allowed for the possibil-ity of intervention and restitution. Henry Stack Sullivan became the first major theorist to develop a systematic psychological treatment for schizophrenia. Contempo-rary literature indicates that about two thirds of all individuals diagnosed with schizophrenia may benefit from treatment.

Essential Features of Schizophrenia

Schizophrenia is a severe disturbance of the brain's functioning. In *The Broken Brain: The Biological Revolution in Psychiatry,* Dr. Nancy Andreasen states:

> The current evidence concerning the causes of schizophrenia is a mosaic. It is quite clear that multiple factors are involved. These include changes in chemistry of the brain, changes in the structure of the brain, and genetic factors. Viral infections and head injuries may also play a role. . . finally, schizophrenia is probably a group of related diseases, some of which are caused by one factor and some by another. (1984, p. 222)

There are billions of nerve cells in the brain. Each nerve cell has branches that transmit and receive messages from other nerve cells. The branches release *neurotransmitters,* chemicals that carry the messages from the end of one nerve branch to the cell body of

another. In the brain afflicted with schizophrenia, something goes wrong in this communication system.

Comparing the brain to a telephone switchboard may be a helpful analogy in understanding the disease. In *Schizophrenia: Straight Talk for Family and Friends,* Maryellen Walsh states:

> In most people the brain's switching system works well. Incoming perceptions are sent along appropri-ate signal paths, the switching process goes off without a hitch, and appropriate feelings, thoughts, and actions go back out again to the world . . . in the brain afflicted with schizophrenia . . . percep-tions come in but get routed along the wrong path or get jammed or end up at the wrong destination. (1985, p. 41)

Schizophrenia may develop so gradually that even the person with the disease may not realize that any-thing is wrong for a long time. This slow deterioration is referred to as *gradual onset of insidious schizophrenia.* A gradual buildup of symptoms may or may not lead to an acute episode or crisis episode of schizophrenia.

An *acute episode* is short and intense, and involves hallucinations, delusions, thought disorder, and an altered sense of self. Sometimes schizophrenia has a rapid or sudden onset. Very dramatic changes in behav-ior occur over a few weeks or even a few days. Sudden onset usually leads fairly quickly to an acute episode. Some people have very few such attacks in a lifetime, others have more. Some people lead relatively normal lives between episodes. Others become very listless, depressed, and unable to function well.

In some, the illness may develop into *chronic schizophrenia*—severe, long-lasting disability charac-terized by social withdrawal, lack of motivation, depression, and blunted feelings. In addition, moderate versions of acute symptoms such as delusions and thought disorder may be present in the chronic disorder.

Symptoms of Schizophrenia

Psychiatrists divide the symptoms of schizophrenia into two broad categories—positive and negative. *Positive* denotes those symptoms that are present but should be absent, and *negative* denotes those symptoms that are absent but should be present. Positive symptoms reflect an excess or distortion of normal functioning. Negative symptoms reflect a diminution or loss of normal functioning.

Positive Symptoms

Delusions are erroneous beliefs that usually involve a misinterpretation of perceptions or experiences. Delusions are steadfastly held by the individual despite obvious evidence to the contrary. The content of delusions may include a variety of themes. *Persecutory delusions*, in which the person believes he or she is being tormented, followed, spied upon, or subjected to ridicule, are most common. A common delusion is that one's thoughts are being broadcast over the radio or television, or that one's thoughts are being controlled by others. *Referential delusions* are also common; the person believes that song lyrics, media messages, or passages from books are specifically directed at him or her. The distinction between a delusion and a strongly held belief is sometimes difficult to make and depends on the degree of conviction with which the belief is held despite clear contradictory evidence.

Hallucinations are sensory perceptions that have a compelling sense of reality, but which occur without external stimulation of the relevant sensory organ. *Auditory hallucinations* are by far the most common. Auditory hallucinations are usually experienced as voices perceived as distinct from the person's own thoughts. Sometimes the voices compliment, reassure, or remain neutral. More commonly, the voices threaten, frighten, and command the individual to do things that may be harmful. The voices may tell the individual that he or she is worthless or stupid, or that he or she has committed horrible acts (e.g., "See that woman? You raped her last night.") The voices may be familiar or unfamiliar. There may be several voices and they may discuss the individual in the third person, commenting critically on the individual's activities.

Thought disorder refers to problems in the way that a person with schizophrenia processes and organizes thoughts. Some psychiatrists claim that disorganized thinking is the single most important feature of schizophrenia. The person may be unable to connect thoughts into logical sequences. Racing thoughts come and go so rapidly that it is not possible to "catch" them. The person may not be able to concentrate on one thought for very long and may be easily distracted or unable to focus attention. Because thinking is disorganized and fragmented, the person's speech is often incoherent and illogical. Thought disorder frequently accompanies inappropriate emotional responses—words and mood do not appear in tune with each other. The result may be something like laughing when speaking of somber or frightening events.

Grossly disorganized behavior may present itself in a variety of ways, ranging from childlike silliness to unpredictable agitation and aggression. The individual with schizophrenia may have difficulty completing any goal-directed behavior, such as organizing meals or maintaining hygiene. The person may appear disheveled, may dress in an odd or unusual manner (e.g., wearing an overcoat on a warm summer day), or may display clearly inappropriate behavior (e.g., public masturbation) or untriggered agitation (e.g., shouting or swearing).

Altered sense of self describes a blurring of the person's feelings about himself or herself. Examples include depersonalization and confused body image. It may be a sensation of being bodiless, or nonexistent as a person. The individual may not be able to tell where his or her body stops and the rest of the world begins.

Negative Symptoms

Apathy is a lack of motivation, energy, or interest in life often confused with laziness. Because the person has very little energy, he or she may not be able to do much more than sleep and pick at meals. Life for the person with schizophrenia can be experienced as devoid of interest.

Blunted feelings or *blunted affect* refer to a flattening of the emotions. Because facial expressions and hand gestures may be limited or nonexistent, the individual seems unable to feel or show any emotion at all. This does not mean that the individual does not feel emotions and is not receptive to kindness and consideration. He or she may be feeling very emotional but cannot express it outwardly. Blunted affect may become a stronger symptom as the disease progresses.

Depression involves feelings of helplessness and hopelessness, and may stem in part from realizing that schizophrenia has changed one's life. *Anhedonia*—the inability to experience pleasant emotions—frequently coexists with these feelings of emptiness. Often the person believes that he or she has behaved badly, has destroyed relationships, and is unlovable. Depressed feelings are very painful and may lead to talk of or attempts at suicide. Biological changes in the brain may also contribute to depression. Individuals may also display avolition—restrictions in the ability to initiate goal-directed behavior.

Social withdrawal may occur as a result of anhedonia, feeling relative safety in being alone, being caught up in one's own feelings, or fearing that one cannot manage the company of others. Individuals with schizophrenia have emotional extremes—aloof and withdrawn or clinging and demanding. They frequently lack the resources needed to show interest in socializing.

Prevalence and Causes of Schizophrenia

The onset of schizophrenia typically occurs between late teens and mid-thirties, with onset prior to adolescence rare. Schizophrenia occurs with equal frequency in females and males, but women are more likely to experience later onset. The peak incidence of onset is between ages 15 and 24 years for males and in the late twenties for females. Gender differences have been noted in the presentation and course of the disease, as women are likely to have more prominent mood symptoms than males, and women generally have a better prognosis (APA, 1994).

The risk of development of schizophrenia in any individual during any one year is 1:2000, and the lifetime risk is 1:100. There are between 100,000 and 200,000 newly treated cases of schizophrenia in the United States each year. An estimated two million Americans have been diagnosed with the disorder. This rate is similar to other countries (Channon, 1993).

Many predisposing factors have been associated with the onset or relapse of schizophrenia—no known single cause of schizophrenia exists. Genetic factors produce a vulnerability to schizophrenia, with environmental factors contributing to different degrees in different individuals. First-degree biological relatives of individuals with schizophrenia have a 10 times greater risk for the disorder than that of the general population (APA, 1994). Environmental factors also clearly contribute to the onset or relapse of the disorder for some individuals. Channon (1993) has identified family environments marked by expressed emotion (i.e., family members exchange critical comments and hostilities or there is emotional overinvolvement) as contributing to a higher relapse rate. Certain personality traits such as being extremely withdrawn, shy, eccentric, suspicious, or overly compliant may also contribute to increased risk for the disorder (Channon, 1993). Just as each individual's personality is the result of an interplay of many factors—cultural, psychological, biological, and genetic—a disorganization of the personality may result from an interplay of similar factors (Shore, 1986).

While research has improved our understanding of the causes of schizophrenia in recent years, its symptoms and associated cognitive abnormalities cannot be isolated to a single region of the brain. In her summation of research directed toward identifying the causation of schizophrenia, Andreasen wrote:

> The working hypothesis shared by most investigators is that schizophrenia is a disease of neural connectivity caused by multiple factors that affect brain development. Our current model of the causation of schizophrenia is very similar to that used to understand cancer. That is, schizophrenia probably occurs as a consequence of multiple "hits," which include some combination of inherited genetic factors and external, nongenetic factors that affect the regulation and expression of genes governing brain function or that injure the brain directly. Some people may have a genetic predisposition that requires a convergence of additional factors to produce the expression of the disorder. (1999, p. 2)

Course of Schizophrenia

The peak incidence of onset of schizophrenia is the late teens and early twenties for men and the late twenties for women. The onset may be abrupt or insidious, often marked by acute psychotic episodes. The first symptoms include loss of interest in school or work, social withdrawal, deterioration in personal care, unusual behavior, and emotional outbursts. Individuals with early onset often have more evidence of structural brain abnormalities and consequently poorer premorbid adjustment. Conversely, individuals with later onset have less evidence of structural brain abnormalities or cognitive impairment and usually display a better outcome (APA, 1994).

The course of schizophrenia is not uniform in every patient, nor is progressive deterioration inevitable. The consensus among researchers is that a return to a state of full premorbid functioning is uncommon. Many individuals will display periods of exacerbation and remission. Negative symptoms usually dominate early in the illness, with positive symptoms developing later on. Because positive symptoms usually respond better to treatment, they often diminish in many individuals. Negative symptoms frequently persist despite therapeutic intervention.

Channon asserts that, although rare, complete recovery from the disorder is possible even after a long period of illness. More commonly, about two thirds of individuals with schizophrenia have chronic social and behavioral impairments, and the other one third will be incapacitated by chronic symptoms and will require long-term or frequent institutionalization (1993, p. 96).

A group of factors associated with a favorable long-term outcome has been identified (Channon, 1993), including:

- Family history of affective disorder but not schizophrenia
- Acute onset of the illness
- Later age of onset
- More affective (mood) signs and symptoms
- Good premorbid functioning in school, vocation, and social adjustment
- Female
- Brief duration of active-phase symptoms

Characteristics related to poor prognosis include:

- Family history of schizophrenia
- Absence of affective symptoms
- Poor premorbid functioning
- Early, insidious onset

According to Channon (1993), the best way to predict an individual's functioning is to look at his or her prior history. The type and duration of symptoms that a person with schizophrenia exhibits tend to repeat in subsequent episodes. The same holds true for social and occupational functioning as well as the likelihood of future hospitalization.

Schizophrenia Subtypes

The *DSM-IV* (APA, 1994) recognizes five subtypes of schizophrenia: paranoid, disorganized, catatonic, undifferentiated, and residual. The diagnosis of a particular subtype is based on the symptoms that predominate at the time of evaluation. It is not uncommon for individuals to have symptoms characteristic of more than one subtype or for a diagnosis to change over time.

Paranoid Type

To warrant a *DSM-IV* (APA, 1994) diagnosis of *paranoid type* schizophrenia, the individual has to fulfill the criteria for schizophrenia and present symptoms dominated by either preoccupation with one or more systematized delusions or frequent auditory hallucinations related to a single theme. Symptoms may include incoherent, disorganized speech, grossly disorganized behavior, catatonic behavior, or flat or inappropriate

affect, although none of these are prominent (Meyer, 1993).

Delusions are typically persecutory or grandiose and are usually organized around a coherent theme. A *persecutory delusion* has as a central theme the belief that the individual or someone close to them is being harassed, attacked, persecuted, or conspired against. An individual experiencing a *grandiose delusion* views himself or herself as having inflated worth, power, or identity. He or she may also believe to have a special relationship to a famous person or deity (APA, 1994). *Hallucinations*, when present, typically associate with the delusional theme. The persecutory themes may predispose the individual to suicidal behavior.

Although persons with the paranoid type of schizophrenia are typically more socially appropriate than those with other types of the disorder, their reactions are usually more stilted or intense than normal responses. This is particularly so if anger and suspicion rather than grandiosity is the predominant symptom (Meyer, 1993).

The onset of this subtype tends to be later in life than for other types of schizophrenia, but usually before 35 years of age. The distinguishing features are often relatively stable over time. The intellectual functioning of these individuals often shows little impairment when cognitive testing is done (Meyer, 1993). *DSM-IV* (APA, 1994) states that this variety of schizophrenia tends to be the least severe of the five subtypes.

Disorganized Type

The diagnosis of *disorganized type* of schizophrenia denotes an individual who displays incoherence, disorganized behavior, loose associations in speech patterns, and markedly flat or inappropriate affect. He or she often displays giggling or random laughter not related to the content of the speech. When present, delusions and hallucinations lack structure or a thematic pattern. Other features commonly associated with this type of schizophrenia include odd facial expressions, peculiar mannerisms, extremely poor social functioning, and the inability to perform activities of daily living (e.g., showering, dressing, food preparation). Cognitive tests generally demonstrate impaired intellectual functioning.

The onset of this subtype usually occurs in adolescence or early adulthood. Overall, chronic adjustment problems and poor long-term remission rates characterize disorganized schizophrenia.

Catatonic Type

Severe psychomotor disturbance is the essential feature of *catatonic type* of schizophrenia. One form of motor disturbance may involve a stuporlike state in which movement is severely reduced and a rigid posture is evident. Some may show waxy flexibility, a condition in which the body passively receives manipulation much like one would move a store mannequin. Another form of motor disturbance is marked by uncontrollable verbal and motor behavior, which is purposeless and not influenced by external stimuli. Individuals of this type can be prone to violent behavior, risking injury to themselves or others. Other symptoms associated with this form of schizophrenia include *echolalia* (the parrotlike repetition of a word or phrase just spoken by another person) and *echopraxia* (the repetitive imitation of the movements of another person).

According to Meyer (1993) two different courses are typically observed in catatonic schizophrenia. The chronic form of this disorder is primarily associated with the stuporlike variety of motor disturbance. The progression of the symptoms are slow and prognosis for remission is low. In its more acute form, this disorder is characterized by an abrupt onset followed by alternating periods of agitation and stupor. Remission is more likely for this form, although recurrences may be common.

Undifferentiated Type

The *undifferentiated type* of schizophrenia category is marked by prominent schizophrenic symptoms; however, either there are mixed symptoms from various subtypes, or the criteria for one specific category is not fulfilled. In recognition of its nonspecific criteria, this subtype is commonly referred to as the "waste basket" variety of schizophrenia.

Residual Type

The *residual type* of schizophrenia diagnosis applies to an individual who has experienced at least one episode of schizophrenia, but who no longer displays any prominent positive psychotic symptoms (e.g., delusions, hallucinations, disorganized speech, or behavior). However, there remains evidence of disturbance as marked by the presence of negative symptoms (e.g., flat affect, the inability to initiate or persist in goal-directed behaviors) or two or more weakened positive symptoms (e.g., eccentric behavior, mildly disorganized speech). The course of the residual type varies, oftentimes remaining stable for many years without acute exacerbation. For some individuals it may represent a transition between one of the other subtypes and complete remission (APA, 1994).

Treatment of Schizophrenia

Current treatment methods for schizophrenia are based on both clinical research and experience. The approaches used are chosen on the basis of their ability to reduce the severity of symptoms as well as to lessen the chances that the symptoms will return. The most common approach to treating schizophrenia usually involves integrating pharmacological and psychosocial treatments.

Pharmacological Approaches

Pharmacological approaches center on the use of antipsychotic medications—*neuroleptics*—first developed in the 1950s. These drugs have proven to be highly effective in dealing with the positive symptoms of schizophrenia. These medications reduce the psychotic symptoms of chronic schizophrenia and often allow the individual to function more effectively and appropriately. For people with recurrent episodes of schizophrenia, neuroleptics prevent relapse into acute symptoms. Unfortunately, the negative symptoms of more chronic schizophrenia, such as depression and apathy, do not respond as well to medications.

Neuroleptics work by blocking receptors for the brain chemical dopamine. *Dopamine* is one of the brain's neurotransmitters and carries messages from certain specific nerve cells to other specific cells in the brain. Evidence suggests that some people with schizophrenia may either have too many dopamine receptors or else have receptors that are overly sensitive to dopamine (Andreasen, 1984; Mostert & Boshes, 1993). Because of this, the brain of the person with schizophrenia may receive too many messages along these pathways. These extra messages may compete with signals transmitted through other chemical pathways and may result in the production of psychotic symptoms.

There are about 30 varieties of neuroleptics currently in use. Although each of the neuroleptics interferes with dopamine, each drug differs in how it affects other brain chemicals. For this reason, as well as physical and sensitivity differences among individuals receiving the medications, people respond somewhat differently to the different neuroleptics. Finding the right neuroleptic at the right dosage requires continual monitoring by medical personnel (Andreasen, 1984).

In addition to attempting to identify and monitor the *maintenance dosage* (i.e., the lowest dosage at which the person's condition is stable), physicians also must try to minimize the unwanted side effects that usually accompany antipsychotic drugs. During the early phase of drug treatment individuals may be bothered by side effects such as restlessness, drowsiness, dry mouth, stiffening of muscles in the neck and jaw, or blurring of vision. These problems are usually cleared up with a change of neuroleptic, a change in dosage, or the addition of another medication to control side effects. The long-term side effects, such as tardive dyskinesia (TD) may be more problematic. *Tardive dyskinesia* is a disorder characterized by involuntary movements affecting the mouth, lips, and tongue, and sometimes the trunk and limbs. It occurs in about 15% to 20% of patients who receive antipsychotic drugs over extended periods of time. Altering the dosage of medication may reduce the symptoms of TD, but for some people the condition may become permanent (Comaty, 1993).

Medications do not "cure" schizophrenia or ensure that psychotic episodes will not occur in the future. For most individuals who experience this disorder, however, the neuroleptics allow them to function more effectively and appropriately. Even with the risk of side effects, persons with the disorder usually benefit from the use of antipsychotic medication.

Psychosocial Approaches

Psychosocial approaches help persons with schizophrenia cope with psychological, social, and occupational problems resulting from the disorder. Even when relatively free of psychotic symptoms, many individuals with schizophrenia experience feelings of dejection, resignation, fearfulness, and the decreased ability to experience pleasure. They commonly have problems establishing and maintaining relationships with others, and often lack the skills necessary to fulfill occupational demands. Psychosocial treatment addresses these problems and aims to help the individual interpret reality, reduce distortions, and improve coping skills.

Psychosocial treatment may include individual, family, and group therapy. The duration of treatment is indefinite, and may take place in a hospital, clinic, halfway house, or home. Several interventions may be used at any one time; the approach used depends on the needs of the person and the available resources.

Individual psychotherapy involves regularly scheduled talks between the individual with schizophrenia and a trained mental health professional. These talks may focus on current or past problems, experiences, thoughts, or relationships. They generally emphasize correcting the person's distorted perceptions regarding themselves and others. Goals of individual psychotherapy include reducing perceptions of isolation and estrangement, avoiding psychotic relapse, and improving social functioning.

Family therapy usually involves the patient, the parents or spouse, occasionally other family members, and the therapist. Involving the family during the early phases of treatment helps to collect information about the person with schizophrenia and his or her environment; to assess the impact of the illness on the family; to educate family members about the illness; and to discuss ways they may help. Once a treatment regimen has been initiated, inclusion of the family helps to reduce stress, to develop an encouraging family social network, and to assist family members in dealing with their own feelings and emotions with respect to the illness. Evidence tends to support the usefulness of family therapy, when the family is available and willing to participate, in decreasing the relapse rate (Naidu, Channon & Woollcott, 1993).

Group therapy sessions usually involve a small number of clients (6 to 10) and one or two trained therapists. Sessions help individuals learn from the experiences of others, test one's perceptions against those of others, and correct distortions and maladaptive interpersonal behavior by means of feedback from other group members. The methods may include recreational activities, social skills training, and psychotherapy. Sessions often focus on coping with problems of daily living, improving interpersonal skills, improving vocational functioning, and coping with community living. This form of therapy may occur in hospitals, day treatment centers, clinics, and home environments. It is usually most helpful after individuals have emerged from the acute psychotic phase of the illness.

Implications for Therapeutic Recreation

Efforts to describe specific roles that therapeutic recreation (TR) might play with individuals with schizophrenia are complex—interventions that may be appropriate at one time might be inconsequential at another time. For instance, during acute, psychotic phases of the illness, when the client is very disturbed and disorganized, TR usually has little practical value. In contrast, during periods of remission TR services may greatly contribute to the fulfillment of a wide range of social, emotional, and leisure needs.

Moreover, individuals who have this disorder often rotate between a variety of settings, ranging from highly monitored clinical environments during acute phases to homogeneous community settings during periods when symptoms are under control. Each setting will dictate the nature of TR services offered.

Due to schizophrenia's complex nature, most scientific investigations to date have focused upon developing a general understanding of the causes and characteristics of the disorder. A very limited quantity of research directed toward treating schizophrenia. An extensive review of TR-related literature focusing upon schizophrenia produced only a handful of published papers. In addition, the majority of these published studies used a single subject, a case study design, or a very limited number of subjects. As a result, caution is advised when attempting to generalize about the use of TR as an intervention strategy with this population.

Participation

In general, the benefits of participation in recreational activities are the same for all individuals. The desire to experience enjoyment, to feel better about oneself, to feel in control, to perceive one has a choice in participation, and to feel challenged do not change as a result of the diagnosis of schizophrenia.

Recreation participation might also hold other benefits of a more therapeutic nature. For individuals with schizophrenia, the chance to try out new behaviors or experiment with ways of interacting with others in a relatively safe environment may be very appealing. Through recreational activities these individuals may get be themselves in situations where they are not closely monitored and their behavior is not scrutinized for its significance and meaning. As Kinney and Kinney (1996) suggest, recreation participation has the potential to improve the individual's perceived quality of life, as well as help the client to feel better about being in a treatment program. This can also lead to greater acceptance of clinical interventions.

Leisure Education

Leisure education serves to address leisure-related skills, attitudes, and knowledge. Perhaps its most direct application to schizophrenia relates to its contributions to the development of independent living skills and community reintegration after hospital discharge. The process of helping the individual with schizophrenia move toward greater independence requires the coordinated efforts of many individuals, including the person with the disorder, his or her family members, and a variety of human services professionals. For the discharged person, diet, exercise, work, housing, and social obligations usually represent considerable challenges. The knowledge, motivation, and skills to use his or her free time in a purposeful and satisfying manner are critical components in making a successful transition to community life. A leisure education program offered by a certified TR professional would logically address this need.

Whether offered through a transition (day) program or a community-based agency like a public recreation and parks department, leisure education programs are ideally suited to assist in the transition to independent living. In addition to increasing leisure competence, such programs may contribute to the development of coping skills and social skills, as well as encourage family interactions. Such skills are particularly useful because people with schizophrenia are highly vulnerable to impulsive behavior such as suicide, as well as temptations such as drugs, alcohol, and unprotected sexual activity (Andreasen, 1999; Torrey, 1988).

Gimmestad (1995) presented an excellent example of the potential contributions of a leisure education program in a case history published in the *Therapeutic Recreation Journal*. This case history summarized the treatment of a 36-year-old woman with schizophrenia. A significant part of the TR treatment program developed for this client was a family-centered leisure education program. The purpose of the family leisure education program was to strengthen the interactions and leisure experiences of the client and her mother. The author described the progress made by the client during her 15-month hospitalization as one of moving "from complete withdrawal and isolation, to weekly trips to a local restaurant, to community outings with other patients" (1995, p. 61) and eventually discharge to a long-term rehabilitation center. The author further suggested that this treatment approach helped the client to learn how to interact and get close to other people, as well as feel more comfortable on the ward and establish trust toward the staff.

Therapy

More than almost any other disorder, schizophrenia warrants a multifaceted treatment plan. Because it is clearly a disease of the brain (Andreasen, 1999), chemotherapy is useful as one component of treatment for most individuals, especially those with a history of remission and hospitalization.

When recreation therapy is employed in work with schizophrenia its focus is most often directed toward helping the individual become more effective in dealing with life crises. Perhaps one of the most valuable contributions of TR involves offering supportive therapy. In *Surviving Schizophrenia*, Torrey (1988) described the role of supportive therapy as:

> providing a patient with friendship, encouragement, practical advice such as access to community resources or how to develop a more active social life, suggestions for minimizing friction with family members, and, above all, hope that the person's life may be improved. (p. 259)

The notion of TR as supportive therapy is consistent with the attributional analysis approach proposed by Iso-Ahola, MacNeil, and Szymanski in 1980. This approach suggested that an essential contribution of TR is its ability to motivate clients toward action by allowing them to perceive themselves as the cause of their own behavior (Iso-Ahola et al., 1980). The authors suggest that the TR specialist work to create situations that ensure clients' sense of perceived control and success.

In conjunction with supportive therapy, TR programs may assist in the development of appropriate social skills needed to help the person with schizophrenia feel comfortable in his or her environment. Toward this end, the TR professional might use structured activities which involve repeated rehearsal and practice of specific social situations (Skalko, 1991). Role-playing activities, for example, could be used to create non-threatening situations which might allow the client to practice previously learned social interaction skills or to help develop new ones. The ultimate goal of such training is to help persons with schizophrenia decrease their sense of social isolation. Although evidence that social skills training can effectively improve social functioning with this population is limited, research conducted by Hayes, Halford, and Varghose (1991) demonstrated that positive improvements in social skills is possible at least on a short-term basis.

Another focus for TR programs may be upon the development of coping strategies to deal with stress in everyday life. While each of us finds certain aspects of our lives stressful, debilitating stress often confronts those with schizophrenia (Health Canada, 1996). In addition to having to deal with "normal" sources of stress, the severely mentally ill individual must cope with a variety of internal sources of stress such as altered perceptions, cognitive confusion, attentional deficits, and impaired sense of identity (Starkey, Deleone & Flannery, 1995).

One approach to helping clients cope with stress might be the development of a stress management program, which may include self-recognition skills, modified breathing exercises, progressive muscle relaxation exercises, mental skills (e.g., cognitive refocusing and guided imagery), and supportive group therapy (Klamen & Doblin, 1993). While the efficacy of stress management programming for persons with schizophrenia remains unproven, results produced in one study suggest that such activities merit further attention (Starkey et al., 1995).

The available literature, although relatively limited, offers a few additional ideas for TR programming for persons with schizophrenia. Physical exercise, known to promote a wide variety of health benefits, is certainly an appropriate focus for some clients with the disorder. Thyer, Irvine, and Santa (1984) demonstrated that a carefully structured exercise program based upon contingency-management procedures (i.e., predetermined award structures based on the completion of behavioral goals) improved levels of fitness among two psychotic residents living in a sheltered group home. Bielanska, Cechnicki, and Budzyna-Dawidowski (1991) used drama therapy to improve emotional self-understanding and social skills of a small group of patients with schizophrenia. In addition, Zagelbaum and Rubino (1991) reported on a combined dance and movement, art, and music therapy program that improved the psychosocial functioning of a 51-year-old woman with a dual diagnosis of mental retardation and schizophrenia.

While therapeutic recreation has much to offer to the person with schizophrenia, this disorder is extremely complex and may manifest itself very differently in different individuals or within the same individual at different times. No matter how benign TR programs may appear, like all interventions they can exacerbate psychosis if started too early or pursued too rapidly. Acquiring as much information as possible about each client with schizophrenia is critical to successful TR programming. Keeping this in mind, we offer the following suggestions for working with clients with schizophrenia:

- Speak slowly and with a low pitch
- Use short, simple sentences to avoid confusion
- Repeat statements and questions using the same words

- Explain clearly what you are doing and why you are doing it
- Establish a structured and regular routine—be predictable
- Offer praise continually
- Avoid overstimulation
- Reduce stress and tension
- One-on-one activities may be more appropriate during initial programming
- Provide activities that your client can successfully complete
- Understand that it may be difficult for a person with schizophrenia to have a conversation with you, and consider listening to music, playing cards, looking at magazines together, or watching a movie
- Encourage, but never push, your client to be part of social gatherings if appropriate
- Help your client to identify sources of stress and to deal with stress in a socially acceptable manner
- Encourage clients to take responsibility

Schizophrenia: What the Future Might Hold

The outlook for people with schizophrenia has improved over the past quarter century. Although no totally effective therapy has yet been devised, many schizophrenic patients improve enough to lead independent, satisfying lives. As we learn more about the causes and treatments of schizophrenia, we should be able to help more individuals afflicted with the disorder to achieve successful outcomes. Studies that have followed people with schizophrenia for long periods, from the first breakdown to old age, reveal a wide range of possible outcomes. A review of almost 2000 patients suggests that 25% achieve full recovery, 50% recover at least partially, and 25% require long-term care (Shore, 1986).

The development of a variety of treatment methods and facilities is of crucial importance because schizophrenic patients vary greatly in their needs for treatment. In particular, better alternatives are needed to close the gap between the lack of intensive treatment offered in outpatient clinics and the highly regulated treatment (including 24-hour supervision) provided in hospitals. With a wide variety of facilities available, mental health professionals will be better able to tailor treatment to the different needs of individual patients. Given the complexity of schizophrenia, many questions about its causes, prevention, and treatment remain unanswered. More rigorous and broad-based research is needed to better understand this mysterious and devastating form of mental illness.

Chapter Summary

This chapter examined schizophrenia and addressed the following issues:

- How the concept of schizophrenia has evolved over time
- Positive and negative symptoms of schizophrenia
- Prevalence and causes of schizophrenia
- Subtypes of schizophrenia: paranoid, disorganized, catatonic, undifferentiated, and residual
- Pharmacological and psychosocial treatments for schizophrenia
- Implications of schizophrenia for therapeutic recreation practice
- Future directions for schizophrenia research

References

American Psychiatric Association. (1994). *Diagnostic and statistical manual of mental disorders* (4th ed.). Washington, DC: Author.

Andreasen, N. C. (1984). *The broken brain: The biological revolution in psychiatry.* New York, NY: Harper & Row Publishers, Inc.

Andreasen, N. C. (1999). Understanding the causes of schizophrenia. *The New England Journal of Medicine, 340*(8), 2–4.

Bielanska, A., Cechnicki, A., and Budzyna-Dawidowski, M. (1991). Drama therapy as a means of rehabilitation for schizophrenic patients: Our impressions. *American Journal of Psychotherapy, 45*(4), 566–573.

Channon, R. A. (1993). Schizophrenia. In J. Flaherty, J. Davis, and P. Janicak (Eds.), *Psychiatry: Diagnosis and therapy* (2nd ed., pp. 91–101). Norwalk, CT: Appleton & Lange.

Comaty, J. E. (1993). Abnormal movements. In J. Flaherty, J. Davis, and P. Janicak (Eds.), *Psychiatry: Diagnosis and therapy* (2nd ed., pp. 449–463). Norwalk, CT: Appleton & Lange.

Davison, G. and Neale, J. (1986). *Abnormal psychology: An experimental clinical approach.* New York, NY: John Wiley & Sons.

Grimmestad, K. (1995). A comprehensive therapeutic recreation intervention: A woman with schizophrenia. *Therapeutic Recreation Journal, 29*(1), 56–62.

Hayes, R., Halford, W., and Varghose, F. (1991). Generalization of effects of activity therapy and social skills training on the social behavior of low functioning schizophrenic patients. *Occupational Therapy in Mental Health, 11*(4), 3–11.

Health Canada. (1996). *Schizophrenia: A handbook for families.* Ottawa, ON: Author.

Iso-Ahola, S., MacNeil, R., and Szymanski, D. (1980). Social psychological foundations of therapeutic recreation: An attributional analysis. In S. Iso-Ahola (Ed.), *Social psychological perspectives on leisure and recreation* (pp. 390–414). Springfield, IL: Charles C. Thomas.

Kinney, J. and Kinney, W. (1996). Psychiatry and mental health. In D. Austin & M. Crawford (Eds.), *Therapeutic recreation: An introduction* (2nd ed., pp. 57–77). Boston, MA: Allyn & Bacon.

Klamen, D. L. and Doblin, B. H. (1993). Stress assessment and reduction. In J. Flaherty, J. Davis, and P. Janicak (Eds.), *Psychiatry: Diagnosis and therapy* (2nd ed., pp. 471–477). Norwalk, CT: Appleton & Lange.

Meyer, T. G. (1993). *The clinician's handbook* (3rd ed.). Boston, MA: Allyn & Bacon.

Mostert, M. and Boshes, R. (1993). Pharmacological treatment of schizophrenia. In J. Flaherty, J. Davis, and P. Janicak (Eds.), *Psychiatry: Diagnosis and therapy* (2nd ed., pp. 101–113). Norwalk, CT: Appleton & Lange.

Naidu, J., Channon, R., and Woollcott, P. (1993). Psychosocial therapy for schizophrenia. In J. Flaherty, J. Davis, and P. Janicak (Eds.), Psychiatry: Diagnosis and therapy (2nd ed., pp. 113–120). Norwalk, CT: Appleton & Lange.

Shore, D. (Ed.). (1986). *Schizophrenia: Questions and answers.* (DHHS Publication No. ADM 86–1457). Rockville, MD: National Institute of Mental Health.

Skalko, T. (1991). Social skills training for persons with chronic mental illness. *Journal of Physical Education, Recreation & Dance, 62*(4), 31–34.

Starkey, D., Deleone, H., and Flannery, T. (1995). Stress management for psychiatric patients in a state hospital settings. *American Journal of Orthopsychiatry, 65*(3), 446–452.

Thyer, B., Irvine, S., and Santa, C. (1984). Contingency management of exercise by chronic schizophrenics. *Perceptual and Motor Skills, 58,* 419–425.

Torrey, F. E. (1988). *Surviving schizophrenia: A family manual.* Markham, ON: Fitzhenry & Whiteside Limited.

Walsh, M. (1985). *Schizophrenia: Straight talk for family and friends.* New York, NY: William Morrow and Company.

Zagelbaum, V. and Rubino, M. (1991). Combined dance/movement, art, and music therapies with a developmentally delayed, psychiatric client in a day treatment setting. *The Arts in Psychotherapy, 18,* 139–148.

CHAPTER 7 SUBSTANCE-RELATED DISORDERS

Throughout history human beings have used a multitude of substances to reduce physical pain, relieve stress, or alter states of consciousness. Almost every culture has discovered some intoxicant that affects the central nervous system, relieving physical or mental anguish or producing a state of euphoria. Whatever the consequences of the use of the substance, its effects (at least initially) are usually pleasing.

Several natural drugs have a long history of use and abuse, including *alcoholic beverages*, derived from the fermentation of fruits and grains; *opium*, the dried milky juice obtained from the immature fruit of the opium poppy; *hashish* and *marijuana*, derived from the hemp plant Cannabis; and *cocaine*, extracted from coca leaves. In recent decades a number of synthetic and synthesized drugs—most importantly the barbiturates, amphetamines, hallucinogens (LSD), and phencyclidine (PCP)—have become increasingly available.

No matter what the source of intoxicating substances, psychoactive agents continue to be the cause of many of modern society's most challenging problems. According to the National Institute on Drug Abuse, substance abuse has an estimated $67 billion per year economic impact on society (1999i). This figure includes costs related to crime, medical care, drug abuse treatment, social welfare programs, and time lost from work.

Substance-related problems occur in both genders and in all racial, socioeconomic, ethnic, and geographic groups. Psychoactive substances produce changes in behavior, perception, cognition, and mood. Many of these substances can produce psychological and physiological dependency among users. In addition to alcohol, the most widely used intoxicating substance, central nervous system stimulants (including cocaine), opioids, hallucinogens, cannabis (including marijuana), phencyclidine, and various inhalants, are among society's frequently abused drugs.

According to the *Diagnostic and Statistical Manual of Mental Disorders* (*DSM-IV*) (American Psychiatric Association, 1994), the pathological use of substances that affect the central nervous system fall into two broad categories: *substance-use disorders* (substance dependence, substance abuse) and the *substance-induced disorders* (substance intoxication, substance withdrawal), as well as a variety of substance-induced states such as delirium, dementia, mood disorder, anxiety disorder, sleep disorder, and sexual dysfunction.

This chapter presents an overview of the nature, extent, and treatment of substance-related disorders. We begin by reviewing a variety of different theories that have been advanced to explain causes of substance-related disorders. Next, we present the main features and criteria for substance dependence, abuse, intoxication, and withdrawal applicable across all classes of substances. We then consider seven separate classes of substances: alcohol, central nervous system stimulants, opioids, hallucinogens, cannabis, phencyclidine, and inhalants. For each class specific aspects of dependence, abuse, intoxication, and withdrawal will be described. In addition, we review the effects, diagnostic criteria, epidemiological information, patterns of use, etiology, and treatment of each substance. The chapter concludes with a discussion of possible implications of the substance-related problems for the field of therapeutic recreation.

Theories of Causation

In trying to understand substance-related disorders, it is important to distinguish between conditions that may induce a person to start using a substance and those that play a central role in maintaining the behavior. Chronic use of many substances can become an addiction; the user eventually begins to use the substance habitually because his or her body demands it. But this physical need does not explain why an individual initially develops the behavior. Efforts to explain the origins of substance-related disorders generally focus upon two broad categories of factors: psychological and physiological.

Psychological Factors

Psychological theories of the origin of substance-related disorders usually emphasize reduction of distress and the pleasant feeling and euphoric state that the substance produces. These theories also attempt to explain why particular kinds of people seem to need these effects. An association has often been noted, for example, between criminality, substance abuse, and antisocial behavior. In this context abuse may be considered as part of the thrill-seeking behavior of individuals diagnosed with antisocial personality disorder (Quay, 1965, 1987).

Similarities in developmental backgrounds have been identified in the life histories of substance abusers. Chein, Gerard, Lee, and Rosenfield (1964) reported a strong correlation between a pathogenic family environment, marked by either the absence of a father or the presence of overtly hostile and distant father, and the increase of likelihood of substance abuse. Chein and his colleagues also recognized the role of peers as the primary source of introduction to a substance. Peer pressure, curiosity, boredom, and aggravation were cited as primary contributing factors in substance-related problems (Chein et al., 1964). Findings such as these suggest the notion that substance-related problems may originate as a learned response to environmental stimuli.

This notion of substance misuse as a learned response has received considerable attention with respect to alcohol abuse. *Learning-based theories* of alcoholism advance the argument that drinking alcohol is a learned response that is acquired and maintained because it reduces distress (Davison & Neale, 1986). Several investigations lend credence to this argument. Sher and Levenson (1982) found evidence that alcohol can dampen tension in otherwise stressful situations for some individuals. Hull (1981) reported that alcohol decreased the self-awareness of highly self-conscious subjects, indirectly reducing tension by helping subjects cope with negative thoughts about themselves. Lubin's (1977) research demonstrated that alcohol helps lessen the awareness of poor performance on an experimental task for a select group of subjects. The established familial pattern of alcohol dependence (APA, 1994, p. 203) may be explained in part by the learning-based theories. The risk of alcohol abuse is likely to be greater for children who have witnessed close relatives deal with stress by consuming large quantities of the substance, than for children who have witnessed other coping mechanisms employed by their relatives.

However, not all children raised in situations where relatives abuse alcohol become alcoholics. If the origin of alcoholism is a learned response, it is likely that some individuals will learn that the reduction in tension associated with consumption is temporary, while many negative effects (e.g., hangovers, problems with relationships, work, the legal system) are long-term. The theory that the alcoholic drinks because alcohol reduces stress does not appear to account for the continuation of drinking over long periods of time. Clearly, other factors are involved.

Psychoanalytic theories of alcoholism often point to fixation at the oral stage of development as the precipitating cause. Early mother-child interactions supposedly either frustrate dependency needs during the stage of maturation or satisfy them to too great an extent. Traditional psychoanalytic explanations for dependency range from overprotective mothers (Knight, 1937), to unconscious homosexual impulses (Fenichel, 1945), to addiction as a means of attempting to destroy one's mother or one's self (Bergler, 1946). Little evidence is available to support the psychoanalytic theories of substance-related disorders.

It has also been proposed that *sociocultural factors* significantly contribute to substance-related problems, especially with alcohol. Cross-cultural analyses show that usually higher rates of alcoholism occur in countries and within ethnic groups that condone drinking, in contrast to countries and cultures that do not. Empirically, a strong relationship exists between the level of the use of alcohol in a culture and the frequency of alcohol problems (Vaillant, 1983).

Although social and cultural factors are clearly important, they obviously cannot be the only ones. First, not all members of societies that condone and promote alcohol drink, nor do all people in alcohol-restricted societies abstain. Second, comparisons of various countries reveal a pattern of alcoholism not entirely consistent with patterns described here (Davison & Neale, 1986). Third, marked differences in the abuse of substances occur within the same society related to such wide-ranging variables as gender, occupation, and marital status (Vaillant, 1983).

Physiological Factors

Physiological theories of causation generally focus upon the effects of a drug on the body. Intoxicating substances cause physiological changes in the body. Because the substance has changed the physiology of the body, the body reacts when the substance is no longer administered. To avoid withdrawal reactions, the individual continues to use the substance. With enough repetition—the amount varies from individual to individual, substance to substance—the person is ensnared by changes in bodily chemistry and the resulting severity of withdrawal reactions.

Scientists increasingly view substance addiction and its related disorders as diseases of the brain. Recent research suggests that all intoxicants have common effects on dopamine, a neurotransmitter involved in the experience of pleasure. Alan Leshner, director of the National Institute on Drug Abuse, stated:

Drugs hijack the mind by hijacking the brain. Scientists have identified molecules in the brain associated with every major drug of abuse. Alcohol, heroin, cocaine, nicotine, marijuana—all modify dopamine function in similar ways. Initially, people take drugs because they like what it does to their brains, but over time, something happens. All of a sudden you're taking drugs not because you like them but because you must. This compulsion is the essence of all addiction. (Leshner, 1999)

Physiological theories also draw support from research that has established a familial pattern to alcoholism. Children of alcoholic parents have four times the risk of becoming alcoholic compared to children from nonalcoholic parents (Janicak, Piszczor & Easton, 1993). While some of this increased risk may be accounted for by learning-based theories, at least some of the transmission can be traced to genetic factors (APA, 1994, p. 203; Vaillant, 1983). The general assumption is that some people, usually men, inherit a genetic predisposition for the disease. This predisposition is characterized by a lower than normal tolerance for the substance, meaning only small amounts of alcohol may be enough to trigger a dependency cycle.

While genetic factors certainly play a role in substance-related problems, they only represent part of the total picture. While physiological risk may be genetically transmitted, environmental and interpersonal factors also clearly contribute to substance abuse. Cultural attitudes toward specific substances, their availability, personal perceptions of stress, and many other nongenetic factors must be recognized as contributing to the formation of a person who abuses this drug.

Substance-Related Disorders

The Diagnostic and Statistical Manual of Mental Disorders (APA, 1994) uses the broad term *substance-related disorders* to refer to disturbances related to taking a drug of abuse (including alcohol). The *DSM-IV* divides substance-related disorders into two broad groups: the *substance-use disorders* and the *substance-induced disorders*. An explanation including key symptoms and criteria for each of these subcategories follows.

Substance-Use Disorders

According to *DSM-IV* (APA, 1994) these disorders constitute the maladaptive behaviors associated with

intoxicating substances. Substance-use disorders are subdivided into two categories: substance dependence and substance abuse.

Substance Dependence

A *substance dependence* diagnosis is characterized by a cluster of cognitive, behavioral, and physiological symptoms associated with continued use of a substance despite serious and recognizable problems. According to the diagnostic criteria established by the *DSM-IV* (APA, 1994), substance dependence refers to a maladaptive pattern of substance use (usually a pattern of repeated self-administration of the substance) which leads to symptoms of distress or significant impairment in the individual's ability to function. The primary symptoms of this disorder include (APA, 1994, p. 181):

- Change in the individual's *tolerance* to the substance, including a need for increased amounts of the substance to achieve intoxication or the desired effect or a diminished effect with a continued use of the same amount of the substance

- Problems associated with *withdrawal* from the substance, including clinically significant physical and emotional distress or impairment in social, occupational, recreational, or other important areas of daily living

- Loss of *control* in terms of the intended amount of the substance used or the period of time it is used

- Increased *time* spent in activities required to obtain the substance or to recover from its effects

- Continued *use* of the substance despite recognition of recurrent problems directly related to its use

Substance Abuse

Substance abuse may be described as a pattern of behaviors that continue despite recurrent and adverse consequences related to the repeated use of the substance. While many of the symptoms of substance abuse are similar to those associated with substance dependence, the criteria for this diagnosis do not include symptoms such as tolerance or withdrawal. Substance abuse focuses on the destructive consequences of repeated use. Although a diagnosis of substance abuse is more common in individuals who do not have a long history of taking the substance, there are some individuals who have repeated substance-related problems but who have not developed evidence of substance dependence. The criteria used to diagnose substance abuse include (APA, 1994, pp. 182–183):

- Recurrent failure to fulfill primary role obligations at work, home, or school
- Persistent use of the substance in potentially hazardous situations (e.g., driving an automobile, operating heavy machinery)
- Repeated instances of legal difficulties (e.g., numerous arrests for operating a motor vehicle under the influence of a substance)
- Continued use of the substance despite frequent social and interpersonal problems either caused by or associated with the effects of the substance

Substance-Induced Disorders

These disorders are caused by the direct effect of intoxicating substances on the central nervous system. Substance-induced disorders are subdivided into two categories: substance intoxication and substance withdrawal.

Substance Intoxication

The essential feature of substance intoxication is the development of a substance-specific condition that is the result of recent ingestion of or exposure to a substance. Critical to this diagnosis is the presence of maladaptive physiological or psychological changes attributable to the substance. Most often the maladaptive changes place the individual at increased risk for adverse effects (e.g., accidents, employment problems). Symptoms of intoxication vary by the substance used as well as characteristics associated with the user. The pertinent criteria used to specify substance intoxication include (APA, 1994, p. 184):

- Development of a reversible substance-specific group of physiological and psychological symptoms which occur together due to ingestion of or exposure to a substance
- Presence of significant maladaptive changes that result from the effect of the substance. These changes often include mood swings, impaired cognitive functioning, diminished judgment, anger or hostility
- Symptoms not caused by another medical or mental condition

Substance Withdrawal

The diagnosis of substance withdrawal refers to the development of a substance-specific maladaptive behavioral change that occurs with stopping or reducing use of a substance. The condition is most often associated with frequent and prolonged use of the substance. The changes that result from withdrawal may cause emotional and/or physical distress and are linked to problems in functional behaviors. Substance withdrawal is usually, but not always, associated with substance dependence. Individuals experiencing withdrawal usually have a craving to readminister the substance to reduce the symptoms. Symptoms of withdrawal vary according to the substance used, most symptoms being the opposite of those observed in intoxication with the same substance. The *DSM-IV* (APA, 1994, p. 185) criteria for substance withdrawal are:

- Development of a substance-specific syndrome due to the cessation of (or reduction in) substance use that has been heavy and prolonged
- Clinically significant distress or impairment in social, occupational, or other areas of functioning
- Symptoms not caused by another medical or mental condition

General Features of Substance-Related Disorders

While the use of intoxicating substances is common, wide cultural variations exist in attitudes toward consumption, patterns of substance use, availability of substances, and the prevalence of substance-related disorders. Alcohol, for instance, is readily available, widely accepted, and commonly consumed in many societies but totally forbidden in others. In contrast, some groups that forbid alcohol openly accept the use of other mind-altering substances.

Age and gender impact prevalence rates for the use of virtually every substance. Individuals between ages 18 and 24 years represent the group with highest prevalence rates for every class of substance. Intoxication is usually the initial substance-related disorder identified, and it frequently begins in the mid to late teen years. Withdrawal can occur at any age as long as the relevant drug has been taken in high enough doses over a substantial time period. Dependence usually has its onset for most drugs of abuse in the twenties, thirties, or forties, but can occur at any age. Substance-related disorders are more commonly diagnosed in males than in females for most classes of substances (APA, 1994, p. 188).

Intoxication usually develops within minutes to hours after a sufficiently large dose of most drugs of abuse. It begins to abate as concentrations of the substance decline in the blood and tissue, but signs and symptoms may last for extended periods. Withdrawal develops with a decline of the substance in the central nervous system. The most intensive reactions to withdrawal usually end within a few days to a few weeks after the cessation of the use of the substance, although some physiological symptoms may last for weeks or even months (APA, 1994, pp. 188–189).

A diagnosis of substance abuse with a particular class of substances often evolves into substance dependence, particularly in substances that have a high potential for the development of tolerance, withdrawal, and patterns of compulsive use (e.g., alcohol, opioids). Substance abuse is more likely to occur in individuals who have begun using the substance only recently. It should be pointed out, however, that some individuals have episodes of substance abuse that occur over extended periods of time without ever developing substance dependence. This is particularly true for substances that have a lower potential for the development of tolerance, withdrawal, and patterns of compulsive use (e.g., phencyclidine). The course of substance dependence varies, although it is usually chronic. There may be periods of heavy intake and severe problems, periods of total abstinence, and times of nonproblematic use of the substance. Many substance users underestimate their vulnerability to developing a pattern of dependence. During periods of remission they may incorrectly assume they have control over the use of the substance and may begin to experiment with the intake of the substance. Unfortunately, such experimentation often leads to a return to dependence (APA, 1994, p. 189).

Some individuals with substance-related problems can function well enough to adequately deal with the demands of everyday life. They may be able to fulfill social, vocational, and recreational responsibilities with a minimum of discomfort. Many others, however, will have severe complications due to their abuse of substances. Substance-related disorders frequently contribute to deteriorating health concerns; accidents at home, at work, or in automobiles; violent and aggressive behavior; and legal problems. Approximately one half of all highway fatalities involve an individual who is intoxicated. Mortality rates among substance-dependent persons are much higher than in the general populations with alcohol abuse involved in an estimated 25% to 35% of all suicides and 50% to 70% of all homicides

(Janicak et al., 1993). In addition, repeated use of substances described in this chapter may have potential adverse effects upon pregnant women, increasing the risk of physiological dependence in the fetus (e.g., fetal alcohol syndrome) and withdrawal syndrome in the newborn (APA, 1994, p. 190).

Classes of Substances Associated With Substance-Related Disorders

Alcohol-Related Disorders

Alcohol is the most frequently used brain depressant in most cultures. An estimated 90% of adults in the United States have had some experience with alcohol. Similar rates of usage occur among Canadian adults (Addiction Research Foundation, 1991a). As many as 14.5 million Americans are thought to be problem drinkers or alcoholics, and some estimates suggest that this figure may go as high as 28 million. Their alcohol-related problems affect countless other individuals, including children of alcoholics. One in three families is affected by problem drinkers (National Institute on Alcohol Abuse and Alcoholism, 1995).

Beverage alcohol (known as ethyl alcohol or ethanol) is produced by fermenting or distilling various fruits, vegetables, or grains. Ethyl alcohol itself is a clear, colorless liquid. Alcoholic beverages get their distinctive colors from the diluents, additives, and by-products of fermentation. Typically, beer is fermented to contain about 5% alcohol by volume (slightly less in light beer). Most wine is fermented to have between 10% and 14% alcohol content; however, fortified wines such as sherry, port, and vermouth contain slightly more. Distilled spirits (e.g., whisky, vodka, rum, gin) are first fermented, then distilled to raise the alcohol content. The alcohol concentration in spirits is approximately 40% by volume, and some liqueurs are slightly stronger. The effects of drinking do not depend on the type of alcoholic beverage, but rather on the amount of alcohol consumed on a specific occasion.

General Effects

Alcohol is not digested—it is absorbed through the stomach and intestinal walls and metabolized in the liver by the process of oxidation. The ethanol breaks down to acetic acid (vinegar), which is then acted upon by enzymes converting it into water and carbon dioxide, which is passed out of the body. The liver can only break down approximately one ounce of 100-proof whiskey per hour, assuming the individual is of average weight. Any excess that cannot be broken down directly affects the brain, causing intoxication. In general, the less an individual weighs, the quicker the impact of alcohol on the brain.

Alcohol acts as a depressant that inhibits the higher brain centers where learned behavior patterns such as self-control are stored. The initial reaction to alcohol consumption is often the loosening of inhibitions, contributing to the common misperception that alcohol is a stimulant. With continued alcohol intake, a loss of the more complex cognitive and perceptual abilities and eventually a loss of simple memory and motor coordination occurs. Continued consumption of the drug can lead to increasingly diminished cognitive functioning, reduced response to stimuli, unconsciousness, and potentially death.

Drinking heavily over a short period of time usually results in a *hangover*—headache, nausea, shakiness, and sometimes vomiting. A hangover is due partly to poisoning by alcohol and other components of the drink, and partly to the body's reaction to withdrawal from alcohol. Although dozens of remedies have been proposed for hangovers, there is currently no known effective cure.

Long-term alcohol abuse is likely to result in central nervous system dysfunction as well as contribute to health-related problems such as heart and liver disease or inflammation of the stomach. Other indirect problems associated with chronic alcohol abuse include loss of appetite, vitamin deficiencies, infections, and sexual impotence. The risk of serious disease increases with the amount of alcohol consumed. Early death rates are much higher for heavy drinkers than for light drinkers or abstainers, particularly from heart and liver disease, pneumonia, some types of cancer, acute alcohol poisoning, accident, homicide, and suicide.

Diagnostic Criteria for Alcohol-Related Disorders

The World Health Organization has defined alcoholism as a chronic behavior disorder manifested by repeated drinking of alcoholic beverages in excess of societal norms for dietary and social use, and to an extent that impairs the drinker's health or social or economic functioning (Janicak et al., 1993). Implicit in this definition is the idea that alcoholism is a disease that

results in the loss of control over drinking regardless of the consequences (Vaillant, 1983). The disease is characterized by an undue preoccupation with the substance to the detriment of one's physical and mental health.

Alcohol-Use Disorders: Alcohol Dependence and Alcohol Abuse

The diagnostic criteria for *alcohol dependence* and *alcohol abuse* are the same as the more general categories, substance dependence and substance abuse. Issues of tolerance and dependence are central to this diagnosis.

People who drink on a regular basis become tolerant to many of the unpleasant effects of alcohol, and thus are able to drink more before suffering these effects. Even with increased consumption, many such drinkers do not appear intoxicated. Because they continue to work and socialize reasonably well, their deteriorating physical condition may go unrecognized by others until severe damage develops or until they are hospitalized for other reasons and suddenly experience alcohol withdrawal symptoms.

Psychological dependence on alcohol may occur with regular use of even relatively moderate daily amounts. It may also occur in people who consume alcohol only under certain conditions, such as before and during social occasions. This form of dependence refers to a craving for alcohol's psychological effects, although not necessarily in amounts that produce serious intoxication. For psychologically dependent drinkers, the lack of alcohol tends to make them anxious and, in some cases, panicky.

Physical dependence occurs in consistently heavy drinkers. Since their bodies have adapted to the presence of alcohol, they suffer withdrawal symptoms if they suddenly stop drinking. Withdrawal symptoms range from jumpiness, sleeplessness, sweating, and poor appetite, to tremors, convulsions, hallucinations, and sometimes death. Alcohol abuse is problem drinking that has never met the criteria for alcohol dependence.

Alcohol-Induced Disorders: Alcohol Intoxication and Alcohol Withdrawal

The essential feature of *alcohol intoxication* is the presence of clinically significant maladaptive behavioral or psychological changes that develop during or shortly after the ingestion of alcohol. These changes may include inappropriate sexual or aggressive behavior, impaired judgment, and impaired social occupational functioning. These changes are accompanied by one or more of the following signs: slurred speech, uncoordination, unsteady gait, nystagmus (involuntary movements of the eyes), impairment in attention or memory, stupor, or coma (APA, 1994, p. 197).

The central characteristic of alcohol withdrawal is the presence of a variety of symptoms that occur in conjunction with the cessation of or reduction in the use of alcohol. Two or more of the following symptoms must be present to meet the criteria for alcohol withdrawal (APA, 1994, pp. 198–199):

- Autonomic hyperactivity (e.g., sweating or pulse rate greater than 100)
- Hand tremors
- Insomnia
- Nausea or vomiting
- Transient visual, tactile, or auditory hallucinations
- Psychomotor agitation
- Anxiety
- Grand mal seizures

These symptoms are significant enough to cause the individual distress or impair his or her ability to perform tasks of daily living.

Natural Course of Alcoholism

The first episode of alcohol intoxication among alcoholics usually occurs in the mid-teens, with the age of alcohol dependence generally peaking in the mid-twenties to mid-thirties The large majority of individuals who develop alcohol-related disorders do so by their late thirties (APA, 1994).

The few longitudinal studies that have addressed alcoholism (e.g., O'Connor & Daly, 1985; Vaillant, 1983) suggest the course of the disease may be different for men and women. Alcohol abuse and dependence are more common in males than in females, with an estimated male-to-female ratio as high as 5:1. In males, onset is usually in the late teens or early twenties; rarely does it occur after age 45. In females, onset tends to be later; however, the symptoms of abuse and dependence may progress more rapidly so that by middle age females may have the same health and interpersonal problems as do males (APA, 1994; Janicak et al., 1993).

Alcoholics commonly experience periods of relapse and remission. A decision to quit drinking, often in response to social, vocational, or legal problems, may be followed by periods of controlled or nonproblematic drinking. However, for the individual who is a problem drinker, once alcohol intake resumes it is highly likely that consumption will eventually escalate and that severe consequences will again be experienced.

Epidemiology

Abuse of alcohol refers to a pattern of behaviors (e.g., legal difficulties, family problems) that continues despite recurrent adverse consequences related to alcohol use. An *alcoholic* is an individual who repeatedly drinks alcoholic beverages in excess of societal norms and to the extent that it impairs one's health or social functioning. Of the estimated 100 million Americans who use alcohol, 14% (1 in every 13 adults) abuse alcohol or are alcoholic (National Institute on Alcohol Abuse and Alcoholism, 1995). This 14% consumes about 50% of all alcoholic beverages in the United States (Janicak et al., 1993). The 1997 National Household Survey on Drug Abuse found that 5.2% of Americans age 12 and over reported heavy alcohol use (i.e., drinking five or more drinks per occasion on five or more days in the past 30 days) in the previous month (U. S. Department of Health and Human Services, 1999). A United States national probability sample of noninstitutionalized adults (18 years and older) reported that approximately 7.41% of adults met standard diagnostic criteria for alcohol abuse or alcohol dependence during 1992. Although more were classified with alcohol dependence (4.38%) than alcohol abuse (3.03%), most persons with alcohol dependence also met alcohol abuse criteria (National Institute on Alcohol Abuse and Alcoholism, 1995).

Men's risk for developing severe alcohol-related problems is three to four times higher than women's. In the United States, although more African Americans than Caucasions abstain from alcohol, the proportions in both groups of light, moderate, and heavy drinkers are similar. Higher rates of alcoholism have been reported among Native Americans, Eskimos, and Latino males. Alcohol-related problems are not prevalent among Americans of Asian descent (U. S. Department of Health and Human Services, 1999).

The incidence of alcoholism in the elderly remains unknown. Older individuals are assumed to be at increased risk of developing alcohol-related problems due to age-related physical changes that may increase their susceptibility to more severe intoxication and subsequent problems at lower levels of consumption. This problem may be exacerbated due to the use of medications taken by older adults.

Adolescents abuse alcohol more frequently than any other drug. The incidence of alcoholism in this age group ranges from 15% to 25% (Janicak et al., 1993). Conduct-related disorders and antisocial behavior often co-occur with alcohol-related problems among adolescents. Alcohol use by teenagers is a major contributing factor in automobile accidents for this age group, adding fuel to many political debates about the legal drinking age in many states. According to Janicak et al. (1993) the number of traffic deaths in the United States have "increased or decreased concomitantly with the lowering or raising of the drinking age in various states" (p. 249).

Risk Factors for Alcoholism

Alcoholism often has a familial pattern, and at least some of the transmission can be traced to genetic factors. The risk for alcohol dependence is three to four times higher in close relatives of people with alcohol dependence (APA, 1994). Higher risk is generally associated with a greater number of affected relatives, closer genetic relationships, and the severity of alcohol-related problems in the affected relative. Although evidence for a genetic predisposition in certain individuals is strong, most experts agree that the development of alcoholism is influenced by environmental factors as well (O'Connor & Daly, 1985; Vaillant, 1983).

Efforts to identify personality factors associated with alcoholism have produced little supportive evidence. Although alcohol dependence has been associated with depression and anxiety disorders, studies have not been able to determine any causal relationship between these conditions. Personality traits and psychosocial stressors may explain specific instances of alcohol-related problems, but they cannot explain the overall vulnerability of an individual for the development of alcoholism (Janicak, et al., 1993).

Social factors may also contribute to the development of alcoholism. Cultural traditions surrounding the use of alcohol in family, religious, or social settings, especially during childhood, can affect the likelihood that alcohol problems will develop. It is well-established that the incidence of alcoholism is higher in societies where alcohol is readily available and its use is socially acceptable.

Morbidity and Mortality

Alcohol-related disorders are one of the most significant health problems in the United States. There are more deaths, illnesses, and disabilities associated with the use of alcohol than from any other preventable health condition. Abuse of alcohol accounts for at least one fourth of all hospitalizations in this country. Alcohol is involved in 25% to 35% of all suicides and 50% to 70% of all homicides. It also is a primary contributor to accidental deaths and domestic violence. Moreover, alcohol abuse is associated with many psychiatric and medical disorders (Janicek et al., 1993).

Treatment

Alcoholism is most commonly treated using a disease model. This approach views the condition as a chronic medical illness, not simply a social or psychological problem. As with any chronic illness, relapse is a normal part of the disease process.

Three primary goals serve as the focus of treatment for the disease. *Detoxification* is the removal of the effects of the drug from the alcoholic's body. Many alcoholics who have been chronically imbibing need an initial period of detoxification, especially in light of the mild confusion and memory and concentration problems commonly found following the cessation of acute drinking. *Abstinence*, the cessation of the use of alcohol, is begun after detoxification has been completed. Alcoholics Anonymous (AA) is the most commonly used means of obtaining abstinence. The third goal, *sobriety*, is the recovery stage of treatment. Sobriety requires the alcoholic to make major psychological and social changes in their life. AA usually plays a major role in maintaining sobriety.

Treatment programs designed to assist individuals with alcohol-related problems include self-help groups (such as Alcoholics Anonymous) and professionally run alcohol treatment programs. *Alcoholics Anonymous* (AA) is a nonprofessional self-help group and the foundation of treatment for most alcoholics. AA views alcoholism as a disease and follows a 12-step program to achieve recovery. Some of the most important principles upon which the AA program are founded include:

- The person is powerless to overcome alcohol addiction on his or her own and needs the group to help him or her abstain from the substance.

- The group setting is a powerful method to confront the problem drinker's denial of illness.

- Acceptance of alcoholism as a disease over which one loses control helps relieve much of the guilt experienced by alcohol-dependent individuals.

- The AA group provides an abstinent social system, role models, and readily available support system needed to achieve and maintain sobriety.

Professionally run alcohol treatment programs often follow the AA model, but are organized and run by individuals professionally trained to provide therapy to persons with alcohol-related problems. Some of these programs offer inpatient treatment involving short-term hospitalization of the alcoholic, while others are run on an outpatient basis. Even when professionally run programs are used, it is generally accepted that all individuals with alcohol-related problems should attend AA if possible. Too little information is available to predict who might better respond to professionally run versus self-help group-oriented treatment.

Pharmaceuticals can be helpful in specific instances for helping to wean the person away from alcohol (Poling, Gadow & Cleary, 1991). However, this introduces the paradoxical problems of treating substance abuse with another substance. The implicit message in any pharmaceutical intervention is that the individual's efforts to change are not of critical concern.

An important component of many treatment programs is *family therapy*. Because alcohol abuse usually causes disruption to family life, relatives need information about the illness for the benefit of the problem drinker and themselves. Such approaches may be extended beyond the nuclear family to friends and associates in an effort to keep them from reinforcing drinking behaviors (Marlatt, Baer, Donovan & Kiviahan, 1988).

Central Nervous System Stimulants (Amphetamines and Cocaine)

Central nervous system stimulants are a class of potent drugs that can produce a variety of psychological and psychomotor effects. The two most commonly abused stimulants are amphetamines and cocaine. Although both of these substances are sometimes used to produce therapeutic effects (e.g., enhance attention span, reduce pain), a great potential for abuse exists with these drugs.

Amphetamine and amphetamine-related drugs (e.g., methamphetamine or "speed") stimulate the central nervous system much in the same way as does adrenaline, one of the body's natural hormones. Amphetamine was first introduced in the 1930s as a remedy for nasal congestion. Later, it was found to be effective in treating such conditions as obesity, hyperactivity in children, and narcolepsy (uncontrollable sleep episodes). College students, truck drivers, and athletes sometimes used amphetamines in efforts to prolong their normal periods of wakefulness and endurance. Studies eventually demonstrated the serious problems of dependency associated with use of the drug. It may still be obtained legally, but only by prescription.

Illicit amphetamines appear on the street under names such as bennies, glass, crank, pep pills, and uppers. A very pure form of methamphetamine is called *ice*. The drug appears as crystals, chunks, and fine to coarse powders. The drug may be sniffed, smoked, injected, or taken orally.

Cocaine is a powerful stimulant that is prepared from the leaf of the coca plant, which grows primarily in South America. Pure cocaine, first extracted in the mid-nineteenth century, was introduced as an elixir in patent medicines. Later, it was used as a local anesthetic for some types of surgery. Currently, it has no clinical application, having been replaced by synthetic anesthetics.

Because of its potent euphoric and energizing effects, many people in the late 19th century took cocaine. In the 1880s Sigmund Freud praised cocaine's potential to cure depression, alcoholism, and morphine addiction. Skepticism replaced this excitement, however, when its addictive power became recognized and documented reports of fatal cocaine poisoning were popularized.

Cocaine is generally sold on the street as a fine, white powder known as coke, C, snow, flake, or blow. Cocaine is usually snorted into the nostrils, but to heighten its intensity users sometimes inject it. Cocaine can also be chemically altered through a process called *freebasing*. The product of freebasing is a purer form of cocaine that is smoked rather than snorted. The drug commonly called *crack* is a crude form of freebase that has become popular in recent years.

General Effects

The short-term effects for both amphetamines and cocaine appear soon after a single dose. With amphetamines the effects disappear within a few hours or days. With cocaine they disappear within a few minutes or hours. At low doses amphetamines produce physical effects such as loss of appetite, rapid breathing, high blood pressure, and dilated pupils. Larger doses may cause flushing, very rapid or irregular heartbeat, tremors, loss of coordination, and collapse. The psychological effects of amphetamine usage include feelings of well-being, heightened alertness, and energy. In higher doses users may become restless or excited, may feel a sense of power, may become hostile and aggressive, and may also behave in an odd, repetitive fashion.

Cocaine taken in small amounts usually produces an accelerated heartbeat, accelerated breathing, and higher blood pressure. It usually makes the user feel euphoric, energetic, and mentally alert to sensations of sight, sound, and touch. Larger amounts of the drug intensify the user's "high," but may also lead to erratic or violent behavior, and may produce tremors, dizziness, and paranoia.

Diagnostic Criteria for Amphetamine-Use and Cocaine-Use Disorders: Amphetamine and Cocaine Dependence and Amphetamine and Cocaine Abuse

Amphetamine-related disorders and cocaine-related disorders are treated as independent categories in *DSM-IV* (APA, 1994). Because both share the common trait of producing stimulating effects to the central nervous system we have chosen to group them together. The diagnostic criteria for these categories are the same as previously identified substance dependence and substance abuse criteria. The distinctive feature for amphetamine and cocaine use concerns issues of tolerance for and dependence on these drugs.

Regular use of amphetamines increases tolerance to some effects, which means that more of the drug is required to produce the desired effects. In contrast, cocaine users may keep taking the original amount of the drug over extended periods and still experience the same euphoria. When users increase their dose it is usually done in an effort to intensify or prolong the effects.

Dependence has both physical and psychological components. Physical symptoms of withdrawal among heavy amphetamine users include fatigue, long but troubled sleep, irritability, intense hunger, and depression. When cocaine users stop taking the drug they usually "crash" and complain of sleep and eating disorders, depression, anxiety, and a strong craving for the drug, which makes the relapse rate for this population high.

Psychological dependence exists when a drug is so central to a person's thoughts, emotions, and activities that the need to continue its use becomes a compulsion. Chronic users of amphetamines *may* experience this compulsion; heavy cocaine users *almost always* develop severe depression if the drug is unavailable.

Diagnostic Criteria for Amphetamine-Induced and Cocaine-Induced Disorders: Amphetamine and Cocaine Intoxication and Amphetamine and Cocaine Withdrawal

The diagnostic criteria for intoxication are the same for both drugs. It includes the development of significant

maladaptive behavioral or psychological changes during or shortly after use of the drug, and two or more of the following physical signs (APA, 1994, pp. 204, 224):

- Tachycardia (abnormally rapid heart rate) or bradycardia (abnormally slow heart rate)
- Dilation of the pupils, raised or lowered blood pressure, perspiration or chills
- Nausea or vomiting
- Weight loss
- Psychomotor agitation or retardation
- Muscular weakness
- Confusion, seizures, or involuntary muscular activity

The diagnostic criteria for withdrawal are also the same for both drugs. When cessation or reduction in use occurs, evidence of a dysphoric mood (an unpleasant mood, such as sadness, anxiety, or irritability) marked by fatigue, vivid unpleasant dreams, sleep disturbances, increased appetite, and psychomotor retardation or agitation results (APA, 1994, pp. 209, 225–226).

Natural Course of Amphetamine-Related and Cocaine-Related Disorders

For some individuals the introduction to amphetamines is the result of efforts to control their weight (e.g., amphetamines and amphetamine-like substances used as appetite suppressants). Others become introduced through the illegal market. Cocaine users are always introduced through the illegal market. The progression from use to abuse to dependence can occur rapidly, especially with cocaine. Dependence is associated with two patterns of administration: *episodic use*, in which substance use is separated by days of nonuse, and daily use (or almost daily use) of the substance. Users may also go on binges marked by continuous high dose use in a short period of time. The *DSM-IV* (1994) reports that there is a tendency for persons who have been dependent on amphetamines to decrease or stop use after eight to ten years due to the development of adverse mental and physical effects. Little information is available on the long-term course of cocaine-use disorders (APA, 1994, pp. 211, 229).

Epidemiology

According to the 1997 National Household Survey on Drug Abuse, an estimated 1.5 million Americans (0.7% of those age 12 and older) were current cocaine users

(U. S. Department of Health and Human Services, 1999). This number has changed little since 1992, although it is a dramatic decrease from the 1985 peak of 5.7 million users (3% of the population). Adults 18 to 25 years old have a higher rate of current cocaine use than those in any other age group. Overall, males have a higher rate of cocaine use than females, and African Americans have a higher rate of current use (1.4%) than do Hispanics (0.8%) or Caucasians (0.6%). The percentage of eighth graders reporting use of crack cocaine at least once in their lives increased from 2.7% in 1997 to 3.2% in 1998 (National Institute on Drug Abuse, 1999a).

A 1996 national survey reported that 4.9 million people age 12 and older had tried methamphetamine at least once in their lifetimes (2.3% of the population). In 1997, 4.4% of high school seniors had used methamphetamine at least once in their lifetimes, an increase from 2.7% in 1990. Methamphetamine is considered to be a growing problem in many metropolitan areas, including Denver, Los Angeles, Minneapolis, Phoenix, and Seattle (National Institute on Drug Abuse, 1999f).

Treatment

Short-term treatment of amphetamine- and cocaine-related disorders usually addresses problems associated with detoxification. General management of the individual focuses on supporting vital functions: reducing central nervous system irritability and sympathetic nervous system overactivity (e.g., fluctuating heart rate, elevated or lowered blood pressure, seizures, hyperthermia), psychotic symptoms, and hastening drug elimination. Medical screening designed to identify other possible causes of these symptoms is usually undertaken at this stage. In addition, pharmacological interventions intended to reduce central nervous system irritability, prevent seizures, reduce psychotic symptoms, and hasten drug elimination may also be used.

Longer-term treatment generally deals with confronting destructive psychological patterns, which often underlie substance use in the first place. Since amphetamine abuse is often an extension of an abuse of prescription pills for dieting, promoting alternative techniques to help with obesity are often helpful to prevent a return to the use of amphetamines. Supportive group therapy, teaching of stress management and relaxation techniques, and cognitive behavior techniques are often useful (Ellis, 1992). For individuals with cocaine-related problems, detoxification is a primary goal. This usually involves the introduction of

agonists (i.e., drugs that substitute for the effects of cocaine) and calcium channel blockers (i.e., drugs that reverse the effects of cocaine toxicity). Intensive psychotherapy with a focus on the avoidance of dependency, followed by involvement in group therapy modeled on AA principles can be effective in helping the individual deal with psychological conflicts underlying the use of the drug (Meyer, 1993).

Opioid-Related Disorders

The *opioids* include both natural opioids derived from the seedpod of the Asian poppy (e.g., morphine), semisynthetics (e.g., heroin), and synthetics with morphinelike action (e.g., codeine, methadone). Opiates have been used both medically and nonmedically for centuries. As early as the 16th century a tincture of opium called laudanum was used as a remedy for "nerves" or to stop coughing and diarrhea. Opioids such as codeine and morphine are still prescribed today as analgesics, anesthetics, antidiarrheal agents, or cough suppressants.

Heroin was introduced in 1898 and declared as a remedy for morphine addiction. Although heroin proved to be a more potent painkiller (analgesic) and cough suppressant than morphine, it also was more likely to produce dependence. Opiate-related synthetic drugs such as methadone were first developed to provide an analgesic that would not produce dependence. Unfortunately, all opioids, while effective as painkillers, can also produce dependence.

Opium appears either as dark brown chunks or in powder form, and is generally eaten or smoked. Heroin usually appears as a white or brownish powder, which is dissolved in water for injection. Most street preparations of heroin contain only a small percentage of the drug, as they are diluted with sugar, quinine, or other substances. Common street names for heroin include horse, H, junk, smack, and shit. Street users usually inject opiate solutions under the skin ("skin popping") or directly into a vein or muscle, but the drugs may also be snorted into the nose or taken orally or rectally.

General Effects

Short-term effects appear soon after a single dose and disappear in a few hours or days. Opioids briefly stimulate the higher centers of the brain but then depress activity of the central nervous system. Immediately after injection of an opioid into a vein, the user feels a surge of pleasure or a rush. This gives way to a state of gratification; hunger, pain, and sexual urges rarely intrude. The dose required to produce this effect may at first cause restlessness, nausea, and vomiting. With moderately high doses, however, the body feels warm, the extremities heavy, and the mouth dry. Soon, the user goes on the nod—an alternately wakeful and drowsy state during which the world is forgotten. Heroin induces a warm, sensual euphoria, usually followed by sleepiness and lethargy.

As the dose increases, breathing gradually slows. With very large doses, the user cannot be roused; the pupils contract to pinpoints; the skin is cold, moist, and bluish; and profound respiratory depression resulting in death may occur. Overdose is a particular risk on the street, where the amount of the drug contained in a hit cannot be accurately gauged. In a treatment setting, the effects of a usual dose of morphine last three to four hours. Although pain may still be felt, the reaction to it is reduced, and the patient feels content because of the emotional detachment induced by the drug.

Long-term effects appear after repeated use over a long period. Chronic opiate users may develop endocarditis, an infection of the heart lining and valves as a result of unsterile injection techniques. Drug users who share needles are also at high risk of exposure to HIV (human immunodeficiency virus).

Diagnostic Criteria for Opioid-Use Disorders: Opioid Dependence and Opioid Abuse

The diagnostic criteria for opioid dependence and opioid abuse are the same as the more general categories of substance dependence and substance abuse. Issues of tolerance and dependence are key. With regular use, tolerance develops to many of the desired effects of the opioids. This means that the user must use more of the drugs to achieve the same intensity of effect. Chronic users are at risk to become psychologically and/or physically dependent on opioids.

Diagnostic Criteria for Opioid-Induced Disorders: Opioid Intoxication and Opioid Withdrawal

The diagnostic criteria for opioid intoxication specifies significant maladaptive behavioral or psychological changes that develop during or shortly after opioid use. Physical indicators include constriction or dilation of the pupils, and at least one of the following signs: drowsiness or coma, slurred speech, or impairment in attention or memory (APA, 1994).

Major withdrawal symptoms peak between 48 and 72 hours after the last dose and usually subside within a week. Opioid withdrawal is diagnosed after meeting the following criteria (APA, 1994):

- Cessation of (or reduction in) opioid use that has been heavy and prolonged, or administration of an opioid antagonist (a drug used to counteract the effects of an opioid) after a period of opioid use
- Development of at least three of the following: dysphoric mood, nausea or vomiting, muscles aches, lacrimation (tearing) or rhinorrhea (discharge from the nose), pupil dilation or sweating, diarrhea, yawning, fever, or insomnia

Natural Course of Opioid-Related Disorders

Opioid dependence is most commonly observed in the late teens or early twenties. Once dependence develops, it usually continues for an extended number of years. Periods of remission (abstinence) and relapse are common. An estimated two thirds of opioid users resume drug use within six months after detoxification (Lahmeyer, Channon & Schlemmer, 1993). Five separate types of opioid users have been identified:

- *Stables* have conventional values, hold legitimate jobs, are generally law abiding, and do not associate with other addicts
- *Hustlers* or *junkies* identify with an addict culture, are not legitimately employed, and subsist on criminal activities
- *Two-worlders* engage in criminal activities and associate with other addicts but are also legitimately employed
- *Loners* are not involved either in the addict subculture or in mainstream culture. They are usually not employed, often live on welfare benefits and may have severe psychological disturbances
- *Analgesic abusers* frequently suffer from chronic pain. They gradually increase the dosage to relieve stress and depression

Epidemiology

Prevalence rates for use of opioids showed a gradual increase throughout the 1990s. The 1996 National

Household Survey on Drug Abuse reported a significant increase from 1993 in the estimated number of current (once in the past month) heroin users. The estimates have risen from 68,000 in 1993 to 216,000 in 1996. Individuals who had ever used heroin in their lives increased from 55% in 1994 to 82% in 1996 (National Institute on Drug Abuse, 1999b).

The 1998 Monitoring the Future Study revealed that prevalence rates for heroin use among 8th, 10th, and 12th graders were approximately two to three times higher than those reported in 1991. The 1997 survey reported that 2.1% of all three groups had used heroin at least once in their life, about 1.3% of each group had used the drug during the past year, and about 0.6% had used it during the past month (National Institute on Drug Abuse, 1999b).

Prevalence rates for opioids are highest among individuals in their late teens and early twenties. Remission generally begins after age 40; however, some persons remain opioid dependent the majority of their lives. Male-to-female ratio of dependency is estimated to be 3:1 or 4:1 (APA, 1994, p. 254).

Opioid dependence is commonly associated with a history of drug-related crime. Medical personnel who have ready access to opioids have an increased risk for abuse and dependence. A history of behavioral disorders in childhood or adolescence has been identified as a significant risk factor for substance-related disorders, especially opioid dependence. In addition, divorce and unemployment or irregular employment, seem to increase the risk of opioid-related problems (APA, 1994).

Treatment

Opioid use, especially heroin, always carries the risk of overdosing. The physical symptoms of opioid overdose include coma, extremely dilated pupils (i.e., pinpoint pupils), and depressed respiration. The individual's skin is usually cold and clammy, skeletal muscles are flaccid, and urine output is decreased. A drug overdose, whether caused by an opioid or other psychoactive substance, is best managed by trained medical professionals.

The two goals of long-term treatment for opioid dependence are detoxification (acute treatment of withdrawal) and maintenance (of nonuse behaviors). The objective in detoxifying an individual is to suppress severe withdrawal symptoms. In most cases, persons going through detoxification will experience physical and psychological discomfort related to the specific drug used and the dose administered. Detoxification involves a carefully monitored program of pharmacological intervention. A common approach used in

inpatient treatment settings is to gradually reduce the dose of the opioid of abuse, while simultaneously introducing nonopioids (e.g., tranquilizers, antidepressants) to ease the symptoms of withdrawal.

Maintenance treatment usually involves a combination of drug therapy and psychotherapeutic techniques. Interestingly, methadone, itself a synthetic opioid, is frequently used to treat heroin addiction both in detoxification as well as in the maintenance phase (Ciraulo & Shader, 1991). When drugs are used in maintenance treatment, however, they are viewed as transitional aids. The long-term goal is to develop coping strategies that provide the individual the strength to avoid relapse. With this intent in mind, supportive group therapy is viewed as important to maintenance. The development of a therapeutic social network, such as provided to the alcoholic by Alcoholics Anonymous, is critical in dealing with persons with opioid-related problems, as they easily return to the destructive settings and circumstances that led to the decision to use in the first place (Herbert, 1987).

Hallucinogen-Related Disorders

The term *hallucinogen* refers to any drug that alters a person's mental state by distorting the perception of reality to the point where (at high doses) hallucinations occur. This diverse group of substances, commonly referred to as *psychedelics* during the 1960s, includes many different drugs ranging from natural plant extracts to wholly synthetic products. Lysergic acid diethylamide (LSD) is the most powerful and most commonly abused hallucinogen. Mescaline and psilocybin (magic mushrooms) are other frequently abused hallucinogens. Both produce effects similar to LSD, but both are far less potent.

Mescaline is prepared from the peyote cactus. The heads of the cactus are dried and then sliced, chopped, or ground, and sometimes put in capsules. It is usually taken orally, but can be inhaled by smoking ground peyote heads.

Psilocybin is the active ingredient in some mushroom species. Pure psilocybin is a white crystalline substance, but the drug is sometimes distributed in crude mushroom preparations. It is usually taken orally.

General Effects

The effects of any hallucinogen and the user's reaction to it can differ significantly among individuals. Users may experience different reactions to the same drug on different occasions—at times the effects may be pleasant and at other times terrifying. Although the differences may be due in part to the variations in the quality of illicit drugs, it also happens when the drugs are known to be pure.

In low doses hallucinogens such as mescaline and psilocybin produce a spectrum of effects, which include alterations in mood and perception. Hallucinations and other severe effects occur at higher doses.

The effects of LSD even in low doses are much more pronounced. Soon after a single dose a spectrum of physical effects usually occur. These include numbness; muscle weakness and trembling; increased blood pressure, heart rate, and temperature; impaired coordination; and nausea. Following the physical effects a variety of dramatic changes in perception, thought, and mood usually begin. These often include vivid hallucinations; distorted perceptions of time, distance, and gravity (e.g., sensations of floating); diminished control over thought processes (e.g., long-forgotten memories resurfacing); and mystical, religious, or cosmic feelings. Many LSD users experience unpleasant reactions (i.e., "bad trips") marked by frightening or depressing thoughts or images, or intense fearfulness and anxiety with dread of insanity or death. In some cases these terrifying hallucinations may result in prolonged depression and anxiety. Also common among chronic users are *flashbacks*—unpredictable, spontaneous recurrences of a previous LSD experience. Typically, flashbacks last only a few minutes or less, but seem to occur more commonly after an LSD user smokes cannabis.

Diagnostic Criteria for Hallucinogen-Use Disorders: Hallucinogen Dependence and Hallucinogen Abuse

The diagnostic criteria for hallucinogen dependence and hallucinogen abuse are the same as the more general categories, substance dependence and substance abuse. Regular use of such hallucinogens as LSD, mescaline, and psilocybin induce tolerance within a few days of consecutive daily doses; little or no effect is experienced with higher doses. After several days of abstinence, however, the effects may again be felt. Cross-tolerance also develops among LSD, mescaline, and psilocybin— a person who has built up tolerance to one of these drugs will be unable to experience the effects of any of the others. Again, normal sensitivity is usually restored after several consecutive days of abstinence (APA, 1994, p. 230).

Chronic users of hallucinogens can become psychologically dependent on the substances and may experience cognitive and emotional cravings for the drug. However, physical dependence does not occur with hallucinogens and there are no withdrawal symptoms after the drugs are discontinued (APA, 1994, p. 231).

Diagnostic Criteria for Hallucinogen-Induced Disorders: Hallucinogen Intoxication and Hallucinogen Persistent Perception Disorder (Flashbacks)

The diagnostic criteria for hallucinogen intoxication specifies significant maladaptive behavioral or psychological changes that develop during or shortly after hallucinogen use. In addition, the disorder is characterized by perceptual changes (e.g., subjective intensification of perceptions, depersonalization, illusions, hallucinations) that occur in a state of full wakefulness and alertness. Physical indicators include pupillary dilation, tachycardia, sweating, palpitations, blurred vision, tremors, and incoordination. At least two of these physical signs must be present during or shortly after a hallucinogen is used for the diagnosis to be made (APA, 1994, pp. 232–233).

Hallucinogen persistent perception disorder (flashbacks) is diagnosed by the reoccurrence of one or more of the perceptual symptoms experienced while previously intoxicated by a hallucinogen. Such flashbacks often involve hallucinations, flashes of color, trails of images of moving objects, or halos around objects. To meet the criteria for this diagnosis the flashbacks must cause clinically significant distress or impairment in the daily functioning of the individual (APA, 1994, p. 234). About one fourth of persons who use hallucinogens will spontaneously experience such flashbacks for months after their last drug use (Lahmeyer et al., 1993).

Natural Course of Hallucinogen-Related Problems

Hallucinogen intoxication usually first occurs in adolescence. It may be a brief or isolated event or it may occur repeatedly. The period of intoxication may be extended if doses are repeated during a particular episode, but frequent dosing reduces intoxication due to the development of tolerance. Depending upon the drug and its administration, peak effects usually occur within a few minutes to a few hours, and intoxication usually ends within a few hours after dosing ends (APA, 1994).

Epidemiology

The peak period of hallucinogen use, especially LSD, occurred during the 1960s. The widespread use of the drugs, often in the name of self-exploration, eventually led to street regulations of hallucinogens in the 1970s. A 1982 survey indicated that 21% of young adults claimed they had used these substances at least once in their lives (Laymeyer et al., 1993). By 1988, the percentage of the population aged 12 and older who had ever used LSD had fallen to 6%. However, the 1996 National Household Survey on Drug Abuse reported an increase in the lifetime prevalence rate to 7.7% (National Institute on Drug Abuse, 1999d).

A 1997 study reported that 13.6% of high school seniors had experimented with LSD at least once in their lifetimes. The percentage of seniors reporting the use of LSD in the past year nearly doubled from a low of 4.4% in 1985 to 8.4% in 1997 (National Institute on Drug Abuse, 1999d).

Use of hallucinogens is most common among those 18–25 years of age (APA, 1994). This suggests that, similar to other substance-related problems, the prevalence of hallucinogen use seems to decline for many individuals as they get older. As with most other drugs of abuse, hallucinogen use and intoxication appear to be more common among males than among females, in this case at a ratio of 3:1. Finally, the risk of serious injury in the form of automobile accidents, physical fights, or decisions made with impaired judgment (e.g., attempts to fly) seem to inevitably increase due to hallucinogen intoxication.

Treatment

Because physical dependence does not occur with hallucinogens and there are no withdrawal symptoms, treatment usually involves dealing with adverse reactions to intoxication. Three categories of adverse reactions are associated with the substance:

"Bad trip" or panic reaction. Usual symptoms of a bad trip include acute extreme panic and a fear of going insane. Treatment entails a combination of talk down therapy (i.e., continual reassurance that the individual is not going crazy and that he or she will return to normal when the effects of the drug wear off) and the use of antianxiety medication. Most bad trips end within 24 hours.

Delirium. Delirium is usually associated with hallucinations. It is marked by agitation, disorientation, paranoia, and delusional thinking. Individuals who experience these symptoms are at high risk for dangerous behavior including inadvertent suicide (e.g., jumping out of windows believing they can fly). Treatment usually includes talk down therapy, the use of physical restraints if necessary, and the use of antipsychotic medication. Hallucinogen-induced delirium usually clears within 24 hours.

Flashbacks. During the flashback individuals experience symptoms they originally experienced while intoxicated with a hallucinogen. The flashback, which lasts for seconds to hours, can be the source of significant distress for the individual. Verbal reassurance that the flashback will pass, advice about future drug use, and small, temporary doses of antipsychotic medication are commonly recommended to deal with this adverse reaction.

Cannabis-Related Disorders

Cannabinoids are substances derived from the hemp plant, *Cannabis sativa. Marijuana* consists of the dried and crushed leaves and flowering tops of the plant, which are usually rolled into cigarettes and smoked. Marijuana is commonly called *pot, weed, herb,* or *Mary Jane*; as a cigarette it is called a *joint* or a *nail*. It is also smoked in a pipe or a bong. In recent years it has been smoked as blunts, cigars that have been emptied of tobacco and refilled with marijuana, often with another drug, such as crack cocaine. Some users also mix marijuana into baked foods or use it to brew tea.

Hashish, a cannabinoid that is much stronger than marijuana, is produced by removing and drying the resin of high-quality cannabis plants. The intoxicating effects of both hashish (hash) and marijuana have been known for thousands of years. Except for a few rare exceptions, the use of cannabinoids has been illegal in the United States since the 1930s. The *DSM-IV* calls cannabis "the world's most commonly used illicit substance" (APA, 1994, p. 219).

The primary active chemical substance in cannabinoids is *tetrahydrocannabinol* (THC). The potency of cannabinoids depends on the concentration of THC, which can vary considerably with the part of the plant used to prepare the drug and the geographic region in which the plant is cultivated. Hashish is usually much stronger than marijuana, for example, because it is extracted from the flowering tops of the plant, where THC is most abundant. The THC content of marijuana has increased significantly since the late 1960s (APA, 1994).

General Effects

Cannabis can induce a wide variety of physical and psychological effects, but rarely causes acute psychiatric or medical emergencies. The physical symptoms associated with cannabis use include tachycardia (increased heart rate), reddened conjunctivas (bloodshot eyes), dry mouth, and increased appetite. Long-term use may cause bronchitis, asthma, and other respiratory problems similar to those commonly experienced by tobacco smokers. In fact, the amount of tar inhaled by marijuana smokers and the level of carbon monoxide absorbed are considerably greater than among tobacco smokers due to the tendency to inhale more deeply and hold the smoke in the lungs.

Cannabis use is also associated with a variety of psychobehavioral effects. Among the symptoms which may result are an initial sense of anxiety giving away to relaxation, friendliness, euphoria, a perception that the passage of time has slowed, and an increased sensitivity to external stimuli (e.g., colors appear brighter, sounds seem louder). The cannabis user experiencing a high is often sedate or serene, in contrast to the LSD user, who is usually restless and intensely alert (Laymeyer et al., 1993).

Recent research suggests that THC may alter the way in which sensory information gets into and is acted upon by the brain. The area of the brain known as the hippocampus seems to be particularly affected by THC. The hippocampus is the area associated with learned behaviors. Studies indicate that THC may suppress the activity of the nerve fibers in the hippocampus. Long-term use of cannabis may produce changes in the brain similar to those seen after long-term use of other major drugs (National Institute on Drug Abuse, 1999e).

Diagnostic Criteria for Cannabis-Use Disorders: Cannabis Dependence and Cannabis Abuse

The diagnostic criteria for cannabis dependence and cannabis abuse are the same as the more general categories, substance dependence and substance abuse. Individuals with cannabis dependence or cannabis abuse have compulsive use, but do not generally develop physiological dependence. Tolerance to most of the effects of cannabis can occur in chronic users. Individuals with cannabis dependence or cannabis abuse may use the drug throughout the day over extended periods of time, and they may spend several hours per day acquiring and using the substance. They may experience problems with family, school, work, or recreational activities, and may also persist in their use despite physical or psychological symptoms (APA, 1994, p. 216).

Diagnostic Criteria for Cannabis-Induced Disorders: Cannabis Intoxication

Intoxication develops quickly (within minutes) if cannabis is smoked, but may take longer to develop if ingested orally. Intoxication typically begins with a high feeling followed by euphoria, inappropriate laughter and grandiosity, lethargy, impaired judgment and/or motor performance, distorted sensory perceptions, sensations of time passing slowly, impairment in short-term memory, and difficulty carrying out complex mental processes. Occasionally, anxiety or social withdrawal can also occur. The diagnosis of cannabis intoxication can be made if these effects accompany two or more of the following signs developing within two hours of cannabis use: reddened conjunctivas (bloodshot eyes), increased appetite, dry mouth, and tachycardia. The effects usually last for about three to four hours, but may vary due to the dose administered, method of administration, and individual characteristics of the user (APA, 1994, p. 218). Withdrawal symptoms, when they occur, tend to be mild and may include irritability, insomnia, sweating, nausea, and vomiting.

Natural Course of Cannabis-Related Disorders

Cannabis dependence and abuse usually develop gradually over an extended period of time. Those who become dependent typically establish a pattern of chronic use that increases in frequency and amount used. With chronic use, some individuals experience a loss of pleasurable effects of the substance. According to *DSM-IV,* individuals with a history of conduct disorder in childhood or adolescence tend to be at higher risk for the development of cannabis-related disorders (APA, 1994).

Epidemiology

Cannabis is the world's most commonly used illicit drug, and marijuana is the most popular form of the substance due to its easy availability. Cannabis-use disorders occur more often in males, and prevalence is most common in persons between 18 and 30 years of age. Cannabis use is common in all socioeconomic and ethnic groups in all areas, rural, suburban, and urban (Laymeyer et al., 1993). According to data from the 1996 National Household Survey on Drug Abuse, more than 68.6 million Americans (32%) 12 years of age and older have tried marijuana at least once in their lifetimes, and almost 18.4 million (8.6%) had used marijuana during the previous year (National Institute on Drug Abuse, 1999f).

Cannabis is often among the first drugs of experimentation for all cultural groups in the United States. Data from the National Institute on Drug Abuse's 1997 Monitoring the Future Study (National Institute on Drug Abuse, 1999e) indicated that marijuana use among 8th, 10th, and 12th grade students continued to rise throughout the 1990s (see **Table 7.1**).

Treatment

An addictive drug causes compulsive craving, seeking, and use even in the face of negative social and health consequences. Cannabis meets this criterion, and more than 120,000 people seek treatment per year (National Institute on Drug Abuse, 1999g). Although the estimate of those seeking treatment is small in comparison to the total number of cannabis users, it does have symbolic significance. No matter how popular a psychoactive substance may be, under certain circumstances it can produce undesirable and dangerous effects.

Among chronic users symptoms of lethargy and anhedonia have been reported. Mild forms of depression, anxiety, or irritability are seen in about one third of individuals who regularly use cannabis (APA, 1994). When taken in extremely high doses, cannabinoids can have effects similar to hallucinogens, potentially causing users to experience mental effects that resemble hallucinogen-induced bad trips. Cannabis is also often used with other substances, especially alcohol and cocaine. Such combinations of substances may produce effects that precipitate the desire to seek treatment. In addition, problems related to cannabis use and impairment in social, occupational, or other important areas or functioning may contribute to the decision to seek treatment.

No standard treatment regimen for cannabis-related disorders exists. Because withdrawal is not an issue with cannabis use, detoxification, a procedure common to the treatment of many other substances, is not needed. When provided, the primary goal of treatment for cannabis use is abstinence.

Phencyclidine-Related Disorders

Phencyclidine (PCP) was developed in the 1950s as an anesthetic for surgery. Because it produced highly undesirable side effects its use was quickly discontinued. In the 1960s it was marketed to veterinarians as an animal anesthestetic and tranquilizer. PCP is no longer used by veterinarians and is produced today only in illicit laboratories.

PCP is a white crystalline powder that is readily soluble in water or alcohol. On the street it is known as *angel dust, ozone, hog, rocket fuel,* or *wack.* Sold in the form of pills, capsules, or powder, it is usually taken orally, intravenously, or smoked.

PCP is difficult to classify accurately, since different doses produce different effects, such as those derived from stimulants, hallucinogens, anesthetics, or analgesics (painkillers). Not all people react the same way to the drug, even after taking the same amount. PCP intoxication is one of the most serious drug abuse syndromes. Paranoia and unpredictable violent behavior are common symptoms. A particular concern with PCP is the frequency with which dealers falsely present it as some other drug such as mescaline or peyote. Thus buyers, expecting the relatively mild effects of these drugs, suddenly experience the stronger and unpredictable effects of PCP.

General Effects

Short-term effects appear soon after taking a single dose of PCP and usually disappear within a few hours or days. At low to moderate doses the physical effects

% using marijuana during the previous year		
Grade Level	1991	1997
8th	6.2	17.7
10th	16.5	34.8
12th	23.9	38.5
% using marijuana daily during the previous month		
Grade Level	1991	1997
8th	0.2	1.1
10th	0.8	3.7
12th	2.0	5.8

Table 7.1: Marijuana use among 8th, 10th, and 12th grade students

of PCP include a slight increase in breathing rate, an increase in blood pressure and heart rate, a rise in temperature, flushing, profuse sweating, and numbness in the arms and legs. Psychological effects include changes in body awareness, similar to those associated with alcohol intoxication.

Higher doses produce a rapid drop in blood pressure, heart rate, and respiration accompanied by nausea, vomiting, blurred vision, dizziness, and decreased awareness of pain. Muscles may contract so intensely they cause jerky, uncoordinated movements and bizarre postures. Heavy doses of the drug can cause convulsions and coma. Psychological effects may include symptoms that mimic the symptoms of schizophrenia, such as hallucinations, delusions, paranoia, and disordered thinking. Most regular users experience occasional bad trips, and some experience unpleasant flashbacks similar to those experienced by LSD users.

People who use PCP for prolonged periods often display symptoms such as persistent speech difficulties, loss of memory (particularly recent memory), long-lasting anxiety, depression, and social withdrawal.

Diagnostic Criteria for Phencyclidine-Use Disorders: Phencyclidine Dependence and Phencyclidine Abuse

The diagnostic criteria for phencyclidine dependence and phencyclidine abuse are the same as for the more general categories, substance dependence and substance abuse. PCP causes no specific physical dependence or withdrawal syndrome; however, heavy users sometimes report craving the drug. Phencyclidine use may continue despite the presence of problems that the individual knows are caused by the substance.

Diagnostic Criteria for Phencyclidine-Induced Disorders: Phencyclidine Intoxication

The diagnostic criteria for phencyclidine intoxication specify significant maladaptive behavioral changes such as belligerence, assaultiveness, impulsiveness, and unpredictability. These changes develop during or shortly after phencyclidine use. For the diagnosis of phencyclidine intoxication to occur, at least two of the following physical symptoms must be present:

- Vertical or horizontal nystagmus (involuntary rhythmic movements of the eye)

- Hypertension or rapid heart rate
- Numbness or diminished responsiveness to pain
- Ataxia (disturbed balance)
- Dysarthria (problems with articulation of speech)
- Muscle rigidity
- Seizures or coma
- Hyperacusis (painful sensitivity to sounds)

These effects can begin almost immediately after an intravenous dose, reaching a peak within minutes. The effects are somewhat slower in oral doses, with peak effects experienced in about two hours (APA, 1994, p. 258).

Epidemiology

Phencyclidine-related disorders occur about twice as frequently in males than in females and occur more frequently among ethnic minorities. The prime age for PCP abuse is between 20 and 40 years old. Medical examiners report that phencyclidine is involved in about 3% of all deaths directly associated with substance use, and it is mentioned as a problem in about 3% of substance-related emergency room visits (APA, 1994).

The most recent data from the National Institute on Drug Abuse (1999h) indicates that about 2.3% of high school seniors had used PCP at least once in the previous year, and 0.7% had used it during the previous month. Compared to data from a similar study conducted in 1979, the number of seniors who have ever used PCP has dropped by about 66% during the past two decades. According to the 1996 National Household Survey on Drug Abuse, 3.2% of the population aged 12 and older have used PCP at least once in their lifetime (National Institute on Drug Abuse, 1999h).

Treatment

PCP causes no specific physical dependence or withdrawal, thus treatment usually involves dealing with problems associated with intoxication. In some individuals PCP may induce psychosis lasting for extended periods of time. Psychosis may be manifested by delusional thinking, paranoia, hyperactivity, depression, or bizarre behavior. Unpredictable assaultive behavior may also be present. In such instances, the primary focus of treatment is upon protecting both the user and those around him or her from physical harm (Laymeyer et al., 1993).

Inhalant-Related Disorders

Inhalants are breathable chemical vapors that produce psychoactive (mind-altering) effects. Almost all commonly abused inhalants are hydrocarbon solvents produced from petroleum and natural gas. These substances have an enormous number of industrial, commercial, and household uses. Common forms of inhalants include cleaning fluids, gasoline, nail polish remover, lighter fluid, model airplane glues, spray paints, spray can propellants, typewriter correction fluids, and plastic cement.

Young people are the biggest group of abusers of inhalants, in part because they are so readily available and inexpensive. Inhaling of intoxicating vapors is most commonly accomplished by soaking a rag with the substance, which is then applied to the mouth and nose, and the vapors are breathed in. Sometimes the substance is placed in a bag and the gasses in the bag are inhaled. Substances may also be inhaled directly from aerosols sprayed in the mouth and nose. Inhalants reach the lungs, bloodstream, and other target sites very rapidly (APA, 1999).

General Effects

Short-term effects appear soon after inhalation. Generally individuals will experience a euphoric feeling, characterized by lightheadedness, exhilaration, and vivid fantasies. Nausea, drooling, coughing, muscular incoordination, slow reflexes, and sensitivity to light may also occur. For some users, feelings of being very powerful may lead to reckless or self-destructive behavior. Inhalant use can also lead to antisocial activities such as property damage or theft.

Intoxication can last only a few minutes or several hours if inhalants are taken repeatedly. Deep, repeated inhalation over short periods may result in a loss of control, culminating in hallucinations, unconsciousness, or seizures. High concentrations of inhalants may cause death from suffocation by displacing oxygen in the lungs and the central nervous system so that breathing ceases. The risk of accidental death increases when dangerous behaviors (e.g., driving an automobile) follow inhalation.

Long-term effects following repeated use over an extended period include reversible physical symptoms such as extreme thirst, weight loss, nosebleeds, bloodshot eyes, and sores on the nose and mouth. Liver and kidney function may be impaired. Irreversible effects caused by inhaling specific substances include hearing loss (paint sprays, glues, cleaning fluids), bone marrow damage (gasoline), and central nervous system or brain damage (glues, gasoline, gas cylinders). Behavioral symptoms in regular heavy sniffers may include mental confusion, fatigue, depression, irritability, hostility, and paranoia.

Diagnostic Criteria for Inhalant-Use Disorders: Inhalant Dependence and Inhalant Abuse

The diagnostic criteria for inhalant dependence and inhalant abuse are essentially the same as the more general category of substance dependence and substance abuse, although some of the generic criteria do not apply. Regular inhalant use induces tolerance, which means increased doses are necessary to produce the same effects (e.g., a regular glue sniffer may need several tubes of plastic cement to maintain the "high" originally achieved by a single tube). However, inhalant dependence is not associated with a characteristic withdrawal nor is there evidence of inhalant use to relieve or avoid withdrawal symptoms. Because inhalants are inexpensive, readily available, and legal, spending a great deal of time attempting to procure inhalants is rare. However, substantial amounts of time may be spent using the substances. Recurrent use may result in the individual giving up or reducing important social, recreational, or occupational activities. Inhalant abuse is associated with continued use of the substance in dangerous situations when judgment and coordination are impaired, or repeated intake of inhalants despite the occurrence of social conflict or school problems. Inhalant dependence and abuse appear to occur only in a small proportion of individuals who use the substances (APA, 1994, p. 241).

Diagnostic Criteria for Inhalant-Induced Disorders: Inhalant Intoxication

Inhalant intoxication is marked by significant maladaptive behavioral or psychological changes associated with the recent use of a volatile inhalant. The most prominent changes include assaultiveness, apathy, belligerence, impaired judgment, and impaired social or occupational functioning. The diagnosis of inhalant intoxication is made when the above changes are accompanied by at least two or more of the following symptoms: dizziness, nystagmus (i.e., involuntary rhythmic movements of the eyes), incoordination, slurred speech, unsteady gait, lethargy, depressed reflexes, psychomotor retardation, muscle weakness, tremor, blurred or double vision, stupor or coma, or euphoria (APA, 1994, p. 239).

Epidemiology

Because of their widespread availability, inhalants are often the first drugs of experimentation for many individuals. Inhalant use may begin during the preteen years and it peaks in adolescence. It appears to be uncommon among persons after age 35. Males use inhalants more often than females, and there may be a higher incidence among those living in economically depressed areas (APA, 1994). Solvent abuse rates are higher among Native Americans than any other ethnic group (National Institute on Drug Abuse, 1999c).

According to data from the National Institute on Drug Abuse's Monitoring the Future Study, the annual rate of inhalant use among seniors in high school has steadily risen from 3.0% in 1976, to 6.7% in 1997. The same study revealed that in 1997 21% of 8th graders and 18.3% of 10th graders had used inhalants at least once in their lives, and 11.8% of 8th graders and 8.7% of 10th graders had used inhalants in the previous year (National Institute on Drug Abuse, 1999c). Similar rates of use were identified among Canadian youth in a 1989 survey of Ontario students in grades 7 to 13 (Addiction Research Foundation, 1991b).

Among 8th, 10th, and 12th graders, the prevalence of inhalant use is exceeded only by the prevalence of alcohol, cigarette, and marijuana use. Inhalant abusers typically use other drugs as well. A recent report published by the National Institute on Drug Abuse (1999c) stated:

> Children as young as fourth graders who begin to use volatile solvents also will start experimenting with other drugs, usually alcohol and marijuana . . . Adolescent solvent abusers are typically polydrug users and are prone to use whatever is available, although they do show a preference for solvents.

Treatment

No standard treatment program for inhalant-related disorders exists. Most efforts aim at prevention. Because inhalant use is usually begun in the preteen or early teen years, this is the target population to which prevention-based educational programs are aimed.

Implications for Therapeutic Recreation

Therapeutic recreation professionals are likely to work with individuals with substance-related disorders in a variety of service settings. These include residential chemical dependency facilities, chemical dependency units within freestanding hospitals, outpatient treatment facilities, and correctional institutions. Services provided at such facilities vary, but often represent a continuum from detoxification programs focused upon acute medical care at one end, to day treatment centers or partial hospitalization programs focused upon adjusting to a life built upon sobriety on the other end. Therapeutic recreation services are most commonly found in the latter type of facilities, which often emphasize psychotherapeutic treatment techniques such as group counseling, stress management, vocational rehabilitation, and family and activity therapies. The most common treatment approach used follows the principles of self-help support groups like Alcoholics Anonymous (AA).

Participation

The use of illicit substances is a major social problem. What motivates individuals to use and abuse potentially harmful and addictive substances? According to Stanton Peele, the author of *The Meaning of Addiction,* "drugs do for abusers what they believe they cannot do for themselves: get rid of anxiety, lead to a good feeling about themselves and make them believe they are competent, in control, and able to master their environment" (cited in Kunstler, 1992, p. 58). This statement is poignant in its characterization of the power of drugs. It suggests that a void often exists in the life of individuals who experience substance-related disorders. Structured leisure participation may be extremely beneficial in filling this void.

Leisure experiences have consistently been identified with anxiety reduction and the promotion of a positive mood (Iso-Ahola, 1994). The sensation of pleasure and a sense of personal well-being have also long been identified with recreational participation (Gunter, 1987; Kraus, 1997). Perhaps most importantly, Neulinger (1981), Iso-Ahola (1994) and Gunter (1987) have suggested that distinguishing features of leisure involvement include the perception of freedom and personal control and involvement motivated by intrinsic rather than extrinsic factors. In other words, an underlying characteristic of a leisure experience seems to be the perception of personal control. Iso-Ahola and Weissinger summarized the evidence as follows:

> Empirical research leaves little doubt about the fact that intrinsically motivated leisure is positively and significantly related to psychological or mental health. Those who are in control of their leisure lives and experiences and feel engaged in and committed to leisure activities and experiences are psychologically healthier than those who are not in control of their leisure lives and feel detached and uncommitted. (1984, p. 41)

It is easy to speculate that those who do not feel in control of their personal lives would be vulnerable to the influences of illicit substances. This view draws further support from characterizations of drug abusers as people who are unable to experience fun and pleasure, who feel inadequate and possess low self-esteem, who see leisure as empty, and who lack stress management and social skills (Kunstler, 1992; Aguilar & Munson, 1991). In a 10-year follow-up study of over 580 subjects, Vaillant (1983) found that the largest percentage of recovered abusers used alternative activities as methods of coping or improving moods.

For such individuals, therapeutic recreation encourages participation in non-drug-related activities that help users cope with issues in their environment and obtain enjoyable states without the use of drugs. According to Francis (1991a), recreational participation may help produce a "flow state" (Csikszentmihalyi, 1975)—experiences of euphoria similar to those which may be produced by mood-altering substances. Francis (1991a) provided helpful recommendations for strategies for facilitating flow states among substance misusers, including:

- Selecting intrinsically motivated activities
- Facilitating creative discovery, exploration, problem solving, and autonomy in recreational programming
- Choosing activities that improve self-confidence, self-knowledge, and realistic goal setting
- Setting up and recognizing successes through immediate and constant feedback
- Choosing and structuring activities that emphasize clear, concrete, and immediately realizable goal attainment

In addition, recreational opportunities provided by therapeutic recreation personnel can help substance users develop the ability to structure their free time, to better manage stress, to enhance their self-esteem, and to help combat loneliness and boredom (Rancourt, 1991a). Through recreational participation TR staff may help abusers deal with self-defeating behaviors like dependency and low tolerance thresholds; develop communication and self-control; enhance independent functioning and physical well-being; and promote sobriety and the prevention of relapse (Carter, Van Andel & Robb, 1995; McCormick & Dattilo, 1995).

Leisure Education

The leisure education component of TR programming is extremely important for individuals with substance-related disorders. Given the fact that most drug abusers have passive and sedentary lifestyles, Kunstler suggested that leisure education can help these individuals better understand "self, leisure and the relationships of their own lifestyles and the fabric of society" (1992, p. 59). She goes on to identify a variety of topics which may be addressed in a leisure education program for this population, including stress management techniques, social skills and assertiveness training, identifying leisure barriers, and developing leisure participation skills.

In a pair of publications, O'Dea Evans (1990a, 1990b) discussed possible goals of a leisure education program for addicted persons. O'Dea Evans believes that individuals who have addiction problems have significant problematic issues with their leisure, including a lack of satisfaction with leisure involvements and a tendency to engage in passive (rather than active) leisure pursuits. She also noted the high incidence of recidivism after treatment for addiction and attributed this in part to the failure to address leisure involvement during the treatment program (1990a). In response, O'Dea Evans (1990b) developed a leisure counseling model for addicted persons. This process-oriented model consists of six components:

1. *Assess*—collect baseline data about the client and his or her situation
2. *Assist*—identify structural and environmental barriers to leisure
3. *Confront*—address attitudinal barriers associated with addiction and leisure lifestyles
4. *Plan*—develop an individualized plan to promote leisure involvement
5. *Participate*—encourage involvement in leisure activities new to the client or reinvolvement in past activities

6. *Recollection*—process leisure involvement emphasizing an awareness of leisure as an essential component in a recovery program

In an effort to test the effectiveness of this model, O'Dea Evans conducted a study using 47 individuals admitted to a chemical dependency program. Preliminary findings demonstrated significant improvement in subjects' perception of leisure. It was theorized that this finding would result in a lower relapse rate for the study's participants (O'Dea Evans, 1990b).

Rancourt (1991b) discussed the idea that leisure education should also address the need to increase opportunities for family socialization and recreation. Efforts toward improving family leisure seems particularly appropriate in light of the fact that family dysfunction appears to be a consistent problem among substance abusers (Malkin, Benshoff, Beck & Toriello, 1996). One response to this situation can be the development of a family-centered leisure education program for persons with substance-related disorders.

Another focus of TR services can be upon the prevention of relapse among individuals who have been treated for substance dependence. Relapse is characterized by setbacks in the substance abuser's ability to maintain sobriety. Many recreational activities are considered high-risk because they place the recovering addict in situations where a substance of abuse is present (e.g., bowling facilities where alcohol is served). In an effort to address relapse prevention, Deiser and Voight (1998) developed the Attribution Retraining Leisure Education Model (ARLEM), a nine-session TR leisure education program for use with substance-dependent individuals with a history of relapse problems. The ARLEM program uses techniques such as recreation activity, experiential education, group discussion, and role-playing to help clients retrain their thought processes to be more optimistic. Similar to the attributional analysis approach to TR programming (Iso-Ahola, MacNeil & Syzmanski, 1980), ARLEM focuses upon helping the substance-dependent individual recognize that they can attribute positive, successful leisure outcomes to their own abilities rather than to external forces such as luck or fate. Through attribution retraining participants may learn to change pessimistic attributions toward leisure experiences into positive ones, thus developing a new coping skill to deal with high-risk leisure situations.

The implementation of a leisure education component in a TR program for a chemically dependent client was detailed in a case study published in the *Therapeutic Recreation Journal* (Hemingway, 1993). The author described the successful involvement of her client in the process of researching recreation opportunities within his home community. This process was made more difficult because the client had limited financial resources and had his driver's license suspended due to his drug-related problems. The leisure education program focused upon helping the client develop the confidence to make his own decisions and to become assertive enough to defend them, especially in situations where he might be tempted to return to his past substance-use habits. Ultimately, the leisure education activities allowed the client to better understand the value of recreation in his life and provided the skills necessary to incorporate various recreation facilities and activities into a new leisure lifestyle (Hemingway, 1993).

Treatment

Clearly, there is no one best way to treat substance abuse. However, the Alcoholics Anonymous (AA) model is generally viewed as a foundation of treatment for many forms of substance-related disorders.

Applying the principles of AA to therapeutic recreation programs designed to treat individuals who abuse substances was the focus of an interpretive study conducted by McCormick and Dattilo (1995). According to the researchers, clients with alcohol problems have been found to have relatively negative attitudes towards leisure and demonstrate some resistance to treatment generally. The authors believed that this resistance could be reduced if services were linked to factors perceived as important to clients such as AA. Upon studying the social world of AA, data collected demonstrated "parallels between the concept of sobriety in AA and philosophical ideals of leisure" (p. 18). The researchers concluded that therapeutic recreation interventions that tie the AA's ideology of the freedom of sobriety to the view of leisure as an opportunity for growth and development would likely enhance the centrality of leisure within the lives of the recovering addict. In making the connection, the therapeutic recreation specialist may then be able to use leisure as a medium to help foster the behavioral changes needed to help substance-dependent individuals overcome their addiction.

Kunstler (1992, p. 59) identified three goals of TR which she described as comparable to the general goals of recovery (see **Table 7.2**).

In an extensive literature review Rancourt (1991b, p. 35) identified a comprehensive list of therapeutic recreation treatment goals that she posits assist the individual during the recovery process. The most salient of the goals she presented include:

- Develop positive ways to structure their free time
- Help them cope with feelings and situations that may have previously been addressed by using or abusing drugs
- Increase their internal locus of control
- Assist them in developing a proactive decision-making style
- Help them to learn to socialize without the use of psychoactive substances
- Promote opportunities for family socialization and recreation

Comprehensive treatment programs for substance abusers usually involve a number of different therapies (e.g., group, art, music) which work together to help promote recovery. According to Hemingway (1993), TR can provide an important and unique contribution to the treatment team. As described in the case study she authored, Hemingway stated:

Recreation activities allowed him (her client) a "starting point" to be comfortable enough to open up with peers and staff and start trusting them. The positive experiences he encountered through recreation encouraged him to express himself in other aspects of treatment. (1993, p. 129)

A broad range of TR activities may be used in treating substance abusers. Kunstler (1992) suggests that both cooperative, group-oriented activities and solitary, individual activities play important roles when working with clients with substance-induced disorders. For the first category, she identified activities such as New Games, ropes courses, putting on a play, or painting a mural, as important sources of promoting trust and developing self-confidence and social skills. Developing recreational interests to pursue by oneself is also very important because "empty time" often presents serious challenges for individuals with a history of substance abuse.

Given the fact that addicts tend to primarily engage in passive leisure pursuits (O'Dea Evans, 1990a), writers view the use of exercise and physical activities as beneficial in treating this population. Based upon data produced in their study of practicing TR specialists, Kremer, Malkin, and Benshoff (1995) noted the evolving significance and contributions of physical activity programs in substance abuse treatment. The researchers reported that at least 50% of the respondents identified walking, active games, sports, weight training, and aerobics as basic components in their TR programs. Physically active programs may encourage

leisure decision making, help to avoid feelings of apathy and withdrawal, and promote healthy lifestyles. Moreover, physical exercise has been shown to decrease depressive symptoms among recovering substance abusers (Palmer, Palmer, Michiels & Thigpen, 1995).

One form of physically active recreation that has received attention in terms of treating individuals with addiction problems is adventure-challenge programming. According to McCormick (1991) adventure-challenge experiences encourage self-assessment and trust building while serving as alternative highs. In a study using a population of adolescents, 44.9% of whom were diagnosed as substance abusers, Whitman (1993) reported that subjects identified positive changes occurring in both personal behavior (e.g., learning to trust others, the ability to express feelings) and group behavior (e.g., working cooperatively) as a result of an adventure program experience. As with other studies using adventure-challenge experiences, this work supports the idea that treatment goals may be addressed at the same time that participants claim to be experiencing pleasurable recreational involvement.

In contrast to physically oriented TR programs, evidence also suggests that some forms of quiet, passive activities may benefit individuals undergoing treatment for addiction. For example, Francis (1991b) explored the use of meditation as a therapeutic activity for substance abusers. In his comprehensive review of related literature, Francis developed a rationale for the use of meditation as a treatment option. Kunstler (1992) supported Francis's view, and identified activities such as guided imagery, yoga, relaxation, tai chi, and silent walking as potentially beneficial for treating individuals with substance-related problems.

Goals of TR	Goals of Recovery
Self-awareness	Believe an addiction is hurting them and wish to overcome it
Self-efficacy	Feel enough efficacy to manage their withdrawal and to manage life without addiction
Self-rewarding recreation	Find sufficient alternative rewards to make life without the addiction worthwhile

Table 7.2 Goals of TR comparable to goals of recovery

Two other treatment activities that may be applicable to TR include drama therapy and visualization. Moffett and Bruto (1990) reported improvement in coping skills and self-expression of chronic substance abusers as a result of the use of a therapeutic theater program. Kominars (1997) described the positive effects on treatment outcomes for chemically dependent subjects in an outpatient treatment program that resulted from the use of visualization techniques.

Family therapy is an important part of most treatment programs for individuals with substance-related concerns. Family members need information about the illness for the benefit of the user as well as for themselves. They need to understand how the substance has become an integral part of their lives and how their relationships with the individual may contribute to the problem.

Finally, the use of therapeutic recreation programs to help treat children of addicted parents has been addressed in a few publications. Ito (1990) discussed problems typically faced by children of alcoholics, and explored possible goals and intervention strategies that could be used by TR personnel to help meet the special needs of these children. In like fashion, Malkin (1994) described a theory-based program of treatment for cocaine-affected infants and children. She described interventions including "baby holders" and family therapy to deal with the physical, emotional, social, and cognitive difficulties experienced by these children.

Chapter Summary

This chapter examined substance-related disorders and addressed the following issues:

- Two broad theories of causation: psychological theories and physiological theories
- Classification system for substance-related disorders adopted by the *Diagnostic and Statistical Manual of Mental Disorders*
- Seven common classes of substances associated with substance-related disorders, including alcohol-related disorders, central nervous system stimulants (amphetamines and cocaine), opioid-related disorders, hallucinogen-related disorders, cannabis-related disorders, phencyclidine-related disorders, and inhalant-related disorders
- Implications for the therapeutic recreation profession for substance-related disorders

References

Addiction Research Foundation. (1991a). *Facts about alcohol*. Available online: http://www.arf.org/isd/pim/alcohol.html

Addiction Research Foundation. (1991b). *Facts about inhalants*. Available online: http://www.arf.org/isd/pim/inhlant.html

Aguilar, T. E. and Munson, W. W. (1991). Leisure education and counseling as intervention components in drug and alcohol treatment for adolescents. *Journal of Alcohol and Drug Education, 37,* 23–34.

American Psychiatric Association. (1994). *Diagnostic and Statistical Manual of Mental Disorders* (4th ed.). Washington, DC: Author.

Baker, J. K., Harding, S. C., and Hadwen, D. K. (1994, Winter). The role of recreation in the treatment of chemical dependency: An analysis of the Homewood Alcohol and Drug Service. *Journal of Leisurability,* 20–26.

Bergler, E. (1946). Personality traits of alcohol addicts. *Quarterly Journal of Studies on Alcohol, 7,* 356–361.

Carter, M. J., Van Andel, G. E., and Robb, G. M. (1995). *Therapeutic recreation: A practical approach.* Prospect Heights, IL: Waveland Press.

Chein, I., Gerard, D. L., Lee, R. S., and Rosenfield, E. (1964). *The road to H: Narcotics, delinquency, and social policy.* New York, NY: Basic Books.

Ciraulo, D. and Shader, R. (1991). *Clinical manual of chemical dependence.* Washington, DC: American Psychiatric Press.

Csikszentmihalyi, M. (1975). *Beyond boredom and anxiety.* San Francisco, CA: Jossey-Boss, Inc.

Davison, G. and Neale, J. (1986). *Abnormal psychology: An experimental clinical approach* (4th ed.). New York, NY: John Wiley & Sons.

Deiser, R. B. and Voight, A. (1998). Therapeutic recreation and relapse prevention intervention. *Parks & Recreation, 33*(5), 78–83.

Ellis A. (1992). Group rational-emotive and cognitive-behavior-therapy. *International Journal of Group Psychotherapy, 42,* 63–80.

Fenichel, O. (1945). *The psychoanalytic theory of neurosis.* New York, NY: Norton.

Francis, T. (1991a). Revising therapeutic recreation for substance misuse: Incorporating flow technology in alternative treatments. *Therapeutic Recreation Journal, 25*(2), 41–48.

Francis, T. (1991b). Meditation as a alternative to substance misuse: A current review. *Therapeutic Recreation Journal, 25*(4), 50–60.

Gunter, B. G. (1987). The leisure experience: Selected properties. *Journal of Leisure Research, 19*(2), 115–130.

Hemingway, V. G. (1993). Therapeutic recreation services for a chemically dependent client. *Therapeutic Recreation Journal, 27*(2), 126,130.

Herbert, M. (1987). *Conduct disorders of childhood and adolescence.* New York, NY: John Wiley.

Hull, J. G. (1981). A self-awareness model of the causes and effects of alcohol consumption. *Journal of Abnormal Psychology, 90,* 586–600.

Iso-Ahola, S. E. (1994). Leisure lifestyle and health. In D. Compton and S. E. Iso-Ahola (Eds.), *Leisure and mental health* (pp. 42–60). Park City, UT: Family Development Resources, Inc.

Iso-Ahola, S., MacNeil, R., and Szymanski, D. (1980). Social psychological foundations of therapeutic recreation: An attributional analysis. In S. Iso-Ahola (Ed.), *Social psychological perspectives on leisure and recreation* (pp. 390–413). Springfield, IL: Charles C. Thomas.

Iso-Ahola, S. and Weissinger, E. (1984). Leisure and well-being: Is there a connection? *Parks & Recreation, 18*(6), 40–44.

Ito, G. H. (1990). A special population: Children of alcoholics and addicts—the role of therapeutic recreation. In G. Hitzhusen and J. O'Neil (Eds.), *Expanding horizons in therapeutic recreation XIII* (pp. 114–131). Columbia, MO: University of Missouri.

Janicak, P. G., Piszczor, J., and Easton, M. S. (1993). Alcohol-related disorders. In J. A. Flaherty, J. M. Davis, and P. G. Janicak (Eds.), *Psychiatry: Diagnosis & therapy* (2nd ed., pp. 247–265). Norwalk, CT: Appleton & Lange.

Knight, R. P. (1937). The dynamics of chronic alcoholism. *Journal of Nervous and Mental Disease, 86,* 538–548.

Kominars, K. D. (1997). A study of visualization and addiction treatment. *Journal of Substance Abuse Treatment, 14*(3), 213–223.

Kraus, R. (1997). *Recreation & leisure in modern society* (5th ed.). Menlo Park, CA: Addison Wesley Longman, Inc.

Kremer, D., Malkin, M. J., and Venshoff, J. J. (1995). Physical activity programs offered in substance abuse treatment facilities. *Journal of Substance Abuse Treatment, 12,* 327–333.

Kunstler, R. (1992). TR's role in treating substance abuse. *Parks & Recreation, 27*(4), 58–60.

Laymeyer, H. W., Channon, R. A., and Schlemmer, R. F. (1993). Psychoactive substance abuse. In J. A. Flaherty, J. M. Davis, and P. G. Janicak (Eds.), *Psychiatry: Diagnosis & therapy* (2nd ed., pp. 266–283). Norwalk, CT: Appleton & Lange.

Leshner, A. (1999, November 21). Addiction: A brain disease. *Parade Magazine,* p. 11.

Lubin, R. A. (1977). Influences of alcohol upon performance and performance awareness. *Perceptual and Motor Skills, 45,* 303–310.

Malkin, M. J. (1994). Recreational therapy and cocaine-affected children. In G. Hitzhusen, L. Thomas, and M. Birdsong (Eds.), *Expanding horizons in therapeutic recreation XVI* (pp. 177–186). Columbia, MO: University of Missouri.

Malkin, M. J., Benshoff, J. J., Beck, M., and Toriello, P. J. (October, 1996). Therapeutic recreation interventions in substance abuse treatment programs. *Parks & Recreation 31*(10), 26–40.

Malkin, M. J., Philips, R. W., and Chumbler, J. A. (1991). The family lab: An interdisciplinary family education program. *Annual in Therapeutic Recreation, 2,* 25–36.

Marlatt, A., Baer, J., Donovan, D., and Kiviahan, D. (1988). Addictive behaviors: Etiology and treatment. In M. Rosenzweig and L. Porter (Eds.), *Annual review of psychology* (Vol. 39). Palo Alto, CA: Annual Reviews.

McCormick, B. (1991). Self-experience as leisure constraint: The case of Alcoholics Anonymous. *Journal of Leisure Research, 23,* 345–362.

McCormick, B. and Dattilo, J. (1995). "Sobriety's kind of like freedom": Integrating ideals of leisure into the ideology of Alcoholics Anonymous. *Therapeutic Recreation Journal, 29*(1), 18–29.

Meyer, R. G. (1993). *The clinician's handbook* (3rd ed.). Boston, MA: Allyn & Bacon.

Moffett, L. A. and Bruto, L. (1990). Therapeutic theater with personality-disorders substance abuses: Characters in search of different characters. *The Arts in Psychotherapy, 17,* 339–348.

National Institute on Alcohol Abuse and Alcoholism. (1995). *NIAAA releases new estimates of alcohol abuse and dependence.* Available online: http://silk.nih.gov/silk/niaal/releases/nlaes.htm

National Institute on Alcohol Abuse and Alcoholism. (1999). *Frequently asked questions.* Available online: http://silk.nih.gov/silk/niaal/questions/q-a/htm

National Institute on Drug Abuse, National Institutes of Health. (1999a). *Cocaine abuse and addiction.* Available online: http://www.nida.nih.gov/Infofax/cocaine.html

National Institute on Drug Abuse, National Institutes of Health. (1999b). *Heroin: Info fax #13548.* Available online: http://www.nida.nih.gov/Infofax/heroin.html

National Institute on Drug Abuse, National Institutes of Health. (1999c). *Inhalants: Info fax #13549.* Available online: http://www.nida.nih.gov/Infofax/inhalants.html

National Institute on Drug Abuse, National Institutes of Health. (1999d). *LSD: Info fax #13550.* Available online: http://www.nida.nih.gov/Infofax/lsd.html

National Institute on Drug Abuse, National Institutes of Health. (1999e). *Marijuana: Info fax #13551.* Available online: http://www.nida.nih.gov/Infofax/marijuana.html

National Institute on Drug Abuse, National Institutes of Health. (1999f). *Methamphetamine: Info fax #13552* Available online: http://www.nida.nih.gov/Infofax/methamphetamine.html

National Institute on Drug Abuse, National Institutes of Health. (1999g). *Nationwide trends: Info fax #13567.* Available online: http://www.nida.nih.gov/Infofax/nationtrends.html

National Institute on Drug Abuse, National Institutes of Health. (1999h). *PCP (phencyclidine): Info fax #13554.* Available online: http://www.nida.nih.gov/Infofax/pcp.html

National Institute on Drug Abuse, National Institutes of Health. (1999i). *Treatment Methods: Info fax #13559.* Available online: http://www.nida.nih.gov/Infofax/treatmeth.html

Neulinger, J. (1981). *To leisure: An introduction.* Boston, MA: Little, Brown, and Company.

O'Conner, A. and Daly, J. (1985). Alcoholism: A twenty-year follow-up study. *British Journal of Psychiatry, 146,* 645–654.

O'Dea Evans, P. (1990a). *Leisure education for addicted persons.* Algonquin, IL: Peapod Publications.

O'Dea Evans, P. (1990b). Leisure education for addicted persons. In G. Hitzhusen and J. O'Neil (Eds.), *Expanding horizons in therapeutic recreation XIII* (pp. 68–88). Columbia, MO: University of Missouri.

Palmer, J. A., Palmer, L. K., Michiels, K., and Thigpen, B. (1995). Effects of type of exercise on depression in recovering substance abusers. *Perceptual and Motor Skills, 80,* 523–530.

Poling, A., Gadow, K., and Cleary, J. (1991). *Drug therapy for behavior disorders.* Elmsford, NY: Pergamon.

Quay, H. C. (1965). Psychopathic personality as pathological stimulus seeking. *American Journal of Psychiatry, 122,* 180–183.

Quay, H. (Ed.). (1987). *Handbook of juvenile delinquency.* New York, NY: John Wiley.

Rancourt, A. M. (1991a). A explanation of the relationships among substance abuse, recreation, and leisure for women who abuse substances. *Therapeutic Recreation Journal, 25*(3), 9–18.

Rancourt, A. M. (1991b). The benefits of therapeutic recreation in chemical dependency. In C. P. Coyle, W. B. Kinney, B. Riley, and J. Shank (Eds.), *Benefits of therapeutic recreation: A consensus view* (pp. 17–67). Philadelphia, PA: Temple University.

Sher, K. J. and Levenson, R. W. (1982). Risk for alcoholism and individual differences in the stress-response-dampening effects of alcohol. *Journal of Abnormal Psychology, 91,* 350–367.

U. S. Department of Health and Human Services. (1999). *National household survey on drug abuse: Main findings 1997 (*DHHS Publication No. SMA 99-3295). Rockville, MD: Substance Abuse and Mental Health Services Administration.

Vaillant, G. E. (1983). *The natural history of alcoholism.* Cambridge, MA: Harvard University Press.

Witman, J. (1993). The distinctiveness of adventure programming in adolescent treatment: Participants; perspectives. In G. Hitzhusen, L. Thomas, and M. Birdsong (Eds.), *Expanding horizons in therapeutic recreation XV* (pp. 150–155). Columbia, MO: University of Missouri.

CHAPTER 8
DISORDERS IDENTIFIED IN CHILDHOOD, ADOLESCENCE, OR LATE ADULTHOOD

This chapter focuses on illnesses usually diagnosed at specific periods in the lifecycle: childhood, adolescence, and late adulthood. The chapter begins with an overview of mental disorders which affect primarily children or adolescents. We discuss general categories of mental disorders associated with the early stages of life and some of the unique problems of assessment, diagnosis, and treatment of mental conditions among young people. We next present a more detailed discussion of a series of specific disorders, including attention-deficit/hyperactivity disorder, oppositional defiant disorder, conduct disorder, autism, anorexia nervosa, and bulimia nervosa. We also highlight dementia, a mental disturbance almost exclusively related to later life. The presentation begins with a general overview of dementia and then moves to a detailed explanation of the most prevalent form of this disorder, Alzheimer's disease (senile dementia of the Alzheimer's type).

Overview of Mental Disorders in Childhood

The roots of mental illness do not lie within the individual alone. Mental disorders are generally considered products of transactions between the individual and his or her environment. Diagnosis of a mental disorder requires systematic assessment of individual attributes such as mood, thought patterns, and behavior, as well as consideration of the environment in which the individual resides. Simply put, our best understanding of mental illness suggests a complex genetic and environ-

mental relationship in which our brain shapes our behavior and learning shapes our brain.

One can appreciate the difficulty inherent in attempting to diagnose mental disorders in children and adolescents. The period of early life is characterized by the development of the brain. This process is associated with change in terms of perception of self, social identity and relationships to others, and understanding of the world. The standard signs and symptoms used to identify mental abnormalities in adults may often be inappropriate when applied to younger populations.

Even with the aid of popular diagnostic classification systems such as the *Diagnostic and Statistical Manual of Mental Disorders* (APA, 1994), the identification of mental disorders is more difficult with children than with adults for several reasons. First, children are often unable to verbalize thoughts and feelings. Thus mental health professionals must frequently rely on other people, such as parents and teachers, to help assess the mental state in children. Second, children's normal development presents an ever-changing framework that complicates evaluation. Some behaviors that may be quite normal at one age may suggest psychological problems at another age (e.g., thumb sucking, bedwetting). Symptoms such as outbursts of anger, difficulty in paying attention, fearfulness or shyness, and difficulties in following directions may be reflective of a child's developmental level rather than an indication of some underlying mental disturbance. Third, the criteria for diagnosing most mental disorders in children and adolescents are derived from those for adults. Relatively little research has been completed to assure the validity of these criteria in children. The expression, manifestation, and the course of a disorder might be very different between younger individuals and adults.

These problems of assessment and diagnosis in children carry over into treatment strategies as well. Most traditional treatment regimens for mental disorders include some combination of psychotherapy and pharmacological intervention. However, research dealing with the efficacy of various treatments has been completed almost exclusively using adult populations. Information about the safety and effectiveness of using various treatments, especially the use of drugs with young children, remains limited. A recent report by the Surgeon General of the United States on mental health (National Institutes of Mental Health, 1999) identified increased research on psychotropic drugs in the treatment of mental disorders in children and adolescents as a priority area of study.

The *DSM-IV* (APA, 1994) classifies mental disorders with onset in childhood and adolescence into nine broad categories:

- Anxiety disorders
- Attention-deficit and disruptive behavior disorders
- Autism and other pervasive developmental disorders
- Eating disorders
- Elimination disorders
- Learning and communication disorders
- Mood disorders (e.g., depressive disorders)
- Schizophrenia
- Tic disorders (e.g., Tourette's disorder)

Several of these categories apply not just to children but to individuals of various ages. Anxiety disorders, mood disorders, and schizophrenia are examples of illnesses which may occur across the entire lifecycle. Other disorders on this list (elimination disorders, learning and communication disorders, and tic disorders) are primarily diagnosed among younger individuals and rarely seen by therapeutic recreation (TR) professionals and consequently not discussed in the present chapter. The remaining three categories (attention-deficit and disruptive behavior disorders, autism and other pervasive developmental disorders, and eating disorders) represent conditions with which TR personnel should be familiar. As a result, these illnesses will be reviewed more extensively.

Attention-Deficit and Disruptive Behavior Disorders

This broad category includes a cluster of disorders almost exclusively diagnosed in individuals between 6 and 17 years. These children share in common limited, inflexible behaviors that inhibit their ability to deal with certain aspects of their environment. While specific behaviors vary with each disorder, individuals display characteristics that impair interpersonal relationships and hinder their ability to display appropriate behavior under normal conditions. In addition, while children diagnosed with these disorders generally have the capacity to learn at normal rates, their behaviors tend to interfere with their ability to learn. This section focuses on three specific disorders: attention-deficit/hyperactivity disorder (ADHD), oppositional defiant disorder (ODD), and conduct disorder (CD).

Attention-Deficit/Hyperactivity Disorder (ADHD)

As the name suggests, *attention-deficit/hyperactivity disorder* (ADHD) is associated with two distinct sets of symptoms: an abnormally short attention span and hyperactivity–impulsivity. In most instances these two problems occur together, although the presence of just one is enough to qualify for a diagnosis of ADHD under *DSM-IV* standards (APA, 1994). The disorder has been called many names over the years, including minimal brain damage, minimal cerebral dysfunction, and hyperactive child syndrome. The term attention-deficit/hyperactivity disorder has evolved as the understanding of this form of dysfunction has improved.

The diagnosis of ADHD is made when a child displays persistent symptoms of inattention or hyperactivity–impulsivity for at least six months and to a degree that it is maladaptive and inconsistent with the individual's development stage. Inattention may not become apparent until the child enters a school environment. According to diagnostic criteria established by the American Psychological Association, *inattention* is diagnosed by the presence of at least six of the following symptoms, which have persisted for at least six months:

- Fails to give close attention to details
- Makes careless mistakes in schoolwork, work, or other activities
- Has difficulty sustaining attention in tasks or play activities
- Does not seem to listen when spoken to directly
- Does not follow through on instructions
- Fails to finish schoolwork, chores, or duties in the workplace (not due to oppositional behavior or failure to understand instructions)
- Has difficulty organizing tasks and activities
- Avoids, dislikes, or is reluctant to engage in tasks that require sustained mental effort (e.g., schoolwork or homework)
- Loses thing necessary for tasks or activities (e.g., toys, school assignments, pencils, books, or tools)
- Easily distracted by extraneous stimuli
- Forgetful in daily activities

Hyperactivity–impulsivity is the second set of symptoms associated with ADHD. Criteria established by *DSM-IV* (APA, 1994) state that hyperactivity–impulsivity may be confirmed by the presence of at least six of the following symptoms, which have persisted for at least six months.

Hyperactivity

- Fidgets with hands or feet or squirms in seat
- Leaves seat in classroom or in other situations when remaining seated is expected
- Runs about or climbs excessively in situations in which it is inappropriate (in adolescents or adults, may be limited to subjective feelings of restlessness)
- Has difficulty playing or engaging in leisure activities quietly
- Talks excessively

Impulsivity

- Blurts out answers before questions have been completed
- Has difficulty awaiting turn
- Interrupts or intrudes on others

In addition to the symptoms of inattention or hyperactivity–impulsivity, the diagnosis of ADHD can be established when all four of the following criteria are met (APA, 1994):

- Some hyperactive–impulsive or inattentive symptoms that cause impairment present before age 7
- Some impairment from the symptoms present in two or more settings (e.g., school, work, home)
- Clear evidence of significant impairment in social, academic, or occupational functioning
- Symptoms do not occur exclusively during the course of a pervasive developmental disorder, schizophrenia, or other psychotic disorder and are not better accounted for by another mental disorder (e.g., mood disorder, anxiety disorder, dissociative disorder, or personality disorder)

Children diagnosed with ADHD usually have difficulty paying attention to details, are easily distracted, and have difficulty following through on tasks and assignments. Individuals affected by ADHD typically display a low tolerance for frustration, lack motivation for all but the most stimulating activities, tend to become bored very easily, and have a relative inability to understand potential consequences of their behavior. They have difficulty learning from their mistakes, which often leads to poor performance at school, unpopularity with their peers, and behaviors which present challenges to parents and teachers (National Institutes of Mental Health, 1999).

These children often experience such difficulties for several years before being correctly diagnosed. Despite these problems, some persons with ADHD have the ability to be highly successful in areas of interest to which they devote their motivation and energy. ADHD occurs in individuals with a range of intellectual and social abilities. Although some have good social skills, many have difficulty due to impairments in reading the nuances of social behavior or inhibiting impulsive responses (Whalen & Henker, 1992).

The characteristics of and the difficulties for a child with ADHD frequently change with age. Although children with hyperactivity often display symptoms during the preschool years, those who are primarily inattentive may not have difficulties until the elementary school years, when the persistent demands of the educational setting tax their limited attention span. Social difficulties and peer rejection are common, especially in less structured situations such as the lunchroom or playground. In the majority of individuals symptoms of ADHD persist to some degree into adolescence and adulthood (Hill & Schoener, 1996). Adolescents may have difficulty with organization and planning for longer-term projects and college work; adults may have concerns about handling the demands of marriage, family, and work (Barkley, 1990; Wender, 1995).

ADHD frequently coexists with other disorders of behavior and learning. Many children with ADHD develop learning difficulties that may not improve with treatment. While variance in the definition of learning disability creates difficulty in establishing a concise estimate of the co-occurrence of ADHD and learning problems, some researchers have suggested that as many as 26% of children with ADHD also have a learning disability (Barkley, 1990; Shaywitz & Shaywitz, 1988). Hyperactive behavior is often associated with the development of other disruptive disorders, particularly conduct and oppositional-defiant disorders. It is estimated that nearly half of all children with ADHD (mostly boys) tend to have these disorders (National Institutes of Mental Health, 1999). In addition, children and adults with ADHD are also at increased risk for mood disorders such as depression and anxiety (APA, 1994; Barkley, 1990).

Prevalence

ADHD is the most commonly diagnosed behavioral disorder of childhood. It affects an estimated 3% to 5% of all children, perhaps as many as 2 million young

Americans. Boys are four times more likely to be diagnosed with the disorder than are girls. On average, at least one child in every classroom in the United States needs help with the disorder (U. S. Department of Health and Human Services, 1996).

Causes

The exact etiology of ADHD remains unknown. The inability to pinpoint an exact cause or set of causes certainly has not been from lack of effort. Over the last several decades researchers have explored a number of possible theories about the causes of ADHD. One of the first theories linked attention disorders to undetectable damage to the brain, perhaps from early infection or complications at birth. Based on this theory, the disorder was called minimal brain damage or minimal brain dysfunction for a number of years. However, upon examination this theory was eventually rejected because it could explain only a limited number of cases of ADHD.

In the late 1970s researchers postulated that the core problem was parental inattention. In 1980 this view led to the adoption in *DSM-III* of the diagnostic label attention-deficit disorder (APA, 1980). Eventually this explanation was abandoned when studies failed to support its basic hypothesis.

Another theory was that refined sugar and food additives make children inattentive and hyperactive. As a result, parents were encouraged to stop serving children food containing artificial flavorings, preservatives, and sugars. Upon a thorough review of data, however, the National Institutes of Health rejected this explanation in the early 1980s (U. S. Department of Health and Human Services, 1996).

Recent etiological research has focused upon natural activity levels in certain areas of the brain. Using new scientific tools and techniques for studying the brain, most scientists now believe that traceable differences exist in brain activity levels between individuals diagnosed with ADHD and those who are not. One popular line of this research views ADHD as caused by the inadequate availability of the neurotransmitter dopamine in the central nervous system of afflicted individuals. *Dopamine* is known to play a key role in initiating purposeful movement and increasing motivation and alertness. The dopamine hypothesis posits that insufficient levels of the neurotransmitter would account for the inattention and hyperactivity associated with ADHD (National Institutes of Mental Health, 1999).

ADHD runs in families, thus inheritance is considered an important risk factor (APA, 1994). Between 10% and 35% of children diagnosed with ADHD have a first degree relative with past or present ADHD. Approximately one half of parents who had ADHD also have a child with the disorder (Biederman, Faraone, and Keenan, 1992). These findings suggest that genes play an important role in the causation of ADHD. Consistent with material identified in the previous paragraph, much of the genetic research is focusing upon genes associated with the transport and reception of dopamine (National Institutes of Health, 1999).

A variety of other conditions known to affect brain development may predispose a child to developing this disorder. These include fetal exposure to cigarettes, alcohol, cocaine, and other drugs. Toxins in the environment may also disrupt brain development, which may lead to ADHD. One such toxin suspected of being a possible contributor to developmental disorders like ADHD is lead, often found in flaking paint in areas where leaded gasoline or lead-based paint once were (U.S. Department of Health and Human Services, 1996).

Oppositional Defiant Disorder

Oppositional defiant disorder (ODD) is diagnosed when a child displays a recurrent pattern of defiance, disobedience, and hostility toward various authority figures, including parents, teachers, and other adults. ODD is characterized by such problem behaviors as persistent stubbornness, resistance to directions, and unwillingness to give in to adults or peers. Children with ODD tend to be defiant and hostile. They are frequently involved in arguments and fights, are deliberately annoying to others, hold grudges and seem to be disposed to revenge (APA, 1994).

Diagnostic criteria used to identify ODD is based on a pattern of negative, hostile, and deviant behavior that persists for at least six months during which four (or more) of the following are present:

- Loses temper
- Argues with adults
- Actively defies or refuses to comply with adults' requests or rules
- Deliberately annoys people
- Blames others for his or her mistakes or behaviors
- Touchy or easily annoyed by others
- Angry and resentful
- Spiteful or vindictive

The disturbance in behaviors associated with the disorder cause clinically significant impairment in social, academic, or occupational function (APA, 1994).

ODD is commonly associated with other childhood psychiatric conditions. It is estimated that between 30% and 40% of children diagnosed with ADHD also have ODD (Chandler, 1999). While ADHD and ODD commonly coexist, they are distinguished by the fact that ODD is characterized by aggressiveness and purposefully annoying behaviors, whereas ADHD is marked by impulsiveness, inattention, and poor social skills. ODD is also associated with childhood mood and psychotic disorders and is sometimes a precursor to conduct disorder (National Institutes of Health, 1999).

Although oppositional behavior is not unusual among children and adolescents, it is most often transient and diminishes as the individual advances in age. In contrast, with ODD the number of oppositional symptoms tends to increase with age. Onset is typically gradual and symptoms most often emerge in the home setting and eventually spread to other settings. The disorder usually becomes evident before age 8, but seldom later than early adolescence (APA, 1994).

Prevalence

The APA (1994) reports rates of ODD at 2% to 16%; however, a recent document published by the National Institutes of Health (1999) estimates the prevalence of ODD at 1% to 6%. Prevalence rates vary depending on the nature of the population sampled and the way the disorder is evaluated. Rates are generally lower when impairment criteria are more strict. Before puberty, the condition is more common among boys, but after puberty the rates in both genders are equal (National Institutes of Health, 1999).

Causes

ODD has no known cause, but a familial pattern seems to exist. The disorder is more common in families in which at least one parent has a history of mental disturbance. In particular, children whose parents have mood disorders, disruptive behavior disorders (e.g., ODD, conduct disorder, ADHD, antisocial personality disorder), as well as substance-related disorders seem to be at higher risk for ODD. Chandler (1999) has written that if a parent is alcoholic and has been in trouble with the law, their children are almost three times as likely to have ODD than a child without this family background. In addition, it appears the disorder is more common in families in which there is serious marital discord (APA, 1994).

Conduct Disorder

In some ways *conduct disorder* (CD) may be thought of as a more severe version of ODD; however, the American Psychiatric Association (1994) views the two disorders as separate and distinct psychiatric disturbances. The primary characteristic of CD is a repetitive and persistent pattern of behavior in which the basic rights of others or major societal norms or rules are consistently violated. The behaviors associated with CD fall into four main categories: aggressive conduct, which threatens or causes physical harm to other individuals or to animals; nonaggressive conduct that results in property loss or damage; deceitfulness or theft; and serious violations of rules and norms.

Diagnostic criteria used to identify CD are based upon the presence of at least three of the following criteria (from any category) during the last 12 months. At least one criterion must have been present in the last 6 months. Diagnosis of CD also requires that these behaviors cause significant impairment in social, academic, or, occupational functioning (APA, 1994).

Aggression to people and animals

- Bullies, threatens, or intimidates others
- Initiates physical fights
- Uses a weapon that can cause serious physical harm to others (e.g., bat, brick, broken bottle, knife, gun)
- Physically cruel to animals
- Physically cruel to people
- Steals while confronting a victim (e.g., mugging, purse snatching, extortion, armed robbery)

Destruction of property

- Engages in fire setting with the intention of causing serious damage
- Destroys property other than by fire setting

Deceitfulness or theft

- Breaks into someone else's house, building, or car
- Lies to obtain goods or favors or to avoid work
- Steals items of nontrivial value without confronting a victim (e.g., shoplifting, forgery)

Serious violations of rules

- Stays out at night despite parental prohibitions, beginning before 13 years of age
- Runs away from home overnight on at least two separate occasions
- Skips school before age 13

Individuals with conduct disorder behave aggressively by fighting, bullying, intimidating, assaulting, or being cruel to people or animals. They may have little empathy for the feelings, wishes, and well-being of others. Vandalism with deliberate destruction of property (e.g., setting fires, breaking windows) is common, as is theft, truancy, precocious sexual activity, and substance abuse. Girls with CD often run away from home and are at higher risk to become involved in prostitution. Behaviors common to CD usually interfere with performance in school; persons with this disorder rarely perform to the level predicted by their age or IQ score. They have difficulty establishing and maintaining healthy relationships with peers and adults. They have injury rates considerably higher than their peers. In addition, they are prone to school expulsion and problems with the law (Shaffer et al., 1996b).

Persons with conduct disorder frequently exhibit characteristics associated with other psychiatric disorders. By far the most common combination is CD coexisting with ADHD. According to Chandler, as many as 30% to 50% of children with CD will also have ADHD (1999). Another 25% to 50% of children with CD will have either an anxiety disorder or depression (Chandler, 1999). Also common are associations with substance-related disorders, learning disorders, and bipolar disorder (Chandler, 1999). The onset of CD may occur as early as age 5 or 6, but is usually evident in late childhood or early adolescence. Onset is rare after 16 years. For many individuals with CD, the symptoms diminish with maturity. Many individuals diagnosed with the disorder achieve adequate levels of social and occupational adjustment as adults. Generally, the earlier the onset of CD the worse the prognosis and the greater the risk in adult life for other psychiatric disturbances, especially substance-related disorders and antisocial personality disorders (APA, 1994).

DSM-IV (APA, 1994) recognizes two subtypes of CD. *Childhood-onset type* is characterized by the onset of at least one criterion behavior prior to age 10. Boys are more commonly afflicted than girls, and boys' behaviors are usually marked by physical aggression and disturbed relationships with peers. Individuals diagnosed with this type of CD usually have symptoms that meet full criteria for conduct disorder prior to puberty. They tend to have persistent symptoms of CD, and are more likely to develop adult antisocial personality disorder than the later developing type of CD (APA, 1994). *Adolescent-onset type* is characterized by the development of symptoms of the disorder after age 10. Individuals with this form of the disorder seem to be less likely to display persistent aggressive behaviors;

they usually develop better social skills, and have a much better overall prognosis than those with the childhood-onset type of CD. The ratio of males to females is lower for the adolescent-onset type of the disorder.

Prevalence

As with ODD, prevalence rates for CD vary widely depending on the definition of the disorder and the nature of the population samples. According to the APA (1994) prevalence rates for persons under age 18 range from 6 to 16% for males and from 2% to 9% percent for females. In contrast, data provided by Shaffer and colleagues (1996a) place rates among 9 to 17 year olds in the 1% to 4% range. The disorder appears to be more common in urban rather rural areas (APA, 1994). Children with an early onset of the disorder have a worse prognosis and a higher risk for personality disorders in adulthood.

Causes

As with ADHD and ODD, the etiology of conduct disorder remains unknown. It is suspected that both biological (including genetic) and psychosocial components may contribute (Raine, Reynolds, Venables, Mednick & Farington, 1998). Children whose biological parents have a history of psychological disturbances, including ADHD, CD, alcohol dependence, mood disorders, or schizophrenia seem to be at a higher risk than peers who do not have a similar family history. Social risk factors for conduct disorder include early maternal rejection, separation from parents with no adequate alternative caregivers, parental marital discord, and family neglect or abuse (Loeber & Stouthamer-Loeber, 1986). Physical risk factors include neurological damage caused by birth complications, low birthweight, learning disorders, and stimulation-seeking/high-risk behavior (National Institutes of Health, 1999).

Treatment of Attention Deficit and Disruptive Behavior Disorders

Although attention-deficit/hyperactivity disorder, oppositional disorder, and conduct disorder are distinct forms of behavioral disturbances, the most commonly accepted approaches to treating the disorders are similar. According to the American Academy of Child and Adolescent Psychiatry (1991), the cornerstone of treatment includes a combination of psychosocial interventions (aimed at helping parents and teachers reduce undesirable and disruptive behavior by means of training in behavioral techniques) and pharmacological interventions (aimed at treating symptoms of these disorders). In many instances a combination of these two forms of treatment is used to help manage problem behaviors. We will briefly discuss each of these two intervention strategies.

Psychosocial Interventions

Psychosocial interventions usually involve training in behavioral management techniques for parents and teachers of youth with ADHD, ODD, or CD. They often include programs geared to help individuals diagnosed with these disorders to develop coping skills to deal with troubling aspects of their environments. Several intervention approaches are available.

Individual psychotherapy is often used with children and adolescents who have the capacity for self-observation and introspection. It helps these individuals to accept themselves despite their disorders. With this intervention clients talk with trained therapists about upsetting thoughts and feelings and explore self-defeating patterns of behavior. Therapists attempt to help their clients to understand their situations and to develop alternative ways to handle their emotions.

Cognitive–behavioral therapy helps people to work on immediate issues of concern. Rather than focusing upon understanding feelings and actions, this approach attempts to develop strategies to directly change behaviors. It may provide assistance in helping to think through tasks and organize one's thoughts, or to develop techniques for controlling impulsive behavior.

Social skill training can help children and adolescents learn new behaviors. In social skills training the therapist displays appropriate behaviors like taking turns, sharing, asking for help, or responding to criticism. The client is then provided the chance to practice each skill. Oftentimes this form of training is used to help the client see how their actions may affect other people. As the name implies, this psychosocial approach emphasizes skills that enhance the individuals' ability to get along with others.

Parenting skills training, which may be offered by therapists or in special classes, provides parents with techniques to manage their child's behavior. Many of these skills are based upon strategies developed in behavior modification programs. One commonly used

technique is time out. *Time out* is used when a child becomes too unruly or out of control. During time outs, the child is removed from the situation and remains alone until calm. Parents are also taught skills for increasing desired behaviors by means of physical or verbal reinforcement. In addition, parents may be taught to provide the child quality time each day, in which they share pleasurable, relaxing moments (U. S. Department of Health and Human Services, 1996).

Pharmacological Interventions

Pharmacological interventions usually involve administering medications to the individual with behavior problems in an attempt to treat the symptoms of the disorder. *Psychostimulants* are drugs that enhance (stimulate) the action of neurotransmitters in the central nervous systems. At present, three psychostimulants—methylphenidate (Ritalin), dextroamphetamine (Dexedrine), and pemoline (Cylert)—are commonly used to treat behavior problems. For many individuals these medicines dramatically reduce their hyperactivity and improve their ability to focus and learn (National Institutes of Mental Health, 1996). Children who do not respond to one stimulant may respond to another. They may also help control the impulsive, destructive behavior that accompanies conduct disorder; however, no drugs have been demonstrated to be consistently effective in treating CD (National Institutes of Health, 1999).

As useful as drugs such as Ritalin have proven to be in helping to treat behavioral disorders, they have also sparked a great deal of controversy. Parameters for establishing appropriate dosage levels for medications used with children remain controversial. Individual monitoring by trained professionals is required to ensure that pharmacological interventions are administered at safe levels for each child or adolescent. A second concern deals with the potential side effects of drug use. Common stimulant side effects include insomnia, decreased appetite, weight loss, headaches, jitteriness, and alterations in growth patterns. While most of these side effects appear to be mild, recede over time, and respond to dose changes, (National Institutes of Health, 1999) it is natural for parents to be concerned about whether taking a medicine is in their child's best interest. Another debate is whether Ritalin and other stimulant drugs are prescribed unnecessarily for too many children. Critics argue that many factors in a young person's environment may cause them to seem overactive, impulsive, or inattentive. Prescribing drugs to children reacting to momentary sources of stress may be unnecessary and potentially harmful. In spite of such controversies, however, evidence supports the fact that as many as nine out of ten children diagnosed with ADHD, ODD, and CD show improvement when carefully treated with medication (U. S. Department of Health and Human Services, 1996).

Pervasive Developmental Disorders

In the past terms such as childhood psychosis, childhood schizophrenia, and atypical development commonly described children with marked impairments in social interaction skills, and communication skills, as well as stereotyped patterns of behavior, interests, and activities. Since 1980 the American Psychiatric Association has labeled this group of symptoms *pervasive developmental disorders* (PDD). The current edition of the *DSM* (*DSM-IV*; APA, 1994) recognizes five separate syndromes under PDD: autistic disorder (autism), Aspergers' disorder, Rett's disorder, childhood disintegrative disorders, and PDD not otherwise specified. We discuss the first three disorders in this chapter.

Autistic Disorder (Autism)

Autism is a perplexing developmental disorder marked by the tendency to turn inward, without interest in formulating relationships with other individuals. *Autistic disorder* is the most pronounced expression of the pervasive developmental disorders, and individual manifestations vary greatly in severity.

Autism existed long before it was systematically studied by Dr. Leo Kanner in the 1940s. Dr. Kanner, a child psychiatrist, published the first description of what he called "autistic disturbances of affective contact" in 1943 (p. 217). He based his description on extensive observations of 11 children who shared similar recognizable traits. According to Kanner, each of these children displayed "an inability to relate themselves in an ordinary way to people and situations from the beginning of life" (1943, p. 242). He also observed several other common traits, including a preference for being alone, an insistence on sameness in their environment, a liking for elaborate and ritualistic routines, and some abilities that seemed remarkable compared with their obvious deficits.

In the 1950s researchers believed autism to be an expression of a psychological disturbance (e.g., psychosis, schizophrenia). Further study, however, demon-

strated that this view of autism was probably inaccurate. Most current research suggests a biological cause, and the syndrome is usually recognized as a pervasive developmental disorder related to deficits within the central nervous system. The currently accepted view as to the nature and diagnostic criteria for autism was first developed by the Autism Society of America in 1977 (Ritvo & Freeman, 1977). The American Psychiatric Association has subsequently revised this view. It is generally accepted that autism is a:

- *Spectrum disorder*—ranging from extremely mild (close to normal) to very severe
- *Developmental diagnosis*—expression of the syndrome varies with age and developmental level of the individual affected
- *Retrospective diagnosis*—diagnosis cannot be made without taking a careful developmental history of the person involved
- *Syndrome*—may coexist with other conditions (e.g., mental retardation)

Diagnostic Criteria

No one specific test identifies autistic disorder. It is usually diagnosed by the presence or absence of certain behaviors. For the diagnosis of autism to be confirmed, a child must have onset of symptoms prior to 3 years of age and meet 6 of the 12 criteria listed in the *DSM-IV* (APA, 1994). These 12 criteria are equally distributed among 3 broad categories: reciprocal social interactions, communication impairments, and behavior abnormalities (APA, 1994, pp. 70–71).

1. Qualitative impairment in *social interactions*, as manifested by at least two of the following:
   - Marked impairment in the use of nonverbal behaviors such as eye contact, facial expressions, body postures, and gestures
   - Failure to develop peer relationships appropriate to developmental level
   - Lack of spontaneous seeking to share enjoyment, interests, or achievements with other people
   - Lack of social or emotional reciprocity
2. Qualitative impairments in *communication*, as manifested by at least one of the following:
   - Delay in or total lack of the development of spoken language (not accompanied by an attempt to compensate through alternative modes of communication such as gesture or mime)

- Marked impairment in the ability to initiate or sustain a conversation with others (in individuals with adequate speech)
- Stereotyped and repetitive use of language or idiosyncratic language
- Lack of varied, spontaneous make-believe play or social imitative play appropriate to developmental level

3. Restricted, repetitive, and stereotyped *patterns of behavior* as manifested by at least one of the following:

- Preoccupation with one or more stereotyped and restricted patterns or interest that is abnormal either in intensity or focus
- Inflexible adherence to specific, nonfunctional routines or rituals
- Stereotyped and repetitive motor mannerisms (e.g., hand or finger flapping or twisting, or complex whole-body movements)
- Persistent preoccupation with parts of objects

Symptoms

As indicated by the diagnostic criteria, the core symptoms of autistic disorder include delays in language development and communication skills, marked limitations in socialization and social behaviors, and unusual and/or aberrant behaviors and interests. Infants with autism often have poor eye contact and are irritable and stiffen when held. In the first and second years of life, they may be unresponsive to caretakers, failing to develop the social bonds that characterize most parent–child relationships. They are often described as both difficult to care for (due to their resistance to change and accompanying temper tantrums) and easy to care for (due to their tendency to entertain themselves for long periods with peculiar interests and activities). They often engage in self-stimulation and self-injurious behaviors such as head banging. They may develop very erratic patterns of sleep, which contribute to the problems experienced by caretakers.

Speech may not develop or develop very slowly. Use and understanding of common nonverbal communication is poor. They may indicate their needs by using the hands of other individuals. They speak infrequently, and when they do speak they often parrot words or phrases or talk incessantly about one topic. They rarely initiate conversation. In addition, children with autism usually have problems understanding the content and timing of communication, have difficulty grasping concepts (especially abstract ones), and often have a hard time answering even simple questions posed to them. In rare instances, some children with autism may speak fluently, but they tend to be overly literal in their understanding of language (e.g., they may have difficulty understanding that an "ear of corn" does not mean that a person's ear is made of corn).

Socially, autistic syndrome is characterized by displays of marked indifference towards others, including primary caretakers. They tend to be slow to develop an understanding of social cues and have much difficulty relating to others. They often seem to avoid contact with others and appear very content to be left alone. It is not uncommon for the child with autism to develop strong, inappropriate attachments to objects rather than people. Their play behavior is solitary, as they seem uninterested in other children. They may use toys in odd ways, such as repeatedly spinning or lining up play objects. They seldom engage in pretend or imaginative forms of play.

Autism is also characterized by the inability to understand the feelings of others. When the child with autism expresses emotions, they tend to be narrow in focus and inappropriate to the situation. The child may frequently giggle or laugh inappropriately, which adds to the discomfort of those around them. Overall, most individuals with the disorder exhibit behaviors that may be classified as socially awkward.

A wide variety of unusual nonsocial behaviors are also common, including *stimulus overselectivity*, whereby an individual focuses only on one aspect of an object or environment while ignoring all other aspects. Caretakers of these children often complain that they frequently seem to act deaf or they continuously stare or fixate on a particular object or aspect of an object (e.g., light reflecting off a spinning object). It is not unusual for the child with this syndrome to have an extreme aversion to change, constantly preferring sameness in their world. They may also frequently express strange fears of nonthreatening objects (e.g., abstract art), while lacking fear of objects that may present real danger (e.g., heavy traffic). Children with autism commonly explore objects in their environment in odd ways, often using such methods as inappropriate licking, mouthing, or smelling. Additionally, many children with autism display the odd habit of relying on peripheral rather than straight on vision when viewing people and objects. Finally, autism is commonly related to the use of many forms of self-injurious behaviors such as head banging, hand biting, and excessive scratching or rubbing.

Prevalence and Associated Features

Autism is relatively rare. According to the criteria used by Kanner, it appears in approximately 4 of every 10,000 births (Frith, 1997). With the more current diagnostic criteria used by APA (1994), the incidence remains about the same at a projected rate of 2–5 cases per 10,000 individuals. Rates of the disorder are four times higher in males than in females (Coleman and Gilberg, 1992). There is also an increased risk of autistic disorder among siblings of individuals with the disorder (APA, 1994).

As identified by diagnostic criteria, the onset of autistic disorder occurs prior to age 3. Parents of children with this syndrome often report concerns about their child at a much younger age, however, because of the infants' lack of interest in parental attention. Children with the disorder commonly demonstrate an indifference or aversion to affection or physical comfort and a failure to respond to eye contact or parents' voices. In a minority of cases, the child may be reported to have developed normally throughout the first year or two (APA, 1994).

As the child develops, improvements in some areas of functioning are common. The presence of communicative speech and overall intellectual level are the strongest predictors of eventual independent functioning. Available data suggest that about one third of individuals with autistic disorder experience full or partial functional independence in adulthood (APA, 1994).

Some individuals with autism have restricted areas of extremely high cognitive functioning. These areas, labeled "islets of ability" by O'Connor and Hermelin, (1991), often include decoding skills, musical skills, exceptional rote memory, the ability to do rapid calculations such as identifying the day of the week for distant dates, and an unusual capacity for jigsaw puzzles. When present, however, these abilities do not seem to help individuals solve problems in their daily lives (Mauk, Reber & Batshaw, 1997).

Autistic disorder is also associated with increased risk for other developmental disabilities, most frequently mental retardation. Approximately 75% of children with autism function at a retarded level (moderate range, IQ 35–50), most commonly requiring extensive services (APA, 1994). Autism can be distinguished from mental retardation by its characteristic social and behavior problems and by a different pattern of cognitive impairment. For instance, whereas children with autistic disorder typically avoid social interactions, socialization is seldom considered problematic for people with mental retardation. Similarly, while language impairments are a prominent feature of autism, delays in language development usually occur within the context of broader cognitive deficits among children with mental retardation. Dr. William Barbaresi of the Mayo Clinic explained this point:

> A mentally retarded child with an IQ of 70 is likely able to carry on a conversation with another person, only at a more simple level (than normal). However, a child with autism and the same IQ may be completely incapable of using language. (1999, p. 2)

Etiology

For many years, autism was thought to be a psychological disorder without an organic basis. In particular, autistic disorder was often believed to be a form of schizophrenia. However, systematic observation found key distinctions between the two disorders. Although the child with autism often behaves in an odd manner, they do not experience the delusions and hallucinations that characterized schizophrenia. In addition, while a child with autistic disorder lacks imagination, a child with schizophrenia may live in a fantasy world of his or her own creation (Mauk, Reber & Batshaw, 1997).

With little evidence to support a psychological cause of autism, psychogenic theories began to emerge. These theories primarily focused on the idea that a child could become autistic because of some existentially threatening experience. At the center of many of these theories was a "refrigerator mother"—a cold and distant mother who failed to bond with her child. Due to the mother's inability to demonstrate affection toward her offspring, the child experienced a severe sense of rejection, which drove them to withdraw into their own inner world that other people could never penetrate. Little evidence exists to support these theories, however, and a growing number of documented cases also exists wherein a child was exposed to severe rejection and deprivation in childhood without the development of autistic disorder (Frith, 1997).

Recent efforts to identify the cause of the disorder have focused upon a potential biological link. Current research seems to indicate that anything that can produce structural or functional damage in the central nervous system can also produce autism. Several recent studies of people with autism have found abnormalities in different regions of the brain, including the cerebellum, hippocampus, and amygdala (Frith, 1997). Neurons in these regions appear to be smaller than normally expected, and the nerve fibers in these regions appear to be physically stunted in appearance (Frith, 1997). The belief among a growing number of scientists studying autism is that eventually neurological mechanisms will be found that underlie the disorder (Mayo Clinic, 1999).

Treatment

Due to the pervasive nature of autism, treatment must be intensive, continuous, and multidisciplinary. The overall treatment goal is lifelong habitation, a process of allowing the individual to gain the necessary skills to function as independently as possible (Hawkins, 1996). According to Mauk and colleagues (1997, p. 436), the main objectives of the treatment of autism include:

- Fostering development
- Promoting learning
- Reducing rigidity and stereotyping
- Eliminating nonspecific maladaptive behaviors
- Alleviating family distress

The interventions most commonly employed include behavioral therapies, education programs, speech-language therapy, pharmacological management, and family support.

Behavioral therapies decrease maladaptive behaviors while increasing adaptive ones. Positive reinforcement is commonly used, although mild punishments such as time out may be required. The efficacy of behavior treatment in leading to improved functioning depends on the severity of the behavior problem, the age treatment is started, and the intensity of the treatment. To produce desired results, behavioral approaches should be integrated into both the home and school environment. Parental involvement in behavioral interventions is essential for successful outcomes (Mauk, Reber & Batshaw, 1997).

Education programs initially focus on teaching social and communication skills. With development, the focus often shifts to skills needed to function in one's present environment or in preparation for functioning in a new environment. Using a functional approach to learning, a natural context usually involving hands-on experiences is most often emphasized (e.g., ordering food in a restaurant is taught at an actual eating establishment). This approach emphasizes teaching very practical skills that the person with autism needs to function in their world (Hawkins, 1996).

Speech-language therapy programs usually emphasize the pragmatics of language. Because children with autism show limited awareness of others, interactive

and meaningful social conversations need to be modeled and practiced. Reinforcement may be necessary to foster language development in young individuals with autism. Sign language may be used, but it is often difficult for autistic children who may have poor fine motor skills. Augmentative communication devices such as a computer or storyboard can be beneficial for some individuals. The use of art and music may also help develop nonverbal communication skills among some children with this disorder (Mauk, Reber & Batshaw, 1997).

A wide spectrum of drugs has been tested in an effort to treat the core symptoms of autism, but none have proved successful. *Pharmacological management* of specific behaviors (e.g., hyperactivity, aggression, self-injury, sleep disturbances) that interfere with a child's global functioning, however, is an intervention commonly used with autistic individuals.

Intervention in the form of *family support* is often an essential part of the total treatment process. Having a child with autism places enormous stress on the family. In addition to the usual difficulties of having a child with special needs, the child with autism presents many additional challenges. These include the need for intense supervision, disrupted sleep patterns, and behaviors that are very difficult to manage. Moreover, the child with autism provides few emotional rewards for their parents (Mauk, Reber & Batshaw, 1997). The intervention strategy for families involves social and emotional support services, services to assist with an autistic child's development, and social services to enable families to experience growth. Common approaches to family support include parent training, family support groups, and respite care programs (Hawkins, 1996).

Asperger's Disorder

Another example of a pervasive developmental disorder is Asperger's disorder. *Asperger's disorder* is a severe developmental disorder characterized by difficulty in social interaction and restricted and unusual patterns of interest and behavior. It shares many similarities with autism, especially in terms of behavioral and social features, but children with this disorder display no significant delays in language development or impairments in cognition (Szatmari, 1991). In fact, some aspects of cognitive development in children with this disorder may appear advanced. Asperger's has been described as "autism without mental retardation" (Klin & Volkmar, 1995).

The major features of Asperger's disorder include the severe and sustained impairments in social interaction and the development of repetitive patterns of behavior, interests, and activities (APA, 1994). For instance, spoken language may be unusually rigid and formal and the nonverbal aspects of communication (e.g., eye contact, body position) may appear abnormal. Older children with Asperger's often exhibit unusual activities and interests in details and statistics (e.g., maps, airplane schedules, sports statistics). Their social ineptitude, however, prevents them from developing friendships and other close personal relationships (Klin & Volkmar, 1995).

Additionally, individuals with this syndrome usually display delays in motor development and often appear clumsily and awkward. Overall, the disorder causes significant impairment in social and occupational functioning, but because of good language and cognitive skills, this disorder is frequently not recognized until later in childhood. Information on the prevalence of this syndrome is very limited, but it appears to be more common in males (APA, 1994).

Rett's Disorder

Rett's disorder is a progressive neurological disorder. The essential characteristic is the development of multiple specific deficits following a period of normal functioning after birth. Individuals with this disorder apparently experience normal early development through the first several months of life, then begin a progressive deterioration of behavior, language, and mental status. They lose purposeful hand movements and characteristically develop stereotypical "hand washing or hand wringing" actions. There is usually a loss of interest in their social environment. Children with this syndrome commonly experience severe impairment in expressive and receptive language development with severe retardation of motor skills and coordination. Rett's disorder is typically associated with mental retardation requiring extensive to pervasive support. By about age 6 the condition generally stabilizes, but recovery of developmental losses is quite limited. Rett's disorder is much less common than autistic disorder and has only been reported in females (APA, 1994; Mauk, Reber & Batshaw, 1997).

Implications for Therapeutic Recreation

Therapeutic Recreation Specialists (TRS) work with children with each of these disorders in both community and private settings. In community recreation settings, TRS provide programs and services focused upon recreation participation (e.g., aquatics, sports, cultural activities). In most instances, children with these disorders can easily be included in existing programs. The only barrier preventing inclusion for some of these children are problems associated with behavior, such as impulsivity and aggressiveness.

In private or nonprofit residential centers, the TRS usually functions as part of a multidisciplinary treatment team. In this setting TRS assist in the identification and treatment of specific problem behaviors. The TRS might use leisure experiences to prevent or remediate disruptive behaviors or the display of inappropriate responses. The development of skills needed to manage socioemotional needs, to facilitate appropriate interactions with others, and to enhance academic performance are also issues commonly addressed by TRS in these settings (Carter, Van Andel & Robb, 1995). When used, leisure education classes typically focus upon recreation and social skill development.

A substantial quantity of research has studied the effects of outdoor/adventure challenge programs upon behavioral problems among youth. Skalko, Van Andel, and DeSalvatore (1991) identified three different studies which produced data supporting a positive relationship between adventure challenge experiences and improved self-confidence, improved sense of personal responsibility, and positive attitudes toward cooperation and trust among emotionally impaired and adjudicated youths. Rawson and McIntosh (1991) also found significant improvement in self-esteem of over 60 children with severe behavior problems as a result of a therapeutic camping intervention. In contrast, Voight (1988) found no significant changes resulting from the use of ropes courses as a treatment modality for emotionally disturbed adolescents.

Some other recreational programs which have been successfully used with children with ADHD, ODD, and CD include physically active games (e.g., tag, Frisbee, golf, football, parachute activities), arts and crafts (e.g., tie-dyeing, sand terrariums, leather works), storytelling, and role-playing activities (Lundgren, 1995).

Given that disruptive behavior is a predominant characteristic of these populations, the TR professional should take precautions to help ensure successful programming. Procedures such as keeping groups small, varying activities frequently, minimizing competition, maintaining consistent rules and boundaries, and limiting distractions help to make individuals with behavioral disorders feel secure, and make it easier for them to maintain their focus. Reinforcement (e.g., praise, instant rewards) for desired behaviors encourages participation and provides opportunities to develop a sense of competence and mastery over the environment (Lundgren, 1995). While these suggestions are probably applicable for work with any group of children, they are particularly crucial for children with ADHD, ODD, or CD who struggle with attention-demanding situations.

Pervasive Developmental Disorders: Autism

In many ways, the role of TRS for individuals with autism is similar to its role for persons with other forms of developmental disabilities. TR's most fundamental goal with these populations is promoting independent functioning to the greatest level possible for each individual. As such, it attempts to facilitate community adjustment by using leisure experiences to develop collateral skills (e.g., self-care skills, social interaction skills, functional academic skills) and to reduce inappropriate or maladaptive behaviors (Dattilo & Schleien, 1991).

For persons with autism, the primary barriers to recreation involvement are cognitive and social–emotional deficits. These may be exhibited by the inability to understand the purpose or the procedures of an activity, inattentiveness, inappropriate personal or social behaviors, and poor communication skills. Like everyone else, however, leisure experiences can add joy and satisfaction to the life of the person with autism. One goal of TRS with this population is to encourage leisure participation by identifying age-appropriate recreational opportunities that are personally meaningful and pleasurable for individuals with this disorder.

According to Hawkins, "Therapeutic recreation can make its greatest contribution in the treatment of people who have autism when the focus is on social and behavioral skills development" (1996, p. 119). This contribution is often achieved by a combination of leisure education activities and treatment-oriented services. The broad focus of leisure education for individuals with autism is usually upon functional skill development needed to promote successful community adjustment. Skills that are needed may be very basic. Henning and Dalrymple (1986, p. 332) have observed

that persons with autism often are unable to differentiate between play and work activities. They suggest that leisure education may be necessary to help these individuals distinguish free time from obligated time, to learn to differentiate between activities commonly thought of as play or work, and to learn to make choices between leisure and work activities.

A variety of other functional skills may be addressed in leisure education classes. Hawkins (1996) stated that teaching social communication skills, such as appropriate ways of interacting socially within situational contexts (e.g., handshakes and hugs) and teaching functional academic skills (e.g., money-management and time-management skills) may be needed by individuals with autism to successfully adjust to community settings. Carter, Van Andel, and Robb (1995) would add self-care (e.g., personal grooming, appropriate manners) and verbal and nonverbal communication skills to this list. Schmidt, McLaughlin, and Dalrymple (1986) have suggested that sport and leisure skill training (e.g., following rules and understanding personal health and fitness) would also be appropriate topics within a leisure education program. While many of these skill components may seem elementary, it may be necessary to teach them when working with persons with autism, owing to this populations' difficulty in learning appropriate behaviors by means of observation (Henning & Dalrymple, 1986).

In comparison to their nonautistic peers, autistic individuals are less efficient in their capacity to learn by means of observing others. However, evidence suggests that the ability to learn through observation is possible, and seems to be enhanced when persons with autism are exposed to their nondisabled peers. For instance, in a study which integrated children with and without autism into a recreation setting, Schleien, Krotee, Mustonen, Kelterborn, and Schermer (1987) found significant increases in appropriate behavior and significant decreases in inappropriate behavior among the disabled subjects. In a second investigation, Schleien, Rynders, Mustonen, and Fox (1990) found that appropriate play behavior exhibited by children with autism significantly increased when they played in the company of nondisabled peers. This research lends creditability claims of potential benefits of inclusive recreation, and reinforces the goal of community adjustment for persons with autism.

TRS also use leisure experiences as a form of therapy for severely involved autistic individuals. TRS professionals may design recreation experiences that help develop fundamental learning skills such as eye contact, attention, compliance, cooperation, expression, directionality, and sensorimotor awareness. For higher functioning individuals, TR interventions may be focused upon improving self-esteem, social interaction, communication skills, or fine and gross motor skills (Henning and Dalrymple, 1986). The use of exercise as a therapeutic intervention has been demonstrated to be effective in decreasing stereotypic inappropriate and maladaptive behaviors among adolescents with autism (Reid, Factor, Freeman & Sherman, 1988; Elliot, Dobbin, Rose & Soper, 1994; Rosenthal-Malek & Mitchell, 1997).

Children with pervasive developmental disorders have a need to experience success, mastery, acceptance, and a sense of well-being. The leisure experience provided by TRS can be enjoyable, educational, and therapeutic for the autistic person. While fun should be emphasized, recreational activities provide an excellent medium to work on other goals.

Eating Disorders

Severe disturbances in eating behaviors are the most fundamental characteristics of eating disorders. These disturbances may take many forms, including the persistent eating of nonnutritional substances (pica), the repeated regurgitation and rechewing of food (rumination disorder), or weighing 20% or more than the standard weight specified with regard to one's sex, height, and body structure (obesity). While each of these conditions are associated in one way or another with disturbances in eating, pica and rumination disorder are seldom diagnosed and obesity is classified by the *DSM-IV* (APA, 1994) as a general medical condition rather than a psychological or behavioral syndrome.

The two most commonly diagnosed eating disorders in North America are anorexia nervosa (AN) and bulimia nervosa (BN). Both conditions produce severe psychological and physical distress, as the symptoms of these disorders often become the most dominant feature in the daily lives of victims. Both AN and BN develop primarily during the teenage years and early 20s, and the incidence of both is significantly higher among females than among males. The incidence of both conditions has increased dramatically in recent decades. Therapeutic recreation specialists are increasingly being asked to work with individuals with AN and BN.

Anorexia Nervosa

Anorexia nervosa (AN) is a disorder of self-starvation that manifests itself in an extreme aversion to food. It almost exclusively affects adolescent girls, with symptoms involving refusal to eat, rapid weight loss, bizarre preoccupation with food, distorted body image and cessation of menstruation. In her best selling book, *Reviving Ophelia* (1994), Mary Pipher suggests that AN is a result of and protest against the cultural role that young women must be beautiful.

> By her behavior an anorexic girl tells the world: "look, see how thin I am, even thinner than you wanted me to be. You can't make me eat more. I am in control of my fate, even if my fate is starving." (1994, p. 174)

In striving for perfection and approval, a person with AN may begin to diet in order to lose a little weight. Dieting does not stop there, however, and the person establishes an abnormal concern with weight. Losing a few pounds is not enough, and the individual becomes increasingly focused on dieting and reducing their weight. It is not uncommon for someone who develops the disorder to starve herself until she weighs just 60 or 70 pounds. Given that the symptoms of AN most often occur during early adolescence when individuals experience a period of rapid physical growth, there is an expectation of weight gain instead of weight loss. AN may be suspected when an adolescent experiences weight loss or fails to gain weight and maintains a body weight less than 85 percent of what is expected for their age and height. Throughout this process of semistarvation, the individual denies hunger and persistently claims to be full after eating a small portion of food (Mental Health Net, 1999). The diagnostic criteria for AN as established by the *DSM-IV* (APA, 1994) include the following:

- Refusal to maintain a body weight at or above a minimally normal weight for one's age and height
- Intense fear of gaining weight or becoming fat, even though the individual is underweight
- Disturbance marked by a distorted view of one's body weight or shape
- Concern that certain parts of their body (e.g., abdomen, buttocks, thighs) are "too fat," regardless of how thin they may be
- Absence of at least three consecutive menstrual cycles

The *DSM-IV* (APA, 1994) also recognizes two subtypes of anorexia: *restricting type* (in which weight loss is accomplished primarily through dieting, fasting, or excessive exercise) and *binge eating/purging type* (characterized by the regular occurrence of binge-eating and purging by inducing vomiting or misusing of laxative, diuretics, or enemas).

Symptoms

Psychological symptoms such as social withdrawal, obsessive–compulsive behavior, and depression often precede and accompany AN. Many individuals with AN have perfectionist traits that are often associated with personality disorders. As was mentioned previously, an extreme fear of gaining weight is usually present, and this fear often is associated with phobic reactions to food. This phobia is coupled with a distorted body image. While most normal teens can give an accurate estimate of their body weight, individuals with AN tend to perceive of themselves as markedly larger than they really are.

Physical symptoms often include the loss of head hair, growth of fine body hair, constipation, intolerance of cold temperatures, and low pulse rate. Their skin often appears dry and has a yellowish appearance. Individuals with AN appear emaciated, but may try to disguise this through loose-fitting, oversized clothing and makeup.

They commonly display poor social and sexual adjustment; however, this situation may coexist with outstanding achievement in such areas as academics or athletics. These achievements are possible due to their sense of perfection as well as the excess of energy many individuals with the condition may have.

In addition, people with AN often display peculiar food behaviors. They may frequently skip meals, take only tiny portions, not eat in front of other people, and eat in ritualistic ways. They may chew mouthfuls of food, but spit it out before swallowing. Frequently, they will grocery shop and cook for entire households, but they refuse to eat the tasty meals they prepare. They may use multiple excuses to avoid eating, including not being hungry, feeling ill or upset, or claiming to have just eaten with friends.

Prevalence

Research suggests that among females in late adolescence and early adulthood about 1% have anorexia nervosa (APA, 1994). That means that about 1 out of every 100 young women between 10 and 25 are starv-

ing themselves, sometimes to death. There are limited data concerning the prevalence of AN among adolescent males, estimates suggests this population accounts for 6% to 10% of all cases of anorexia (Mental Health Net, 1999). Most researchers agree that the number of individuals with his disorder is increasing.

The primary age of onset of symptoms of AN is between 12 and 18 years, with a mean age of onset at 17 years (APA, 1994). The onset of this disorder grows increasingly rare with age—very rarely is it diagnosed in females over 40 years of age. The onset of the illness often corresponds to a stressful life event. The course the disorder takes varies markedly, as do outcomes. Some individuals with AN recover fully after a single episode, some exhibit fluctuating pattern of recovery and relapse, and others experience chronic deterioration of health over many years. The long-term mortality rate for AN is over 10% (APA, 1994). When death results, it most often is caused by starvation, suicide, or electrolyte imbalance (APA, 1994). In addition, individuals (especially females) who have a first-degree biological relative with AN are at increased risk of the disorder.

Bulimia Nervosa

Bulimia nervosa (BN) is an eating disorder that also primarily affects young women. In contrast to the self-starvation associated with AN, the central feature of bulimia is the intermittent and seemingly uncontrollable episodes of rapid ingestion of large quantities of food in a short time (binging), which may be followed by self-induced vomiting or the misuse of laxatives, diuretics, or enemas (purging). To qualify, an episode of binging must take place within 2 hours and the amount of food consumed considered definitely larger than most people would eat during a similar period of time and under similar circumstances. Coexisting with this binge behavior is the self-perception of loss of control over eating. Purging may consist of self-induced vomiting, misuse of medications, or excessive exercise. While on the surface individuals with BN often appear to be well-adjusted socially, this serious disease is particularly hard to overcome because it usually has been a pattern of behavior for a long time. The *DSM-IV* (APA, 1994) has identified the following diagnostic criteria for bulimia nervosa:

- Recurrent episodes of binge eating

- Recurrent and inappropriate form of compensatory behavior marked by efforts to purge oneself

- Binge eating and compensatory behaviors both occur twice a week for 3 months on average

- Body image and self-assessment are unduly influenced by body shape and weight

The *DSM-IV* (APA, 1994) recognizes two subtypes of BN: *purging type* (in which the person regularly engages in self-induced vomiting or the misuse of medications) and *nonpurging type* (in which the individual uses inappropriate compensatory behaviors such as fasting or excessive exercise, but does not engage in self-induced vomiting or the misuse of medications).

Symptoms

Individuals diagnosed with BN regularly engage in binge behavior. Although the food consumed varies, it commonly involves foods that are high in carbohydrates and fats and easily available and ingested (without cooking). Foods such as ice cream, cookies, candy, doughnuts, and bread are typically eaten during binges. Diagnosis of the disorder, however, depends more on the abnormality in the amount of food consumed, rather than a craving for a specific nutrient such as carbohydrates (Flaherty & Andrianopoulous, 1993).

Individuals with BN are typically ashamed of their eating problems and usually make an effort to conceal their symptoms. Both food buying and ingestion is commonly done in secret. An episode may or may not be planned in advance. Binge episodes may occur at any time of day, although they seem more common when the individual comes home in the evening. Termination of eating usually occurs when the individual is uncomfortably full. While binging, individuals experience feelings of loss of self-control or being in a frenzied or trance-like state (APA, 1994).

Most individuals with bulimia terminate each binge episode with inappropriate compensatory behaviors to help prevent weight gain. As mentioned previously, the most common method of purging is self-induced vomiting—a procedure employed by 80% to 90% of persons with BN (APA, 1994). The motivation to vomit is a combination of attempting to relieve physical discomfort as well as to avoid gaining weight. In the early stages of the disorder, the use of fingers or instruments to stimulate the gag reflex may be used to induce vomiting. As the disorder progresses individuals often become adept at inducing vomiting and it may become almost a reflex action.

Other methods of purging may be used, including the misuse of laxatives, diuretics, and enemas. It is not uncommon for people with bulimia to attempt to compensate for binging by fasting for a period of time or by engaging in exercise excessively. Among individuals

with bulimia there is an increased incidence of emotional difficulties. Minnesota Multiphasic Personality Inventory (MMPI) profiles reveal high scores on measures of depression, impulsivity, anger, anxiety, and social withdrawal (Flaherty & Andrianopoulous, 1993). The *DSM-IV* (APA, 1994) reports an increased frequency of depressive symptoms (e.g., low self-esteem) or mood disorders (e.g., dysthymic disorder and major depressive disorder) in persons with BN. Substance abuse or substance dependence, especially use that involves alcohol and stimulants, occurs in an estimated one third of individuals with bulimia. Between one third and one half of this population also have personality traits that meet criteria for one or more personality disorders (APA, 1994).

Prevalence

The prevalence of bulimia nervosa among adolescent and young adult females is approximately 1% to 3% (APA, 1994). College students have received considerable attention in studies dealing with eating disorders. Among this population it has been reported that almost one half of those surveyed have engaged in a binge-eating episode (Flaherty & Andrianopoulous, 1993), and that about 4% of college-aged women have bulimia (Anorexia Nervosa and Related Eating Disorders, Inc., 1999a). As with anorexia, about 90% of all diagnosed cases of BN occur in females.

Bulimia has been reported to occur with roughly similar frequency in most industrialized nations of the world. In the United States, individuals diagnosed with BN are primarily Caucasian, but the disorder has also been identified among other ethnic groups (APA, 1994). There is no proven cause of BN, but as with other eating disorders, an increased frequency of bulimia occurs in the first-degree biological relatives of individuals with the disorder.

Causes of Anorexia and Bulimia

Specific causes of anorexia and bulimia are unknown. A combination of factors—biological, psychological, family, and social—likely are woven together to trigger the development of the disorders.

Biological Factors

Research suggests that abnormal levels of certain chemicals in the brain predispose some people to anxiety, perfectionism, and obsessive–compulsive thoughts and behaviors (Anorexia Nervosa and Related Eating Disorders, Inc., 1999b). Such personality types seem to be more vulnerable to eating disorders. Also, once a person begins to starve, this behavior can alter brain chemistry and exacerbate the condition.

Researchers have discovered that the section of the brain containing the hypothalamus begins to work improperly after the onset of anorexia or bulimia. This improper functioning may result in lower blood pressure, lower body temperature, lack of sexual interest, and hormonal changes resulting in abnormalities of menstrual cycles (Mental Health Net, 1999).

Psychological Factors

People with AN or BN tend to be perfectionists, often having unrealistic expectations of themselves and others. In spite of achievements, they may feel ineffective, inadequate, and worthless. They often seem to have a narrow perspective of reality and see things in black and white terms. Thus, if fat is bad and thin is good, then thinner is better, and thinnest is best.

It has been posited that people with AN use eating behaviors to attempt to take control of their lives. While they may be strong-willed, they feel they are weak, powerless, and victimized. They also may feel angry and turn their anger toward themselves. They may lack a sense of identity, and may use their eating habits to help manufacture an identity which they feel will be socially approved and admired (Anorexia Nervosa and Related Eating Disorders, Inc., 1999b).

Family Factors

Some researchers believe that certain characteristics are common to the families of persons who develop anorexia or bulimia. These families often appear to be warm and loving on the surface, but this loving atmosphere may mask underlying problems in which family members are excessively involved in each other's lives and overly dependent on one another. People with AN may feel smothered in their families or feel misunderstood and abandoned. Parents who overemphasize the importance of physical appearance or who appear critical of their children's bodies may unwittingly contribute to eating disturbances.

These families also tend to be overprotective, rigid, and ineffective in resolving conflicts that occur within the household. Parents may hold unrealistic expectations of achievement for their offspring, which contributes to

feelings of doubt, fear, and anxiety. As a result, an adolescent may try to resolve their problems by manipulating their weight and eating behaviors (Anorexia Nervosa and Related Eating Disorders, Inc., 1999b).

Social Factors

The media in contemporary society bombards us all with messages that promote the advantages of being thin. Impressionable people are told—either directly or indirectly through actors and models—that success, popularity, romance, and power require physical beauty in general and thinness in particular. Less often stated but clearly understood is the corollary: people who are not thin and beautiful are rejected, lonely, failures.

Young females are disproportionately affected by eating disorders. Never before in history have females been subjected to the cultural demands for thinness as they are today. Mary Pipher (1994, pp. 183–184) calls this a "national cult for thinness" and states:

> Beauty is the defining characteristic for American women. It's the necessary and often sufficient condition for social success. It is important for women of all ages, but the pressure to be beautiful is most intense in early adolescence. Girls worry about their clothes, makeup, skin, and hair. But most of all they worry about their weight. Peers place an enormous value on thinness.

> In 1950 the model who portrayed the White Rock mineral water girl was 5 feet 4 inches tall and weighed 140 pounds. Today she is 5 feet 10 inches tall and weighs 110 pounds.

In contrast, males are encouraged to be strong and powerful. For males, thin is often equated with skinny or weak. Instead of thinness being equated with being glamorous or sexy as it usually is with females, males view thinness as an undesirable shape for their bodies. Perhaps this explains, at least in part, why less than 10% of people with eating disorders are males.

Triggers and Eating Disorders

Both anorexia and bulimia appear most commonly in bright, attractive young women between 12 and 25 years. Often these individuals seem to have everything going for them. If someone is vulnerable to an eating disorder, sometimes all it take to initiate the chain reaction of behaviors that characterize these disturbances is a trigger event which they do not know how to handle. A trigger could be something as seemingly innocuous as teasing or as traumatic as rape.

Triggers often are associated with difficult life transition or loss—divorce, family problems, a new school, or the breakup of an important relationship. Such situations may place increased demands on the individual, which may seem overwhelming. The individual may feel helpless or out of control.

People vulnerable to eating disorders may also feel lonely, feeling they have few friends and that they do not fit into social situations. They may feel that they have no confidants with whom they can share their thoughts, feelings, or fears. Often they seek healthy connections to others but fear criticism and rejection if their perceived shortcomings become known.

Wanting to take control and repair their lives, and under the influence of a culture that glorifies thinness, the person may focus on his or her body instead of broader problems. Dieting, binging, purging, exercise, and other behaviors may be misguided efforts to take charge in a world that seems overwhelming.

Treatment

Without treatment, it has been estimated that up to 20% of people with serious eating problems die. With treatment, that number falls to 2% to 3% and about 60% of people with AN or BN recover (Anorexia Nervosa and Related Eating Disorders, Inc., 1999a). They maintain a healthy weight, retain a positive self-concept, and develop meaningful relationships with others. Even with treatment, about 20% of people with eating disturbances make only partial recoveries. Their lives may be characterized as fluctuating between periods of normal behavior and other periods in which their focus on food and weight predominate. They are seen repeatedly in emergency rooms, eating disorder programs, or mental health centers (Flaherty & Andrianopoulous, 1993; Anorexia Nervosa and Related Eating Disorders, Inc., 1999a).

Treatment for anorexia and bulimia usually begins when the affected individual visits a physician, usually at the insistence of a parent, friend, or school official. Before specific treatment of anorexic or bulimic behavior can be undertaken the individual must be assessed for medical problems. Hospitalization may be required to medically stabilize the individual. Criteria used to determine the need for hospitalization include:

- Rapid weight loss in the previous six months
- Severe loss of energy
- Fluid and electrolyte imbalance
- Cycle of binging, vomiting, and restriction of eating that cannot be broken

The basic hospital treatment program usually involves ongoing management of medical concerns, bed rest with supervised feedings to increase weight (for patients with anorexia), and nutrition stabilization programs. The treatment program usually attempts to address the psychiatric dimensions of these disorders by means of personal, nutrition, and family counseling programs (Flaherty & Andrianopoulous, 1993).

Outpatient treatment for eating disorders occurs at specialized clinics, public or private psychiatric facilities, or community mental health programs. Treatment for AN and BN usually consists of nutrition education, individual psychotherapy, and family counseling. Nutrition education is a crucial part of any program designed to treat individuals with eating disorders. The person must be taught about nutrition in general (food types, fat metabolism) and should also learn about food and body weight. One goal of nutrition education programs for persons with eating disorders is to have each individual establish a realistic weight goal for themselves as well as a meal and activity schedule designed to maintain their desired body weight. Such a program should allow the client to actively participate in treatment in order to allow them to develop a sense of personal control over their situation.

Individual psychotherapy is necessary to help the individual understand the disease process and its effects. *Cognitive therapy* can be helpful in getting the client to focus on issues such as the obsession with weight and being thin, their low self-esteem, and the tendency toward dichotomous thinking, (e.g., fat versus thin, right versus wrong). A basic psychotherapeutic dilemma is whether to concentrate on weight and eating habits or explore underlying psychological issues. The therapist must generally be prepared to do both.

Family counseling helps to develop a supportive home environment. Persons with anorexia or bulimia often become a source of family tension because their eating behaviors cause frustration for the entire family unit. Family therapy helps family members relate more effectively with one another and to work together for the well-being of all members of the family.

For some individuals with AN or BN who are also diagnosed with serious psychiatric conditions, *pharmacological interventions* may be employed. In cases such as severe depression, for instance, antidepressants may be an important part of therapy. Behavior may improve rapidly in these situations and the individual can then respond more quickly to treatment aimed at resolving their eating disorder.

As with other psychiatric disturbances we have discussed, however, immediate success in treating

eating problems does not guarantee a permanent cure. Persons with anorexia and bulimia may experience relapses. Experts usually recommend follow-up therapy lasting 3 to 5 years. In addition, as eating disorders have become increasingly more prevalent, self-help groups and various voluntary organizations dedicated to working with persons with eating disturbances have increased. These groups and organizations can play an increasingly important role in helping to prevent the likelihood of a relapse for individuals with anorexia or bulimia.

Implications for Therapeutic Recreation

After immediate health issues have been dealt with and a plan to address weight gain/restoration (anorexia nervosa) or abstinence from compulsive use of food (bulimia nervosa) has been developed, therapeutic recreation (TR) may be used to deal with the physical and emotional consequences of these conditions. TR Specialists working with this population often focus upon the feelings repressed by addictive eating disorders. Goals commonly addressed by TR include (Mitchell, 1999):

- Develop self-esteem
- Subordinate the role of physical appearance to self-esteem
- Convince affected individuals of the need to develop other sources of values
- Provide strategies/activities to help gain a sense of control
- Use leisure interests as an alternative to the self-control expressed by eating behaviors
- Develop a healthy lifestyle through participation in leisure experiences

Participation

There are few activities in which individuals with eating disorders are unable to participate. While TR professionals must be cautious not to allow individuals with anorexia to overdo calorie-demanding physical activities, in most cases few restrictions are required. Some commonly used activities include weightlifting (which helps individuals increase bone density and build calcium levels), relaxation and stress management techniques, and socialization activities such as storytelling, name games, board games, charades, or life-history talks. Team and individual sports such as

Frisbee golf, badminton, and table tennis may also be used to teach physical skills, provide a sense of competition, and encourage socialization. In addition, arts, crafts, and musical activities are appropriate for this population. For persons with anorexia, activities that encourage public eating (e.g., visiting restaurants) can be helpful in achieving program goals (Mitchell, 1999).

Leisure Education

Leisure education programs help educate the individual about using their free time in a healthy and satisfying manner. In addition to exploring personal leisure attitudes and leisure behaviors, these programs may be particularly beneficial in helping persons with eating disorders to learn to use community recreation resources such as theaters, shopping malls, parks, and recreation centers (Mitchell, 1999). When absorbed in their addictive behaviors, these individuals often forgot how to enjoy themselves. Through values clarification and self-awareness experiences, techniques taught to facilitate leisure education, individuals can become aware of the relationship between their beliefs and attitudes and their past and present behaviors. As clients explore leisure experiences as an alternative to eating (or avoiding food), they may become increasingly aware of the true nature and rhythms of their bodies and are less likely to distort their body images (Carter, Van Andel & Robb, 1995).

Therapy

Treatment programs for individuals with eating disorders usually include a combination of behavior therapy, supportive and insight-oriented psychotherapy, and family therapy. Specific techniques vary, but often include group discussion and feedback on goal setting and personal relationships, cognitive restructuring related to beliefs about thinness and body image, education about eating disorders and nutrition, relaxation training, and assertiveness training (Kraus & Shank, 1992).

Within this eclectic approach to treating eating disorders, the use of TR has numerous applications. For example, the observation of individuals' involvement in activities might help expose behaviors, such as excessive exercising or unusual rituals surrounding food, which are indicative of dysfunctional eating habits. Kaufman, McBride, Hultsman, and Black (1988) observed that persons with anorexia and bulimia experience fewer benefits from recreational activities than their peers without this disorder. Consequently, the use of leisure assessment instruments may be useful in helping to diagnose specific eating-related problems. Because eating is a leisure experience, TR professionals have the opportunity to demonstrate how the individual's feelings and self-perceptions affect food consumption (Carter, Van Andel & Robb, 1995).

TR may also be beneficial in treating the emotional disturbances experienced by persons with anorexia or bulimia. As we stated, feelings such as isolation, guilt, loneliness, and loss of control are common among these individuals. For many of these persons, control over their eating behaviors makes up for the lack of control that they feel over other aspects of their lives. The use of planned, structured leisure experiences by the TR professional may contribute to promoting feelings of self-control and personal decision making. Through TR programs, persons with eating disorders can explore ways of gaining control of their lives as an alternative to defining self-control by their eating habits. The attributional approach to therapeutic recreation, as outlined by Iso-Ahola, MacNeil, and Szymanski (1980) would seem particularly appropriate for enhancing feelings of personal control and self-efficacy.

In addition, TR may be used to simply add enjoyment and pleasure to the lives of individuals with eating disorders. These individuals often are so obsessed with food and their bodies that they seldom find enjoyment in the daily lives. As Sumpter has written:

> It's quite common among eating disorder or chemically dependent patients to have forgotten how to enjoy spare time. Obsessive thoughts of food or drugs preoccupy their leisure activity. A big part of treatment is retraining people to develop healthy and constructive leisure. (1989, p. 3)

While the content of TR programs for anorexia and bulimia must be determined on an individual basis, common activities include creative and expressive pursuits as well as programs of physical exercise. Creative activities (e.g., art, music, writing, pottery) can be used to foster self-control and enhance self-esteem, and may also help individuals express feelings and emotions (Wolf, Willmuth & Watkins, 1989).

Exercise activities, including weightlifting, walking/hiking, swimming, active games, and sports maintain overall physical fitness, maintain normal bone development, tone muscles, and encourage an active lifestyle (Mitchell, 1999). Of course, exercise activities, especially for individuals with anorexia, must be closely monitored to avoid excessive exertion. For individuals with bulimia, a recent study produced

evidence that suggests that exercise intervention may be an important deterrent to binge eating (Levine, Marcus & Mouton, 1996).

Whatever activities are used, it is important that they be approached in a calm and relaxed manner. Such an approach helps to avoid feelings of anxiety and loss of control, and to decrease the obsessive attitude about perfection common to many individuals with eating disorders.

Dementia

In contrast to the disorders previously reviewed in this chapter, dementia overwhelmingly affects individuals after the age of 50. *Dementia* is associated with the loss of intellectual and social abilities severe enough to interfere with the individual's ability to function independently. Dementia usually robs individuals of their ability to remember things, to think in a clear organized fashion, and to understand information basic to daily life. It accounts for more than one half of all new nursing home admissions and is the one condition most feared by older adults (Merck, 2000). For the estimated 20% or more of the 85 and over population affected by dementia, the later stages of life are often spent in a state of total dependence (APA, 1994). Given that we are an aging society, the actual number of individuals affected by dementia is expected to rapidly grow over the next several decades.

The expected relationship between cognitive decline and advanced years has become a part of the image surrounding later life in our society. For centuries people called cognitive failure among the aged *senility* and considered it to be an inevitable part of the human aging process. Despite the fact that disorders that negatively impact cognitive performance are more common among older adults than people at earlier stages in the life cycle, it is now understood that dementia *is not* a normal or expected part of aging. Dementia is a condition usually caused by diseases (e.g., Alzheimer's, Parkinson's) or infection (e.g., Creutzfeld–Jacob, HIV) that result in the loss of cells within the brain. This cell loss produces the characteristic symptoms of dementia.

Dementia is characterized by a deterioration of intellectual functioning and cognitive skills, leading to a decline in the ability to perform activities of daily living. According to the *DSM-IV* (APA, 1994), the development of multiple cognitive deficits associated with dementia may be due to physiological effects of a general medical condition, the persisting effects of a substance, or multiple factors (e.g., combined effects of two or more diseases). Although dementia may be caused by many conditions (e.g., Alzheimer's disease, cerebrovascular disease, Parkinson's disease, Pick's disease, Creutzfeld–Jacob disease), persons with the disorder share a common presentation of symptoms.

The predominant feature of dementia is the development of multiple cognitive deficits, including impairment of memory and disturbances in language, motor abilities, sensory recognition, and/or executive functioning (e.g., the ability to think abstractly and to plan, initiate, sequence, monitor, and stop complex behavior). Impairment in short-term memory (the inability to learn new information) may be characterized by the inability to memorize the names of a few common objects and to repeat them after a brief interval of time. Long-term memory impairment (inability to remember information that was known in the past) may be indicated by the inability to recall information of personal relevance (e.g., date of birth, place of birth, names of family members) or facts of common knowledge (e.g., dates of well-known events, past presidents).

While short-term and long-term memory losses may be formally tested, early symptoms of dementia often take the form of disturbances in previously learned skills. Individuals may increasingly begin to lose wallets and keys, forget to turn off the stove, or become lost in familiar environments. In advanced stages of dementia, memory deficits may become so severe that the person forgets critical personal information such as their birthday, anniversary, or occupation, or they may have no sense of where they are.

Aphasia—deterioration of language function—is also a symptom common to dementia. The speech of persons with aphasia is vague, with excessive use of indefinite terms such as "thing" and "it." Comprehension of spoken and written language also deteriorates.

Apraxia—disturbance in the ability to carry out motor activities despite intact comprehension and motor function—is also symptomatic of the disorder. Individuals may be impaired in their ability to pantomime the use of objects (e.g., brushing one's teeth) or to execute previously learned motor acts (e.g., writing one's name). Apraxia certainly contributes to declines in activities of daily living such as dressing, cooking, or grooming.

Individuals with dementia also commonly display disturbances in the ability to think abstractly or to cope with situations that require novel ways of thinking. They may have difficulty shifting from one topic to another or following a sequence of instruction. Often even relatively simple cognitive tasks such as counting,

reciting the alphabet, or assembling blocks prove too difficult for some people with dementia to complete. As with other symptoms, the decline in executive functioning usually compounds the functional problems associated with daily living skills.

Individuals with dementia may display poor judgment in decision making. They often seem unable to understand more than one dimension of a problem/situation. They commonly make unrealistic assessments of their abilities and may underestimate the risks involved in everyday activities such as driving a car or cooking a meal. They may experience changes in their personality, behave oddly, or become anxious, obstinate, or aggressive.

The age of onset of dementia varies, but it usually occurs late in life. The frequency of new cases for those 65 years and older is approximately 1% (Sharma & Gierl, 1993). The total number of individuals affected in this age group may be as high as 15% (Merck, 2000). Estimates of the prevalence of dementia among those 85 years and older range from 20% (APA, 1994) to up to 50% (Merck, 2000). The wide range in estimates may reflect variance in the severity of symptoms, as well as differences in diagnosed versus self-reported or family-reported cases. Nonetheless, prevalence of the disorder increases with age and is highest in the 85+ age group, the fastest growing segment of the population in North America.

Historically, dementia has been considered to be a progressive disorder that is irreversible after onset. With the publication of the most recent edition of the *DSM* the American Psychiatric Association (1994) has altered their opinion and state that the course of dementia is not always progressive, but may be static or even remitting. They suggest that the reversibility of the illness is a function of the underlying pathology as well as the application of effective treatment. The APA has stated, "the level of disability depends not only on the severity of the individual's cognitive impairments but also on the available social supports" (1994, pp. 137–138).

Dementia of the Alzheimer's Type

The underlying etiology of dementia is an important consideration in determining the course and prognosis of the disorder. Of the various causal factors associated with dementia, *Alzheimer's disease* is the most common, accounting for over 50% of dementias in the elderly (Merck, 2000). The disease was named after German physician Alois Alzheimer. In 1906, Dr. Alzheimer noticed changes in the brain tissue of a woman who had died of an unusual mental illness. He found abnormal clumps (plaques) and tangled bundles of fiber (tangles). Other changes in the brains of people with Alzheimer's disease include a loss of nerve cells in the areas vital to memory and other mental functions and lowered levels of chemicals that carry complex messages back and forth between billions of nerve cells important to thinking and memory.

The first sign of Alzheimer's disease may be mild forgetfulness. The disease progresses to affect language, reasoning, understanding, reading, and writing. Eventually, people with Alzheimer's disease may become anxious or aggressive and may even wander from home. The disease is considered irreversible. Eventually, the failing nervous system affects all body functions. The person may become completely incapacitated. Death often comes from a complicating problem, such as pneumonia or an infection.

Diagnosis Criteria and Symptoms

The diagnostic criteria established by the *DSM-IV* (APA, 1994) clearly associates Alzheimer's disease with the broader diagnosis of dementia. Because dementia is the primary symptom of Alzheimer's, diagnostic criteria focus upon multiple cognitive deficits. These include impairment in memory as well as cognitive disturbances in language (aphasia), motor function (apraxia), the ability to recognize and identify common objects (agnosia), or the ability to plan, organize, or understand sequencing (executive functioning). These cognitive deficits must be severe enough to cause impairment in social or occupational functioning, and represent a significant decline from a previous level of functioning. In addition, the onset of dementia of the Alzheimer's type is gradual and progressive. The diagnosis should only be made when other established causes of dementia (e.g., central nervous system conditions such as cerebrovascular disease, Parkinson's disease, Huntington's disease), systemic conditions (e.g., hypothyroidism, HIV infection), or persisting effects of a substance (e.g., alcohol) have been ruled out (APA, 1994, pp. 139–140).

While these symptoms represent the formal diagnostic criteria used to identify Alzheimer's disease, recognition of subtle changes in cognitive functioning by individuals with the disease or by their family usually marks the first step in the identification of the condition. While no two people experience Alzheimer's in exactly the same way, classic signs that signal losses shared by people in the early stages of the disease include difficulty in the following areas:

- Short-term memory loss
- Learning and retaining new information
- Reasoning and abstractive thought
- Judgment and planning
- Language skills
- Inhibition and impulse control

Biological Changes

These functional changes obviously do not occur without a cause. In the case of Alzheimer's disease, the source of cognitive decline is a biological change in the brain. The path of change is marked by the degeneration of neurons, which progressively lose their ability to communicate and eventually die. Because the human brain cannot replace nerve cells, some brain function is lost.

Alzheimer's disease appears to result from the degenerative loss of cells from the cerebral cortex and hippocampus regions of the brain. While the specific cause of neuron degeneration is not known, changes in levels of certain neurotransmitters—chemicals that bridge synapses between neurons—may play a role. Autopsies performed on individuals with the disease consistently reveal lower than normal levels of certain neurotransmitters. However, it is still unclear whether the decrease in neurotransmitters in the brains of people with Alzheimer's is the cause of cell loss or just the result of the disease process.

Much of the current research focuses on the abnormal structures found throughout the brains of people with Alzheimer's. These structures, known as *senile plaques* and *neurofibrillary tangles*, are telltale markers of the disease.

Plaques are mainly composed of a protein called amyloid beta, a by-product of a larger protein involved in cell membrane function. Amyloid beta protein is secreted by cells throughout the body but produced in particularly large amounts in the brain. The plaques develop in the spaces between neurons. Researchers are intrigued by amyloid beta plaques because they seem to occur early in the disease process—before any surrounding neuron damage is evident and often 10 to 20 years before symptoms develop. Although the ultimate cause of neuron death is not known, mounting evidence suggests that a form of amyloid beta protein may be the culprit (Merck, 2000).

The internal support structure for nerve cells depends on the normal functioning of a protein called tau. In people with Alzheimer's disease, threads of tau protein undergo alterations that cause them to become *tangled*. Researchers suspect that as neurons in the brain die, the symptoms associated with Alzheimer's disease increase (Merck, 2000).

The diagnosis of Alzheimer's disease is usually based on medical history, a physical examination, and mental status tests. As indicated in the diagnostic criteria established by the *DSM-IV* (APA, 1994), efforts are made to identify other possible causes of thinking and behavior change before a conclusion of Alzheimer's is reached. Even when the evidence seems to clearly point to Alzheimer's as the source of dementia in an individual, a confirmed diagnosis is only possible when an autopsy reveals the presence of the pathological structures identified as plaques and tangles.

Prevalence

It is estimated that 2% to 4% of people over the age of 65 have dementia of the Alzheimer's type (APA, 1994). Over 4 million Americans have Alzheimer's disease (Merck, 2000). It accounts for over 50% of the dementia in the aged, and an estimated 60% of people in long-term care facilities have the disease (Merck, 2000). The prevalence increases with age. According to the Alzheimer's Disease and Related Disorders Association (2000), approximately 20% of adults between the ages of 80–84 have the condition, while 47% of those 85 or older are affected. It is more common in women than men, perhaps because women live longer. It is expected to be a growing public health issue in the future as the 76 million baby boomers reach later adulthood during the next 30 years.

Course

The course of dementia of the Alzheimer's type tends to be progressive. Individual variations are extremely common. The symptoms in some affected persons may progress very steadily, in others they may progress slowly and may seem to plateau. The following clinical stages—early, intermediate, late, and terminal—often measure the progress of the disease:

The *early stage* is characterized by forgetfulness and increasing problems of retention of information. The individual misplaces common objects and forgets familiar names, dates, or phone numbers. They have progressive difficulty performing activities of daily living (missing appointments, balancing their checkbook). They may become lost while traveling in familiar environments. Recognizable changes in personality,

especially growing irritability and agitation, may accompany the growing sense of loss of personal control.

The *intermediate stage* is marked by the total inability to learn and recall information. The individual increasingly loses their orientation to time and place, forgets personal history, does not recognized familiar people. Assistance with basic skills such as bathing, dressing, and toileting becomes more common. Wandering, uncooperativeness, hostility, or physical aggressiveness often characterize behavioral disorganization. Aphasia, apraxia, and agnosia are increasingly evident. Although they may remain ambulatory, risk for falls and accidents increases due to their confusion.

The *late stage* is characterized by the loss of recent and remote memory. Current events may be entirely meaningless. Individuals become totally unaware of their surroundings. By this stage, most individuals require total care and placement in a long-term care facility is often necessary.

The *terminal stage* of Alzheimer's is marked by the inability to perform any activity of daily living. Most individuals at this stage are bedridden and totally incontinent. Unable to recognize their spouse or significant others, they eventually become mute and unable to communicate their needs. The final phase of Alzheimer's is coma and death, usually from infection.

Familial Pattern

Alzheimer's disease is thought to have a familial pattern. The *DSM-IV* (APA, 1994) reports that first-degree biological relatives of individuals with the disease are more likely to develop the disorder compared to the general public. In about 20% of cases, dementia of the Alzheimer's type has been shown to be inherited as a dominant trait with linkage to several chromosomes (Merck, 2000). Studies of the genetic aspects of Alzheimer's are difficult to undertake because family members in the past may not have lived long enough for the disease to be expressed. Other causative agents such as infections or environmental contaminants may also contribute.

Treatment

Although Alzheimer's disease is not curable, treatment is essential to help maintain self-care and adaptation for as long as possible. The rate of impairment progresses differently in each individual, therefore careful monitoring is necessary to deal with complications that may arise quickly. Treatment usually involves five components: drug therapy, behavioral management, individual psycho-therapy, environmental support, and caregiver support.

No effective drug for the treatment of memory deficits or cognitive impairment exists. Drugs primarily attempt to correct neurochemical dysfunctions. For example, drug therapy is commonly used to help treat symptoms of depression often evident in the early phases of Alzheimer's. Pharmacotherapy may also play an important role in helping to decrease agitation, belliger-ence, or aggressive behavior that often accompanies the disease.

Behavioral management techniques are also impor-tant in dealing with disruptive and inappropriate behav-ior of persons with dementia. The use of reinforcement and other behavior modification strategies, commonly used in institutional settings, help to moderate antisocial behavior.

The use of psychotherapeutic techniques such as reality orientation and remotivation are common with confused or disoriented individuals. These techniques may be used for individuals with Alzheimer's disease to help maximize new learning and recall. They also may help to decrease agitation associated with feelings of disorientation and to combat depression.

Environmental supports reinforce skills needed to maintain activities of daily living. Examples include grab bars in bathrooms, appropriately placed stools and chairs, and clothing that is easy to put on and remove.

Finally, caregiver support is recognized as a critical component in the treatment of person's with Alzheimer's. Regular meetings with other dementia caregivers provide emotional and practical sustenance important for the endurance of many family caregivers. These groups enable caregivers to share experiences, feelings, and useful methods of dealing with difficult behaviors of their family members with Alzheimer's disease.

Non-Alzheimer's Dementias

Alzheimer's is suspected to be the primary cause of over half of all cases of dementia. A variety of other diseases and conditions however, are also known to be sources of dementia. The more commonly occurring non-Alzheimer's dementias include vascular (multi-infarct) dementia, the dementia associated with Parkinson's disease and Huntington's disease, Pick's disease, and dementias associated with infections (e.g., Creutzfeld–Jacob disease and AIDS).

A person with non-Alzheimer's dementia usually displays similar symptoms to those seen in individuals

with dementia of the Alzheimer's type. Like those with Alzheimer's, individuals with non-Alzheimer's dementia often exhibit impairments in areas of cognitive func-tioning, such as speech (aphasia), motor activity (apraxia), interpretation of sensory input (agnosia), judgment, and memory. They may also experience changes in personal habits and interests, and may undergo alterations in their personality marked by agitation, anxiety, or irritability. In contrast to the cognitive and behavioral changes associated with Alzheimer's dementia, these changes in non-Alzheimer's dementias can occur suddenly and do not necessarily progress.

Vascular dementia (formerly called *multi-infarct dementia*) has a structural or intrinsic cause. In this condition, small strokes, called lacunae, destroy enough brain tissue to impair function. Vascular dementia occurs more commonly among individuals with hypertension, but can often be avoided with blood pressure manage-ment. Some degree of vascular dementia is found in up to 20% of autopsies in older adults (Merck, 2000).

Parkinson's disease is a slowly progressive neuro-logical condition characterized by tremor, rigidity, and instability. The dementia associated with Parkinson's disease includes impairments in memory retrieval, deficits in executive functioning, and declines in cognitive and motor skills. It has been estimated that more than 25% of all individuals with Parkinson's disease have demen-tia (Merck, 2000).

Huntington's disease is an inherited progressive degenerative disease that affects the body and the mind. It stems from a disorder within the brain that causes nerve cells to waste away. Difficulties with memory retrieval, executive functioning, and judgment may occur in the early stages of the disease. As the disease progresses, changes in personality and declines in intellect, memory, speech, and judgment occur. Demen-tia may develop in the later stages of Huntington's (APA, 1994).

Pick's disease, a less common form of dementia, involves the frontal and temporal regions of the cerebral cortex. Pick's disease is characterized by disturbances in behavior, personality, and eventually memory. Affected individuals have prominent apathy and memory disturbances. They often show visible declines in terms of carelessness, poor personal hygiene, and decreased attention span. The disease is relentless in its progression, and may ultimately include language impairment and very erratic behavior. Like Alzheimer's disease, a diagnosis is usually only confirmed at autopsy (APA, 1994).

Infectious diseases may also cause dementia. The most well-known infectious cause is *Creutzfeld–Jacob disease*, a rare and fatal brain disorder thought to be caused by a slow virus and rarely diagnosed in individuals younger than 60. Persons with this disease experience memory impairment and behavior changes in the early stages, but the disease progresses rapidly with mental deterioration and involuntary movements (muscle jerks) increasingly occurring. The late stages of the disease are marked by increased risk of incontinence, seizures, blindness, and eventually coma. The course is more rapid than that of Alzheimer's disease and usually lasts less than two years before death (Merck, 2000).

Persons with *human immunodeficiency virus* (HIV) can also develop dementia. Dementia associated with HIV infection is typically characterized by forgetfulness, slowness of movement, poor concentration, and problem-solving deficiencies. Dementia due to HIV disease is often associated with behavioral problems as well, such as apathy and social withdrawal. The development of tremors, rapid repetitive movements, imbalance, hypertonia, delusions, and hallucinations are often present with this form of dementia (APA, 1994).

Implications for Therapeutic Recreation

Participation

Senile dementia among older adults results in dramatic changes in cognition, personality, and behavior. Recreational activities that were meaningful and brought pleasure at earlier periods in their life may hardly be recognized by persons with Alzheimer's disease. However, this does not dismiss the need for offering leisure experiences for this population. Indeed, while the Alzheimer's patient's reaction to a once-enjoyed activity may not reflect enjoyment, many researchers believe that involvement in recreation experiences continues to enhance their quality of life (Hawkins, May & Rogers, 1996).

In their comprehensive review of TR interventions in gerontology, Riddick and Keller (1991) documented a wide variety of activities that have been used with persons with dementia. Among the programs identified were arts and crafts, board games, bible study, drama, dance and movement, exercise and fitness, gardening, music, video games, and water aerobics (p. 195).

While pleasurable participation may be the primary objective of offering such activities, these experiences may also serve to contribute to treatment goals as well. As one example, Buettner (1999) designed an innova-

tive study that used sensorimotor recreation activities to deal with boredom and motor restlessness among a sample of nursing home residents with dementia. The recreation program, which the author labeled *Simple Pleasures*, adapted common and familiar items and used them as props to alter disturbing behaviors. Items such as purses and fishing boxes filled with preselected safe objects—polar fleece covered hot water bottles, sewing cards, squeezies, tetherballs, and message magnets—attracted the attention of residents, thus encouraging interaction and participation and decreasing undesirable behaviors such as screaming, wandering, restlessness, and motor and verbal repetitiveness.

Weiss and Kronberg (1986) described a second example of how a TR program focused mainly on participation might be used for broader goals. *Time-Oriented Programming* attempts to reinforce a sense of the flow of life with residents with dementia. Using this approach, the TRS attempts to personalize interactions with severely disoriented individuals in an effort to facilitate self-awareness, self-esteem, and orientation to reality.

Leisure Education

Since leisure education is generally regarded as preparation for independent leisure functioning, its purpose for older adults with dementia may have limited relevance. In one of the few published papers that addressed this topic, Weiss and Kronberg (1986) claimed that leisure education programs can facilitate reminiscence, which leads to self-awareness and reduced confusion. The authors' claim that the topic of leisure may be used as a focal point to stimulate conversation and increase the attention span of individuals with dementia. Leisure is an appropriate trigger due to highly personalized nature and association with pleasant past experiences (1986, p. 39).

Weiss and colleagues elaborated upon this idea further in 1987 and 1990 publications. The first paper described the use of a mapping project to facilitate reminiscence among nursing home residents (Weiss & Thurn, 1987). The second paper, "Meals, Memories and Memoirs: A Culinary Odyssey," described how the use of a culinary theme produced positive responses, including increased attention span and verbal interaction among confused older adults. The application of this program for addressing the therapeutic recreation goals of this population is also described in this work (Weiss, Markue-Patch & Thurn, 1990).

Mobily and Hoeft (1985) and Weiss and Thurn (1990) provided different perspectives on the use of leisure education with confused older adults. Both papers advanced the idea of providing leisure education training to the families of person's with dementia. The results of this intervention may encourage greater leisure interactions between Alzheimer's patients and their caregivers (Mobily & Hoeft, 1985) and facilitate reminiscing with older disoriented individuals (Weiss & Thurn, 1990).

Therapy

The overwhelming majority of literature dealing with the use of TR among older adults with dementia has been focused upon using leisure experiences to help maintain or improve cognitive functioning. A variety of approaches are used to enhance mental abilities of individuals with dementia. A few of the most common approaches—reality orientation, remotivation, reminiscence, validation therapy, and others—will be summarized.

Reality orientation (RO) supports confused individuals by orienting them to their caregiver's sense of reality. The fundamental assumption of RO is that some of the disorientation found among persons with dementia can be alleviated through the constant reiteration of basic personal and current information. One method used with RO is a 24-hour-a-day, individualized approach in which all interactions with the confused individual emphasize current reality (e.g., self-identity, sense of time and place). The second approach of RO consists of classes held to help small groups of disoriented individuals become aware of the present and the reality their life situation (Teague & MacNeil, 1992). While RO remains a very popular intervention, studies designed to investigate the efficacy of this approach have produced contradictory findings (Riddick & Keller, 1991).

Remotivation is a technique of small group interaction most often used with individuals in the early to middle stages of dementia. Remotivation classes are provided to groups of people who are functioning at about the same cognitive level. Remotivation sessions are usually highly structured and consist primarily of group discussion about topics of shared interest. Remotivation groups ordinarily meet once or twice a week, for about 30 to 60 minutes per session (Dennis, 1994).

Reminiscence has been defined as the reexperiencing of past events as current memory alive with affect—having a "you are there" quality (Clements, 1982, p. 342). Butler and Lewis (1973) have suggested that the process of reminiscing is a healthy adaptation mechanism, particularly important during the last phases of the life cycle when life review is common.

Reminiscence provides emotional development, establishes sense of time, and reduces cognitive dissonance (Clements, 1982). Unlike RO and remotivation, the use of reminiscence usually does not have a formalized structure or routine. Several excellent suggestions for the development and use of reminiscence in TR programs for confused older adults were provided by Weiss and her coauthors in a series of publications (Weiss & Thurn, 1987, 1990; Weiss, Markue-Patch & Thurn, 1990).

Validation Therapy is a humanistic approach for providing confused older adults with the opportunity to resolve emotional conflicts through the expression of their feelings. Validation therapy does not judge, analyze, or intend to change the disoriented person, nor does it emphasize orientation. The TR professional using this approach attempts to assist the older individual in attaining their own goals by allowing them to express unmet needs and reflecting upon their personal feelings. Guidelines for the use of the validation therapy approach have been developed by Feil (1989).

The use of *music* as a therapeutic aid has also been studied. Music is generally regarded as an anxiety-reducing agent, often used to calm an agitated person (Sandel, 1986). Music also improves attending skills and active participation (Christie, 1992), increases the effectiveness of reality orientation sessions (Bumanis and Yoder, 1987; Smith-Marchese, 1994), stimulates memories, and triggers recall of words (Smith, 1990). It has long been recognized that even individuals in the later stages of Alzheimer's may remember every word of a song they were familiar with many years before. The use of *pets* has also been shown to be effective in increasing the social behaviors of institutionalized Alzheimer's clients (Garlock-Kongable, 1988) and reducing agitation among individuals with dementia at an adult day care site (Damon & May, 1986). *Aerobic exercise programs*, such as regular walking, have been shown to decrease behavioral problems for older adults experiencing dementia (Bonner & Cousins, 1996; Holmberg, 1997). Arakawa-Davies (1997) has reported that the effectiveness of a reminiscence program for persons with senile dementia was enhanced by the use of a *dance and movement intervention*. Improvements in strength and flexibility and a decline in agitation were attributed to a *sensorimotor intervention* in a case study of an 80-year-old woman with Alzheimer's type dementia (Buettner, 1995). Similar results were reported in a study using *sensory stimulation* with Alzheimer's patients (Mobily & Hoeft, 1985). Other possible techniques which have been demonstrated to be effective with confused older adults include *horticulture/gardening* (Burgess, 1990), *intergenerational programs* (Ward, Kemp & Newman, 1996), and *craft projects* (White, Anderson-Laser, Ganz-Imphong & Mattiko, 1992).

Chapter Summary

This chapter examined disorders identified in childhood, adolescence, or late adulthood and addressed the following issues:

- Assessment and diagnosis of mental disturbances among younger populations
- Disorders characterized by inattentiveness and disruptive behaviors
- Pervasive developmental disorders, focusing on autism
- Eating disorders, including anorexia nervosa and bulimia nervosa
- Dementia, including dementia of the Alzheimer's type
- Implications for the therapeutic recreation profession for disorders of childhood, adolescence, and late adulthood

References

Alzheimer's Disease and Related Disorders Association. (2000). Understanding Alzheimer's Disease. Available online: http://www.alz.org/people/understanding

American Academy of Child and Adolescent Psychiatry. (1991). Practice parameters for the assessment and treatment of attention deficit/hyperactivity disorders. *Journal of American Academy of Child and Adolescent Psychiatry, 30,* 1–3.

American Psychiatric Association (1980). *Diagnostic and Statistical Manual of Mental Disorders* (3rd ed.). Washington, DC: Author.

American Psychiatric Association. (1994). *Diagnostic and Statistical Manual of Mental Disorders* (4th ed.). Washington, DC: Author.

Anorexia Nervosa and Related Eating Disorders, Inc. (1999a). Treatment and recovery. Available online: http://www.anred.com/tx.html

Anorexia Nervosa and Related Eating Disorders, Inc. (1999b). What causes eating disorders? Available online: http://www.anred.com/causes.html

Arakawa-Davies, K. (1997). Dance/movement therapy and reminiscence: A new approach to senile dementia in Japan. *The Arts in Psychotherapy, 24*(3), 291–298.

Barkley, R. A. (1990). *Attention Deficit Hyperactivity Disorder: A Handbook for Diagnosis and Treatment.* New York, NY: Guilford Press.

Biederman, J., Faraone, S. V., and Keenan, K. (1992). Further evidence for family-genetic risk factors in attention deficit hyperactivity disorder. *Archives of General Psychiatry, 49,* 728–738.

Bonner, A. P. and Cousins, S. O. (1996). Exercise and Alzheimer's disease: Benefits and barriers. *Activities, Adaptation, & Aging, 20(4),* 21–29.

Buettner, L. L. (1995). Therapeutic recreation as an intervention in persons with dementia: A case study of Mrs. M. *Therapeutic Recreation Journal, XXIX*(1), 63–69.

Buettner, L. L. (1999). Simple pleasures: A multilevel sensorimotor intervention for nursing home residents with dementia. *American Journal of Alzheimer's Disease, 14*(1), 41–52.

Bumanis, A. and Yoder, J. W. (1987). Music and dance: Tools for reality orientation. *Activities, Adaptation, & Aging, 8*(3), 23–27.

Burgess, C. W. (1990). Horticulture and its application to the institutionalized elderly. *Activities, Adaptation & Aging, 14(3),* 51–57.

Butler, R. N. and Lewis, M. J. (1983). *Aging and Mental Health.* St. Louis, MO: C. V. Mosby Company.

Carter, M. J., Van Andel, G. E., and Robb, G. M. (1995). *Therapeutic recreation: A recreational approach* (2nd Ed.). Prospect Heights, IL: Waveland Press.

Chandler, J. (1999). Oppositional defiant disorder (ODD) and conduct disorder (CD) in children and adolescents: Diagnosis and treatment. Available online: http://www.klis.com/chandler/pamphlet/oddcd/oddcdpamphlet.htm

Christie, M. E. (1992). Music therapy applications in a skilled and intermediate care nursing home facility: A clinical study. *Activities, Adaptation, & Aging, 16*(4), 69–75.

Clements, W. M. (1982). Therapeutic functions of recreation in reminiscence with aging persons. In M. L Teague, R. D MacNeil, and G. L. Hitzhusen (Eds.), *Perspectives on leisure and aging in a changing society* (pp. 338–351). Columbia, MO: University of Missouri.

Coleman, M. and Gillberg, C. (1992). The autistic syndromes. In A. M. Donellan (Ed.), *Classic Readings in Autism* (2nd ed., pp. 370–382). New York, NY: Teachers College Press.

Damon, J. and May, R. (1986). The effects of pet facilitative therapy on patients and staff in an adult day care center. *Activities, Adaptation, & Aging, 7*(2), 117–120.

Dattilo, J. and Schleien, S. (1991). The Benefits of therapeutic recreation in developmental disabilities. In C. P. Coyle, W. B Kenny, B. Riley, and J. W. Shank (Eds.), *Benefits of therapeutic recreation: A consensus view* (pp. 69–150). Ravensdale, WA: Idyll Arbor.

Dennis, H. (1994). Remotivation Groups. In J. M. Burnside and M. G. Schmidt (Eds.), *Working with older adults: Group processes and techniques* (3rd ed., pp. 153–162). Boston, MA: Jones & Bartlett Publishers, Inc.

Elliott, R. O., Dobbin, A. R., Rose, G. D., and Soper, H. V. (1994). Vigorous, aerobic exercise versus general motor training activities: Effects on maladaptive and stereotypic behaviors of adults with both autism and Mental Retardation. *Journal of Autism and Developmental Disorders, 24*(5), 565–572.

Feil, N. (1989). Validation therapy with late-onset dementia populations. In G. M. M. Jones and B. M. L. Miesen, (Eds.), *Caregiving in dementia: Research and applications* (pp. 199–218). New York, NY: Routledge.

Flaherty, J. A. and Andrianopoulous, G. D. (1993). Eating disorders. In J. A. Flaherty, J. M. Davis, and P. G. Janicak (Eds.), *Psychiatry: Diagnosis & therapy* (2nd ed., pp. 196–211). Norwalk, CT: Appleton & Lange.

Frith, U. (1997). Autism. *Scientific American, 7*(1), 92–98.

Garlock-Kongable, L. R. (1988). *The effects of pet therapy on the social behaviors of institutionalized Alzheimer's clients.* Unpublished master's thesis, University of Iowa, Iowa City.

Hawkins, B. A. (1996). Autism. In D. R. Austin and M. E. Crawford (Eds.), *Therapeutic recreation: An introduction* (2nd ed.). Boston, MA: Allyn and Bacon, 112–129.

Hawkins, B. A., May, M. E., and Rogers, N. B. (1996). *Therapeutic activity intervention with the elderly: Foundations and practices.* State College, PA: Venture Publishing, Inc.

Henning, J. and Dalrymple, N. J. (1986). A guide for developing social and leisure programs for students with Autism. In E. Schopler, and G. B. Mesibov (Eds.), *Social Behavior in Autism* (pp. 321–350). New York, NY: Plenum Press.

Hill, J. C. and Schoener, E. P. (1996). Age-dependent decline of attention deficit hyperactivity disorder. *American Journal of Psychiatry, 153,* 1143–1146.

Holmberg, S. K. (1997). A walking program for wanderers: Volunteer training and development of an evening walker's group. *Geriatric Nursing, 18,* 160–165.

Iso-Ahola, S. E., MacNeil, R. D., and Szymanski, D. J. (1980). Social psychological foundations of therapeutic recreation: An attributional analysis. In S. E. Iso-Ahola, (Ed.), *Social psychological perspectives on leisure and recreation* (pp. 390–414) Springfield, IL: Charles C. Thomas.

Kanner, L. (1943). Autistic disturbances of affective contact. *Nervous Child, 2,* 217–280.

Kaufman, J. E., McBride, L. G., Hultsman, J. T., and Black, D. R. (1988). Perceptions of leisure and an eating disorder: An exploratory study of bulimia. *Therapeutic Recreation Journal, XXII*(1), 55–63.

Klin, A. and Volkmar, F. (1995). *Asperger Syndrome: Some Guidelines for Assessment, Diagnosis, and Intervention.* New Haven, CT: Learning Disabilities Association of America.

Kraus, R. and Shank, J. (1992). *Therapeutic recreation service: Principles and practices* (4th Ed.). Dubuque, IA: William C. Brown.

Levine, M. D., Marcus, M. D., and Moulton, P. (1996). Exercise in the treatment of binge eating disorder. *International Journal of Eating Disorders, 19*(2), 171–177.

Loeber, R. and Stouthamer-Loeber, M. (1986). Family factors as correlates and predictors of juvenile conduct problems and delinquency. In M. Tonry and M. Morris, (Eds.), *Crime and justice* (Vol. 7). Chicago, IL: University of Chicago Press.

Lundgren, M. K. (1995). *Attention deficit hyperactivity disorder in children and therapeutic recreation implications.* Unpublished Honors Thesis, University of Iowa, Iowa City, IA.

Mauk, J. E., Reber, M. and Batshaw, M. L. (1997). Autism and other pervasive developmental disorders. In M. L. Batshaw (Ed.), *Children with disabilities* (4th ed., pp. 425–447). Baltimore, MD: Paul H. Brookes.

Mayo Clinic (1999, May 10). Autism: A confusing childhood disorder. Available online: http://www.mayoclinic.com

Mental Health Net (1999). Eating disorders: Anorexia nervosa. Available online: http://www.mentalhealth.net/factsfam/anorexia.html

Merck & Company, Inc. (2000). Cognitive failure: Delirium and dementia. In *The Merck Manual of Geriatrics.* Available online: http://www.merck.com/pubs/mm_geriatrics

Mitchell, J. (1999, November 22). (CTRS). University of Iowa Hospitals and Clinics, Interview.

Mobily, K. E. and Hoeft, T. M. (1985). The family's dilemma: Alzheimer's disease. *Activities, Adaptation, & Aging, 6*(4), 63–70.

National Institutes of Mental Health (1999). Mental health: A report of the Surgeon General (Chapter 3, Children and Mental Health). Available online: http://www.surgeongeneral.gov/library/mentalhealth/toc.html#chapter3

O'Conner, N. and Hermelin, B. (1991). Talents and preoccupations in idiot savants. *Psychological Medicine, 21,* 959–964.

Pipher, M. (1994). *Reviving Ophelia: Saving the selves of adolescent girls.* New York, NY: Ballantine Books.

Raine, A., Reynolds, C., Venables, P. H., Mednick, S. A., and Farington, D. P. (1998). Fearlessness, stimulation-seeking, and large body size at age 3 years as early predisposition's to childhood aggression at age 11 years. *Archives of General Psychiatry, 55,* 745–751.

Rawson, H. E. and McIntosh, D. (1991). The effects of therapeutic camping on the self-esteem of children with severe behavior problems. *Therapeutic Recreation Journal, XXV*(4), 41–49.

Reid, P. D., Factor, D. C., Freeman, N. L., and Sherman, J. (1988). The effects of physical exercise on three autistic and developmentally disordered adolescents. *Therapeutic Recreation Journal, XXLL*(2), 47–56.

Riddick, C. and Keller, J. (1991). The Benefits of Therapeutic Recreation in Gerontology. In C. P. Coyle, W. B. Kenny, B. Riley and J. W. Shank (Eds.), *Benefits of Therapeutic Recreation: A Consensus View* (pp. 151–204). Ravensdale, WA: Idyll Arbor.

Ritvo, E. R. and Freeman, B. J. (1977). National Society for Autistic Children definition of the syndrome of autism. *Journal of Pediatric Psychology, 4,* 146–148.

Rosenthal-Malek, A. and Mitchell, S. (1997). Brief report: The effects of exercise on the self-stimulatory behaviors and positive responding of adolescents with autism. *Journal of Autism and Developmental Disorder, 27*(2), 193–199.

Sandel, S. L. (1986). Expressive group therapy with severely confused patients. *Activities, Adaptation, & Aging, 7*(4), 117–127.

Schaffer, D., Fisher, P., Dulcan, M. K., Davies, M., Piacentini, J., Schwab-Stone, M. E., Lahey, B. B., Bourdon, K., Jensen, P. S., Bird, H. R., Canino, G., and Regier, D. A. (1996a). The NIMH Diagnostic Interview Schedule for children Version 2.3 (DISC-2.3): Description, acceptability, prevalence rates, and performance in the MECA Study. Methods for the Epidemiology of Child and Adolescent Mental Disorders Study. *Journal of the American Academy of Child and Adolescent Psychiatry, 35,* 865–877.

Schaffer, D., Fisher, P., Dulcan, M. K., Davies, M., Piacentini, J., Schwab-Stone, M. E., Lahey, B. B., Bourdon, K., Jensen, P. S., Bird, H. R., and Canino, G. R. D. (1996b). The second version of the NIMH Diagnostic Interview Schedule for Children (DISC-

2). *Journal of the American Academy of Child and Adolescent Psychiatry, 35,* 865–877.

Schleien, S. J., Krotee, J. L., Mustonen, T., Kelterborn, B., and Schermer, A. D. (1987). The effect of integrating children with autism into a physical activity and recreation setting. *Therapeutic Recreation Journal, XXI*(4), 52–62.

Schleien, S. J., Rynders, J. E., Mustonen, T., and Fox, A. (1990). Effects of social play activity on the play behavior of children with autism. *Journal of Leisure Research, 22*(4), 317–328.

Schmidt, G., McLaughlin, J. and Dalrymple, N. J. (1986). Teaching students with Autism: A sport skills specialists' approach. *Journal of Physical Education, Recreation and Dance, 57*(7), 60–63.

Sharma, R. and Gierl, B. L. (1993). Dementia. In Flaherty, J. A., Davis, J. M., and Janicak, P. G. (Eds.), *Psychiatry: Diagnosis and therapy* (2nd ed., pp. 235–246). Norwalk, CT: Appleton & Lange.

Shaywitz, S. E. and Shaywitz, B. A. (1988). Attention deficit disorder: Current perspective. In J. F. Kavanagh, and T. J. Truss, Jr., (Eds.), *Learning Disability: Proceedings of the National Conference* (pp. 369–523). Baltimore, MD: York Press.

Skalko, T., Van Andel, G., and De Salvatore, G. (1991). The benefits of therapeutic recreation in psychiatry. In C. Coyle, W. B Kinney, B. Riley, and J. W. Shank, (Eds.), *Benefits of therapeutic recreation: A consensus View* (pp. 289–337). Ravensdale, WA: Idyll Arbor.

Smith, S. (1990). The unique power of music therapy benefits Alzheimer's patients. *Activities, Adaptation, & Aging, 14*(4), 59–64.

Smith-Marchese, R. (1994). The effects of participatory music on the reality orientation and sociability of Alzheimer's residents in a long-term care setting. *Activities, Adaptation, & Aging, 18*(2), 41–47.

Sumpter, S. (1989, Fall). Leisure time: Fun or work? *Health Scene,* 3.

Szatmari, P. (1991). Asperger's Syndrome: Diagnosis, treatment, and outcome. *Psychiatric Clinics of North America, 14,* 81–93.

Teague, M. L. and MacNeil, R. D. (1992). *Aging and Leisure: Vitality in Later Life* (2nd ed.). Dubuque, IA: Brown & Benchmark.

U. S. Department of Health and Human Services (1996). *Attention Deficit Hyperactivity Disorder.* (NIH Publication No. 96-3572) Washington, DC: U. S. Government Printing Office.

Voight, A. (1988). The use of ropes courses as a treatment modality for emotionally disturbed adolescents in hospitals. *Therapeutic Recreation Journal, XXII*(2), 57–64.

Ward, C. R., Kamp, L. L., and Newman, S. (1996). The effects of participation in an intergenerational program on the behavior of residents with dementia. *Activities, Adaptation, & Aging, 20*(4), 61–69.

Weiss, C. and Kronberg, J. (1986). Upgrading TR service to severely disoriented elderly. *Therapeutic Recreation Journal, XX*(1), 32–42.

Weiss, C. and Thurn, J. (1987). A mapping project to facilitate reminiscence in a long-term care facility. *Therapeutic Recreation Journal, XXI*(2), 46–53.

Weiss, C., Markue-Patch, M., and Thurn, J. (1990). Meals, memories and memoirs: A culinary odyssey. *Therapeutic Recreation Journal, XXIV*(4), 10–22.

Weiss, C. R. and Thurn, J. M. (1990). Perceived effects of a training program to enhance family members' ability to facilitate reminiscing with older disoriented residents. *Therapeutic Recreation Journal, XXIV*(1), 18–31.

Wender, P. H. (1995). *Attention-Deficit Hyperactivity Disorder in Adults*. New York, NY: Oxford University Press.

Whalen, C. K. and Henker, B. (1992). The social profile of attention-deficit hyperactivity disorder. *Child and Adolescent Psychiatric Clinics of North America, 1*, 395–410.

White, C. L., Anderson-Laser, C., Ganz-Imphong, J., and Mattiko, M. (1992). In G. Hitzhausen, (Ed.), *Expanding horizons in therapeutic recreation XV* (pp. 204–211). Columbia, MO: University of Missouri.

Wolf, J., Willmuth, M., and Watkins, A. (1986, November). Art therapy's role in the treatment of anorexia nervosa. *American Journal of Art Therapy, 25*, 39–46.

CHAPTER 9 PSYCHOMOTOR DOMAIN

The psychomotor domain represents a collection of behaviors characterized by observable physical activities and inferred from actions executed by the musculoskeletal system and guided by the nervous system. The psychomotor domain depends on all physiological systems for its integrity. As Harrow (1972) points out, "to facilitate development of explicit objectives . . . the writer must have some basic understandings regarding the functioning of the organism" (p. 30). Hence, this text takes a broader view of the psychomotor domain than is typically represented in other textbooks.

One caveat should be mentioned before proceeding. The division of human behavior into cognitive, affective, and psychomotor domains gives the false impression of clear and distinct demarcations between behaviors; however, these divisions are quite arbitrary. For example, observable physical activity, particularly of a skilled nature, requires cognition (e.g., a good soccer player is always thinking about game tactics while executing the physical aspects of soccer skills). Likewise, observable physical behavior is often used as evidence of learning (e.g., demonstration of a learned skill such as typing or playing a musical instrument). Keeping the arbitrary nature of dividing human behavior into domains in mind will be even more crucial when discussion in subsequent chapters turns to specific disorders.

This is aptly demonstrated in Berryman, James, and Trader's (1991) discussion of physical disabilities and TR. They remind TR practitioners that much of the impact of a physical malady pertains to patient characteristics other than physical symptoms (e.g., a frequent response to a spinal cord injury is depression). Treating the whole person is essential to the success of any TR program. We only divide behavioral domains for our own convenience—to make aspects of TR practice (e.g., making assessments, writing goals and objectives, completing evaluations) easier to comprehend.

Following a description of the components of psychomotor domain, the chapter turns to an overview of physical disabilities and afflictions frequently treated in TR programs. Mortality and morbidity statistics and chronic conditions are reviewed, along with he impact

of physical disabilities on the person, his or her family, and his or her leisure lifestyle. A brief overview of normal development provides basis for the specific discussions found in the chapters that follow. The next section provides definitions and basic anatomical principles that are prerequisite to the understanding of information contained with chapters 10–15. A description of the four basic tissue types is also provided. The chapter concludes with important practical and programming information pertaining to wheelchair safety and lifting patients.

Components of the Psychomotor Domain

The psychomotor domain, first described in detail by Harrow (1972), has been a useful tool for educators concerned with learning and classifying observable behaviors. Because they are frequently called upon to develop measurable and observable markers for patient improvement, program effectiveness, and quality assurance reviews, TR practitioners should find knowledge of the psychomotor domain useful. Harrow's description of the psychomotor domain is a hierarchy— each of the components function as a prerequisite for the next, more advanced level of activity (see **Table 9.1**, p. 160).

Reflex movements represent the most basic level of the psychomotor domain. Reflex movements are not subject to conscious control. The reflexes persist throughout life, are generally protective in nature, and are not generally regarded as modifiable. Therefore, only unusual circumstances would require the writing of treatment objectives in TR at this level of the psychomotor domain.

An example of this classification level is a *stretch reflex*. When you visit the physician for a routine physical examination, the doctor will test your reflexes to determine the integrity of the peripheral nervous system, the muscle system, and some parts of the central nervous system. The doctor will tap on your patellar tendon between your patella (kneecap) and tibia (shin). This stimulus typically elicits a slight knee jerk caused by the contraction of the quadriceps femoris muscle group on the front of the thigh. The stretch reflex prevents the muscle fibers in the quadriceps femoris from being overstretched and damaged. Hence, it is regarded as a protective reflex.

The first level of the psychomotor domain that may attract the attention of a therapeutic recreation specialist

(TRS) is *basic fundamental movements*. Basic locomotor patterns (e.g., walking) are represented at this level along with normal developmental accomplishments pertaining to limb movements (e.g., throwing) or manipulative movements (e.g., grasping). Although basic movement patterns are not present at birth, in normal development they appear during the first year of life. As many of the reflexes present at birth are integrated, the basic movements begin to appear. Clearly, these fundamental movement capabilities are prerequisite to subsequent levels of psychomotor behavior, such as skilled movements.

Although educators in public schools usually are not especially concerned about basic movement patterns because they are already present when children enter schools, the TRS may have several clients that have treatment and intervention issues that encompass basic movement patterns. Candidates include persons with developmental disabilities who have not acquired basic movement skills at all (e.g., difficulty with ambulation is common among children with cerebral palsy) and persons with acquired disabilities who have lost some basic movement capabilities (e.g., persons

with head injuries who exhibit difficulty with ambulation or manipulative skills on one side of the body).

An example of using the psychomotor domain at the level of basic movement patterns for patient who has had a stroke could be:

Treatment Team Goal: to improve dexterity of the affected hand

TR Treatment Objective: the patient will complete three craft projects of his choosing using fine motor skills (e.g., grasping, holding, handling, drawing) within three weeks

Perceptual abilities and physical abilities represent the next two levels of the psychomotor domain, suggesting that perceptual abilities are prerequisite to physical abilities. But developmental literature suggests that perceptual abilities and physical abilities develop at about the same time in early childhood and continue to develop into adolescence.

Perceptual abilities refer to the interpretation and understanding of stimuli from various sources. Kinesthetic stimuli relate to head, trunk, and limb position (proprioception or joint sense) and are essential to

Level	Components	Definition
Reflex Movements	Segmental Intersegmental Suprasegmental	Subconscious movements in response to a specific stimulus
Basic Fundamental Movements	Locomotor Nonlocomotor Manipulative	Movement patterns that form a basis for skilled movements (e.g., running, jumping)
Perceptual Abilities	Kinesthetic Visual Auditory Tactile Coordinated Abilities	Interpreting of stimuli from various modalities needed to make adjustments to changes in the environment
Physical Abilities	Endurance Strength Flexibility Agility	Functional characteristics of organic health also needed for skilled movements
Skilled Movements	Simple Compound Complex	Efficiency in performing complex movements based on basic fundamental movements
Nondiscursive Communication	Expressive Interpretive	Communication through bodily movements

Table 9.1 Taxonomy of the psychomotor domain

maintaining balance and equilibrium. Visual and auditory perception refer to the understanding of stimuli detected by the retina of the eye and the inner ear. Tracking and recalling images and sounds are examples of visual and auditory perception.

Tactile discrimination relies on touch stimuli from a variety of receptors distributed mostly in the skin and its accessory structures (e.g., hair follicles). Being able to recognize a familiar object (e.g., a pencil) when placed in the hand without the aid of vision is accomplished through tactile perception—recall of what an object feels like from previous experience and recognition of the present stimuli as a match.

Coordinated abilities refer to the use of two or more perceptual components and movement patterns. (e.g., eye-hand coordination). For example, seeing a soccer ball, tracking it, and kicking it combines perception with a basic movement.

An example of using the psychomotor domain at the level of basic movement patterns for patient who has had a stroke could be:

Treatment Team Goal: to improve right visual neglect

TR Treatment Objective: during a game of "in the news," the patient will correctly name pictures of popular figures when spread on a table in front of him 75% of the time in the right visual field (i.e., on the right half of the table) without prompting from the TRS

Note that the behavioral data gathered in this objective provide inferential evidence that the correct perception has occurred. Otherwise, the person would not be able to execute the behavior at a satisfactory level of performance. The evidence for the achievement of a treatment objective based on a perceptual ability is therefore indirect and inferred from a behavior linked to the perception of the stimulus of interest (i.e., if the patient did not see and understand the images accurately, he would not be able to correctly name the popular figures).

Physical abilities include items familiar to most readers as some of the essential elements of physical fitness. Indeed, low fitness is a common problem among persons with both congenital and acquired disabilities. Some of the newer models of practice (Austin, 1998; Van Andel, 1998) include physical fitness and function as an important outcome of TR practice. In addition, low fitness and physical ability attract increased attention from practitioners because of emerging emphasis in TR practice on the prevention of secondary problems. Hence, physical abilities will be among the more common focuses of TR programs.

Endurance includes both muscular endurance and cardiovascular endurance. *Muscular endurance* is commonly measured by the number of repeated events one can execute at a submaximal level with one or more muscle groups (e.g., push-ups or sit-ups to fatigue). *Cardiovascular endurance* requires some muscle endurance plus sustained submaximal effort by the heart, lungs, and vascular system. It is commonly assessed through the use of large muscles groups over a protracted period of time (e.g., jogging or swimming for a half hour).

Muscular strength is usually distinguished from muscular endurance as a matter of degree. *Muscular strength* refers to a single maximum effort, whereas muscular endurance refers to repeated submaximal efforts. Hence, muscle strength is commonly assessed through the use of weights. The TRS should be cautious in assessing strength, as many clients with chronic conditions may put themselves at risk for injury by attempting a maximum effort to assess strength. Manifest or latent cardiovascular disease presents the most serious risk during the execution of a maximum effort.

However, the good news is that training to improve muscle strength does not require maximum effort. In fact, the training programs for improving muscle strength and improving muscle endurance look very similar. This means that the assessment of muscle endurance usually yields a satisfactory estimate of muscle strength in at-risk groups (e.g., persons with heart disease).

Flexibility refers to the range of motion at a joint. It is often assessed through the use of a goniometer (a large protractor) in field settings. Other tests of flexibility involve stretching and measuring the length of the stretch.

The final component of the physical abilities category, *agility*, refers to the ability to change direction without losing balance. As such, agility is a variant of kinesthetic perception, one of the components at the perceptual abilities level of the psychomotor domain. The difference is that balance under the kinesthetic perception category is static, whereas the balance under agility refers to dynamic balance (i.e., balance while in motion). Agility is vital for older adults if they are to avoid falls and potential injury (see the following statistics on falls). Agility is easily assessed by having the client negotiate an obstacle course for time. The obstacle course may be adapted for the particular disability (e.g., ambulatory versus wheelchair), but the crucial component remains the same—requiring the subject to change direction.

An example of using the psychomotor domain at the level of physical abilities for a patient who has osteoarthritis could be:

Treatment Team Goal: to improve balance and decrease the risk of a fall

TR Treatment Objective: during exercise group, the patient will practice rising from a seated position, walking around a cone placed 5 meters away, turning 180 degrees, and returning to sit in the chair at least 5 times each exercise period so that at the end of four weeks the patient will decrease the amount of time needed to execute the task by at least 10% when compared to baseline

Skilled movements require a certain level of proficiency in tasks that are not inherent (basic) movement patterns, such as sports. Skilled movements may also include tasks that are close to those in the basic movements level, but the level of proficiency expected is greater (e.g., everyone can run, but not everyone can run track well enough to compete).

The skilled movements comprise three components: simple, compound, and complex. *Simple skilled movements* are level two movements that have been changed to respond to a specific circumstance. For example, recreational dances are adaptations of basic locomotor movements. *Compound skilled movements* represent the next component under the skilled movements level. Compound movements are adaptations of basic movements that include the use of some external implement or tool. Tennis and golf are good examples of compound movements.

Complex skilled movements require application of physical laws by the person performing the skill. Gymnastics events or tumbling activities often require the participant to make subtle body adjustments to perform the desired stunt. Complex activities characteristically involve the entire body and not just one segment of the body.

An example of using the psychomotor domain at the level of skilled movements with a patient who has paraplegia as a result of a spinal cord injury is as follows:

Treatment Team Goal: to assist the patient in learning activities for the meaningful use of free time

TR Treatment Objective: the patient will acquire proficiency in two sport activities that he will select from a list of available activities at the facility. Proficiency will be demonstrated by average performance (50th percentile) when compared to standardized performance norms for the two activities selected

The final level of the psychomotor domain is that of *nondiscursive communication*. Movements frequently

communicate messages to others. From facial expressions of delight and sorrow to the wave of a hand signaling a greeting or farewell, body language is full of information. The two subcategories of nondiscursive movement include expressive communication and interpretive communication.

Expressive communication refers to posture, facial expressions, and movements that occur on a routine, day-to-day basis. The expressive component is developed through habit, culture, and socialization. Expressive communication becomes quite automated by adulthood (e.g., we often cannot hide our emotions). *Interpretive communication* is of greater interest to the TRS because at this level the actor plans the movement with the intent of communicating a specific message, often of a creative or aesthetic nature. Figure skating and dance require the interpretive level of nondiscursive communication. Interpretive communication movements must be invented, practiced, and even modified to assure that the intended message is being sent.

An example of using the psychomotor domain at the level of nondiscursive communication for a patient who has cerebral palsy is as follows:

Treatment Team Goal: to assist the patient in acquiring creative skills for use in leisure time

TR Treatment Objective: the patient will learn how to figure skate well enough to participate in the end of winter skating jamboree held at the local ice arena

As demonstrated here, the psychomotor domain is a useful tool for developing treatment and learning objectives for TR practice. Harrow's (1972) taxonomy of the psychomotor domain helps the TRS understand and plan outcomes that relate to observable behavior and delineate the boundaries of physical disabilities. The latter topic is taken up in greater detail in the next section.

Overview of Physical Disabilities

Mortality Statistics

Table 9.2 lists the leading causes of death in the United States. This table shows that most people in the United States die of disorders that have to do with a combination of the effects of aging, exposure to adverse environmental stimuli (e.g., pollution), and negative lifestyle habits (e.g., sedentary lifestyle, smoking). These data mark a departure from a few generations ago, when infectious diseases and childhood diseases accounted for a large percentage of deaths.

More people are living longer because of the scientific breakthroughs that have eradicated or controlled many of the leading causes of death at the beginning of the twentieth century. Antibiotics, better nutrition and sanitation, and improved healthcare have allowed most people in Western societies to live nearer to the maximum expected human life span (about 80 years). However, this trend has uncovered the more contemporary pattern of morbidity and mortality—the diseases of lifestyle and aging illustrated in Table 9.2.

Chronic Conditions

Along with the change in the leading causes of death has emerged a new class of health concerns, the chronic condition. Chronic conditions cause the person to live in a more limited manner. They affect quality of life and the ability to carry on the day-to-day functional activities necessary for independent living. **Table 9.3** (p. 164) lists the leading chronic conditions in the United States in order of prevalence. Many of the leading chronic conditions contribute to the leading causes of death (e.g., high blood pressure is a risk factor for heart attack and stroke). Many of the leading causes of death are also chronic conditions if the disorder is not immediately fatal (e.g., a person may suffer a nonfatal heart attack and then live with the limitations imposed by the associated weakness).

One of the most significant changes in healthcare over the last 50 years is the type of patient being seen. Patients tend to be older, sicker, and more debilitated as a result of the increased prevalence of chronic conditions. Most chronic conditions increase in frequency and rate in the older age groups; many relate to the eventual cause of death.

Rank/Cause	Rate per 100,000
1 Diseases of the heart	280.7
2 Malignancies (cancer)	204.9
3 Cerebrovascular diseases (stroke)	60.1
4 Chronic obstructive pulmonary diseases	39.2
5 Accidents	35.5
6 Pneumonia and influenza	31.6
7 Diabetes mellitus	22.6
8 HIV/AIDS	16.4
9 Suicide	11.9
10 Chronic liver disease and cirrhosis	9.6

Table 9.2 Ten leading causes of death in the United States for 1995

Many chronic conditions make the individual more susceptible to secondary problems. For instance, persons with arthritis and orthopedic disorders are apprehensive about ambulation and exercise because of pain. The musculoskeletal system then deteriorates further as a result of the inactivity, which puts the person at greater risk for a fall. A National Safety Council report (1991) indicated that after the age of 75, the leading cause of accidental death is falls, not automobile accidents. And the mortality data are conservative because they do not tell how many nonfatal falls resulted in fractures that further impacted the person's independence and quality of life.

Hence, the TRS in both clinical and community settings is apt to see a much different client than those seen a generation ago. For example, whereas 30 years ago clinical TRS often worked with spinal cord lesions, now the TRS is more likely to work with a person with arthritis accompanied by one or more other chronic conditions. Most patients do not have just one problem. Likewise, clients seen by the community TRS 30 years ago were predominantly school-age students with developmental disabilities. Nowadays the community TRS is apt to service older adult clients with chronic conditions not severe enough to require inpatient clinical treatment, but significant enough to require ongoing attention from outpatient- and community-based services. In addition, Beaudouin and Keller (1994) observed that more patients being discharged from inpatient agencies have a need for indefinite rehabilitation and maintenance services. Often the patient discharged from an inpatient rehabilitation situation is assumed to be "cured." Nothing could be further from the case: a person with a diabetes mellitus will require lifelong exercise, for example, if he is to avoid or delay the onset of significant secondary health problems. The person with a head injury may continue to improve for up to two years, well after discharge. Yet, he is afforded only a relatively short time in active, inpatient rehabilitation.

Chronic Disability and Quality of Life

Limited data exist pertaining to the impact of disability and chronic conditions on quality of life. Coyle and Kinney (1990) surveyed 790 community-dwelling persons with physical disabilities 18–55 years of age. They asked about leisure satisfaction, accessibility of recreation facilities, barriers to leisure, and functional impairment. The average age of the respondents was 37 years. Only 21% were employed full-time, with another 10% employed part-time. The subjects were also described as "financially impoverished," on the average. The results speak to serious quality of life issues associated with chronic conditions.

Reading and watching television were the most popular activities reported by the subjects—hardly the activity profile conducive to improving or maintaining health in the presence of a chronic condition. Subjects reported that the most significant barriers to more active participation were weather, transportation, facility factors (access, availability, and distance), having the skills and abilities to participate, and safety concerns. The typical subject's leisure profile was sedentary, homebound, low skill, and low social involvement (Coyle & Kinney, 1990). Not surprisingly, the same study revealed a negative relationship between leisure satisfaction and severity of disability—the more severe the disorder, the lower the score on the leisure satisfaction measure. Furthermore, more impaired persons had more difficulty identifying places where they could go for recreation in the community.

Coyle and Kinney (1990) reached several conclusions about persons with physical disabilities residing in the community. First, they maintained that many persons with physical disabilities residing in communi-

ties were isolated, according to the typical leisure profile reported. Many were unemployed, stayed at home, were physically inactive, and had little social involvement. Almost half could not name more than three accessible facilities in the community. This "hidden population" needed more leisure education and community reintegration programs to develop meaningful leisure pursuits.

Earlier, Lyons (1987) reported findings similar to those of Coyle and Kinney (1990). She surveyed 150 adults with spinal cord lesions, multiple sclerosis, and stroke about their leisure. Lyons' subjects reported very little leisure outside the home, passive leisure activity, and social isolation. The subjects who adjusted most successfully reported returning to work and having transportation. Presumably, the income that resulted from work and the availability of transportation combined to counteract the tendency toward social isolation observed in so many cases of persons with physical disabilities. However, Lyons (1987) did not conclude that successful adjustment to disability is entirely determined by employment and car ownership. Instead, because she also found a positive relationship between leisure satisfaction and adjustment to disability, Lyons argued that a satisfying lifestyle could be established

Type	All ages	Under 45	45–64	65 and over
Arthritis	128.8	32.8	239.0	501.5
Deformity or orthopedic impairment	119.7	97.4	170.0	165.6
High blood pressure	108.8	32.2	222.3	364.0
Hearing impairments	86.3	36.8	137.9	286.4
Heart disease	85.8	30.1	135.7	324.9
Asthma	56.1	58.6	50.8	50.5
Chronic bronchitis	54.0	50.1	63.9	60.5
Migraine headaches	43.4	44.5	52.5	21.8
Visual impairments	33.1	21.2	45.1	82.2
Diabetes	29.9	8.1	63.1	101.2
Tinnitus	27.1	10.7	46.3	90.1
Cataracts	24.9	2.5	17.3	166.2
Intervertebral disk disorders	23.1	13.8	50.7	31.7
Anemias	18.0	17.6	17.6	20.4
Ulcer	17.1	12.3	25.2	31.6
Bladder disorders	14.4	9.3	16.9	39.7
Kidney trouble	13.5	10.9	17.2	22.4
Cerebrovascular disease	11.5	1.6	18.2	57.4
Glaucoma	10.0	1.9	11.8	53.9
Hardening of the arteries	8.6	0.2	11.1	52.9
Rheumatic fever	8.0	5.3	12.4	16.1
Emphysema	7.8	0.7	9.9	45.5
Paralysis of extremities	5.5	2.8	9.1	15.0
Absence of extremities	5.4	2.6	7.8	17.8
Epilepsy	5.4	5.5	4.7	5.7

Table 9.3 Selected chronic conditions for 1994 per 1000 by age

based on leisure, with adjustment for the limitations imposed by the illness and abilities discovered or learned after onset. She further stated that "we must think of the experience of leisure not in isolation but in the context of overall adjustment to disability" (p. 4). Hence, Lyons suggested that the person experiences a leisure adjustment to the disability.

Two other small sample studies have confirmed the impact of disability on the leisure of persons with physical disabilities. Perry (1995) examined the leisure constraints on families with children with physical disabilities. She interviewed 16 families and the list of constraints followed a familiar pattern. The leading constraints reported by families who had children with physical disabilities were lack of time, lack of money, mobility issues, lack of accessible facilities, extra planning requirements, and lack of community resources. When asked how they solved the problems associated with the reported constraints, subjects reported three strategies: take action, decrease participation, or no solution. Unfortunately, the latter two had detrimental consequences on leisure.

Caldwell and Lee (1994/1995) took a different approach to the investigation of TR and persons with spinal cord injury (SCI). They asked patients with SCI about their interpretation of the role and significance of TR during and after rehabilitation (after return to the community). In general, the patients had very favorable evaluations of the importance of TR services in their rehabilitation. However, some of the patients reported one negative aspect of TR after discharge: inpatient TR raised their expectations of what was possible in terms of a satisfying leisure lifestyle. The problem, reported the patients, was that the raised expectations made adjustment more difficult in the community because many of the advantages and opportunities afforded them during rehabilitation were unavailable in the community after discharge. A supportive, accepting environment filled with peers with similar injuries and positive-thinking professionals were more important factors than the physical infrastructure necessary for participation.

Rehabilitation for Persons with Physical Disabilities

Berryman et al. (1991) reported on significant issues in the rehabilitation process. They listed five crucial issues for practically all persons with physical disabilities: retaining or reclaiming a sense of mastery and control over one's life, controlling stress, finding purpose to life, changing attitude toward disability, and improving body image. All of these issues, argued Berryman and associates, were addressed by TR. Choice and competent performance in recreational pursuits enhance mastery. Recreational activities, especially those requiring some physical exertion, help relieve or control stress. Discovering new leisure interests or adapting preinjury leisure pursuits provide a measure of purpose to life. Understanding potentials and possibilities in leisure is apt to change attitudes toward disability in a favorable direction. Last, improved physical ability and skills during recreation may lead to an improvement in body image.

Normal Development

This section presents a general overview of growth and development, including, prenatal development, birth, postnatal development, and perceptual motor development. It reviews basic developmental principles to help the reader prepare a context for the disorders covered in subsequent chapters. Only through knowledge of normal growth and development can the TR student come to appreciate the extent of the impairment and the impact of the disorder on the client. Subsequent chapters treat specific topics in growth and development that pertain to the systems being covered in each chapter.

Prenatal Development

Growth and development begins with conception. Fertilization occurs in the *fallopian tubes* of the female. It represents the union of a single male reproductive cell, a *sperm cell*, and a single female reproductive cell, an *egg cell*. Each reproductive cell carries one half of the offspring's future genetic profile. The equal contribution of maternal and paternal *chromosomes* results in an offspring with a complete set of 46 total chromosomes (23 pairs) that represent an individual's complete genetic makeup. Following this union, the newly formed cell is referred to as a *zygote*.

Over the next three days the zygote travels down the fallopian tube toward the *uterus* for implantation. As the zygote migrates down the fallopian tube it experiences rapid cell division. This rapid mitotic division is referred to as the *cleavage* stage, and the resulting ball of cells is called a *morula*.

As the morula nears the end of its trip down the fallopian tube and prepares to enter the uterus, its cells begin to differentiate. The resulting structure is known as a *blastocyst*. A blastocyst consists of an outer layer of cells called the *trophoblast,* a *cavity* on the inside, and an inner layer of cells known as the *embryoblast.* Eventually the inner cells will differentiate into the embryo and the outer cells will become part of the *placenta.*

As the blastocyst moves into the uterus, it begins the next stage of prenatal development—*implantation.* This refers to the activities surrounding the attachment of the blastocyst to the uterine wall. This step is essential to the viability of the embryo because it establishes a mechanism for respiration and nutrition through the placenta. The blastocyst literally eats its way into the uterine wall through the use of powerful enzymes and implantation is accomplished. By the end of the stage of implantation about two weeks have passed since conception.

During the second week, the *embryo* (the inner cells) begins to differentiate and form the three *germ layers.* The three germ layers are initially in the form of a flattened, *embryonic disk.* Later cells from the layers will migrate to different locations to form all of the anatomical structures necessary to life (see **Table 9.4**). When the last germ layer is formed, the beginning of the *embryonic period* is signaled, which will continue for the next 6 weeks.

During the embryonic period, the anatomy necessary to support the growing infant is established. During the 6 weeks of embryonic life the placenta and *fetal membranes* form. Also, the germ layers differentiate into the structures listed in Table 9.4.

The formation of two membranes is particularly vital to life in the womb—the *placenta* and the *amnion* are essential to the developing embryo. The placenta is formed from a portion of the outer layer of the blastocyst, called the *chorion,* and a portion of the uterine wall, called the *decidua.* Fingerlike projections of the chorion, known as *chorionic villi,* penetrate into the decidua. Hence, the placenta has both an embryonic contribution and a maternal contribution. The placenta is a highly vascular structure that brings maternal and embryonic blood into close proximity. Although blood from mother and infant do not mix in a normal pregnancy, they are close enough to allow for the diffusion of nutrients and oxygen from mother to child. Therefore, the placenta is the mechanism for respiration and nutrition in the prenatal period.

Connecting the placenta to the embryo is the *umbilical cord.* The umbilical cord contains arteries and veins responsible for carrying oxygen and nutrient rich blood from the placenta to the embryo in exchange for waste products and carbon dioxide.

Another protective structure derived from the embryo is the *amniotic sac.* It is formed when the amnion surrounds the entire embryo. It is filled with fluid, which offers added protection for the growing embryo.

By the end of the embryonic period most of the anatomical structures necessary for life are in place. The next seven months of gestation are referred to as the *fetal* period. The infant begins to look human, and much of the remaining seven months is spent growing and maturing so that life can be sustained outside the womb.

Birth

Labor can be divided into three distinct stages: dilation, expulsion, and placental. The *dilation stage* is usually the longest. It refers to the enlargement of the *cervix,* the opening to the uterus, to a diameter of 10 centimeters. This is customarily regarded as the minimum diameter for the infant's head to pass through the birth canal. The *expulsion stage* is the actual childbirth—expelling the infant from the uterus. Last, in the

Germ Layer	Derivatives
Ectoderm	Epidermis of skin Nervous system Pituitary gland Outer part of adrenal gland Sensory receptors
Mesoderm	Muscle system Skeletal system Connective tissue Circulatory system Dermis of skin Kidneys Ureters Part of adrenal gland
Endoderm	Liver Pancreas Respiratory system Digestive system Bladder Urethra Parathyroid Thymus Thyroid gland

Table 9.4 Structures derived from the 3 germ layers

placental stage, the placenta separates from the uterine wall and is passed down the birth canal.

Postnatal Development

Postnatal development represents the remainder of life. It includes the neonatal period (birth to 1 month), infancy (1 month to 2 years), childhood (the end of infancy to the onset of puberty, about age 12), adolescence (the onset of puberty until adulthood and the cessation of growth, about age 20), and adulthood (20 years to death). Each period has important themes the TRS should be aware of—some developmental, which represent maturation, and some degenerative, which represent the aging process.

Following birth, the newborn is typically assessed for vitality and given an Apgar score (Malina & Bouchard, 1991). The *Apgar score*, a system of scoring an infant's physical condition 1–5 minutes after birth, was developed by anesthesiologist Virginia Apgar. Scores may range from 0–10, with a higher score indicating better health. Two points are possible for heart rate, breathing, muscle tone, reflex response, and color.

The *neonatal period* is marked by reflexive movements on the part of the infant. He is not in control of his motor capabilities and must establish two crucial functions—respiration and heart rate. Otherwise, the neonate's behavior is governed by reflexes aimed at enhancing his chances for survival (e.g., rooting and sucking reflexes for feeding).

The nervous system is anatomically complete at birth, but immature. As the infant's nervous system develops, primitive reflexes become inhibited or incorporated into voluntary movement patterns (Malina & Bouchard, 1991). In the case of an infant with a developmental disability (e.g., cerebral palsy), some of the primitive reflexes may persist into later life and constrain the development of normal movement patterns.

Infancy is characterized by a distinct increase in motor control and mastery of many basic movements, most notably ambulation. Infants increase substantially in length and weight, and the brain is near adult size by the end of the infancy period.

The so-called "brain growth spurt" (Malina & Bouchard, 1991) continues until around age four. It is marked not only by growth in the size of the brain, but also notable development of the cerebellum, whose major functions are to regulate coordination, balance, and equilibrium. Development of the cerebellum, along with completion of the myelination process in the central nervous system, facilitate walking and all

movements that are derived from a basic, upright, ambulation posture (e.g., running).

Head control is accomplished early during the infancy period. Next the trunk and upper extremities are controlled and reflexes regulating the limbs are integrated. Sitting posture is followed closely by various forms of prone progression (e.g., creeping, crawling). Standing independently gives the infant the confidence to try assisted walking by holding on to a parent's hand. Finally independent walking is observed somewhere between 10 and 14 months. Walking is the major developmental task of infancy; it depends on a series of postural changes that lead to the development of motor control (Malina & Bouchard, 1991).

Harrow (1972) reminds readers of several long-standing principles of psychomotor development that hold throughout infancy and childhood. Development tends to progress from head to toe. Proximal parts of the body are brought under control before distal parts of the body. Infants learn how to control their trunks, shoulder girdles and hip girdles before their upper and lower extremities. Control of the digits is the next task to be accomplished. Grasp precedes the ability to manipulate objects in a meaningful manner (e.g., writing). Reciprocal capabilities are the last to develop (e.g., climbing steps using alternating gait and arm swing). The cumulative effect of these principles of psychomotor development is that most fundamental motor skills are present by ages 6 to 7.

Childhood is marked by significant intellectual development not only attributable to maturation, but also environmental stimulation accessed through the added capacity for exploring the environment. Consistent growth with marked improvement in motor control over the period from 2 to 12 years of age is another theme. Children separated by a year or less demonstrate marked differences in psychomotor capabilities.

The onset of puberty, slightly earlier in girls than boys, signals the beginning of adolescence. Puberty is characterized by an increase in the amount of sex hormones in the bloodstream. The sex hormones stimulate the development of many secondary sex characteristics that serve to distinguish males and females (e.g., the distribution of muscle and fat, height, hair, the thickness of bones) As the sex organs mature, they become functional. Puberty is also a time of continued intellectual and emotional development.

Adulthood begins around the age of 20, marked by a cessation of growth in stature and strength. Also, adulthood means that the aging process has begun. Degeneration of systems is a constant theme over the following decades. The aging process varies considerably from person to person. Although aging and deterioration are somewhat genetically determined, people can do a great deal to slow the deterioration of physiologic systems and retain significant vigor, health, and intellectual capability well into their 80s and 90s.

Perceptual-Motor Development

Perception refers to the understanding and interpretation of sensory information by the central nervous system, specifically the brain. The term *perceptual motor* establishes an association between understanding and interpreting sensory information and the act of making a motor response. Even though sensory and motor systems are commonly studied as separate entities, they interact. Motor responses deteriorate if sensory information is not delivered to the central nervous system in an appropriate fashion, not interpreted correctly, or not associated with the appropriate motor responses.

Children need visual, auditory, and kinesthetic information to learn proper motor responses and skills (Haywood, 1993). Sensory systems continue to improve throughout childhood, with visual, auditory, and kinesthetic perception reaching near adult levels of sophistication by the end of the childhood period (around age 12). Likewise, as people age during the adult period, sensory systems deteriorate and perception slows, resulting in motor performance decrements.

The relationship between perception and motor performance illustrates an important point made earlier in this chapter. Evidence for perceptual ability cannot be observed directly—it must be inferred from motor performance. If perceptual mechanisms begin to fail, performance decrements are usually observed. This is clearly the case with older adults who run an increased risk of falling. One significant risk factor for falling is the deterioration of visual and kinesthetic mechanisms that help maintain balance and adjust equilibrium to environmental circumstances.

As children develop individual sensory and perceptual abilities in visual, auditory, and kinesthetic modalities, the next step is to be able to integrate multiple systems. This is called intersensory integration (Haywood, 1993). More complex skills require the use of two or more sources of sensory information. These sources must be integrated in a coherent manner to be interpreted correctly and facilitate a rapid, smooth, and coordinated movement. For instance, when fielding a ground ball in softball, better players use visual (seeing the ball), auditory (hearing the bat hit the ball), and kinesthetic (feeling the ball enter the glove) to execute a complex motor skill. Integration of these sensory modalities does not occur immediately, but it does improve as the child matures toward adolescence.

Balance is both a simple and a complex skill. Balancing on one foot in a low stimulus environment with adequate lighting is not difficult for most people. But balancing while executing another complex movement under competitive and rapidly changing conditions (e.g., dribbling a basketball) is a challenge that causes even elite players to error on occasion. Balance generally improves throughout childhood (Haywood, 1993) and into adolescence.

However, as with perception in general, balance capabilities gradually deteriorate as the person ages, and loss of balance is an especially dangerous development for adults over the age of 75. Haywood (1993) noted that falls are the leading cause of accidental deaths among older adults. Moreover, Haywood maintained that fear of falling leads to enough anxiety and concern among older adults that it causes them to change their lifestyles. Fear of falling may result in even less motor activity, which, will further exacerbate the risk of falling.

Just as motor development depends on perception, so too does perceptual development depend on early childhood motor experiences (Haywood, 1993). Diversified movement experiences in childhood contribute measurably to the development of visual, auditory, and kinesthetic perception and the integration of the three modalities later. Varied movements challenge sensory and perceptual systems; movement provides practice for perceptual mechanisms and enhances their capacity to meet a broad array of sensory challenges presented by the environment.

Anatomical Terminology and Basic Concepts

Terminology

Figure 9.1 represents the anatomical position. The anatomical position is an assumed, neutral starting position for all movement. The head is erect, with eyes forward and feet about shoulder width apart. The fingers are pointed down, the palms face forward, and the shoulders are square.

The *regional terminology* used to label Figure 9.1 is fixed. This means that the word *brachial* always refers to the arm, the word *carpal* always refers to the wrist, and so on. The more commonly used terms are known as directional terms. *Directional terms* are more diffi-cult because they are relative and not fixed. This means that the reader must always be given at least two anatomical locations to determine the accuracy of the term selected. For example, the term *lateral* means toward the outside. But it is not possible to judge whether the term was being used in a correct manner unless one knew what structure was to be lateral to a second structure. To say that the hip is lateral in the anatomical position means nothing unless we add that the hip is in a lateral position relative to the navel. But relative to the thumb in the anatomical position, the hip is medial.

Table 9.5 (page 170) summarizes the directional terms. Note that anterior and posterior mean the same as ventral and dorsal, respectively. Sometimes three terms are necessary to understand three-dimensional space. The terms superficial, intermediate, and deep describe the depth dimension. *Superficial* refers to structures close to the surface (e.g., skin), *deep* refers to structures positioned in the central core (e.g., heart), and *intermediate* refers to structures found in between (e.g., muscles).

Three imaginary planes of reference cut the body into different halves. One plane divides the body into a front and a back half, the frontal plane. A second plane cuts the body into a top and a bottom half, the trans-verse plane. And finally, the *saggital* plane divides the body into a left and right half. The planes describe the different views provided in diagrams that portray the body or an organ after it has been sectioned. Planes also describe specific movements. For example, flexion and extension refer to decreasing and increasing the angle at a joint in the saggital plane. Movements may increase or decrease the angle at a joint in a different plane, but they are not labeled flexion and extension.

Cavities

Large cavities, naturally occurring spaces in the body, are commonly used to divide the body into two or more compartments. The *dorsal body cavity* is composed of the *cranial cavity* and the *vertebral cavity*. The dorsal body cavity contains the central nervous system, the brain, and the spinal cord. The *ventral body cavity* is bordered posteriorly by the vertebral column (spine),

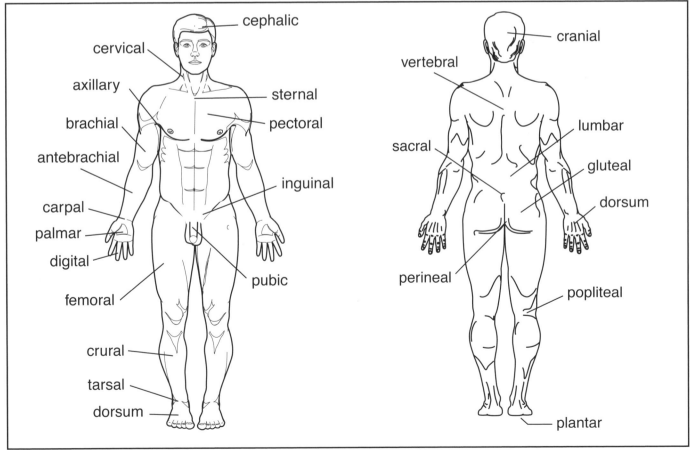

Figure 9.1 Anatomical position

laterally by the ribs, and anteriorly by the sternum (breastbone). The inferior border of the ventral body cavity is represented by the floor of the bony pelvis. The ventral body cavity is not closed completely on its anterior border below the ribs and sternum. The ventral body cavity can be further divided into an *upper thoracic cavity* containing the heart and lungs, and a *lower abdomino-pelvic cavity* containing the digestive, urinary, and reproductive systems. Collectively, all of the contents of the ventral body cavity are called *viscera.*

Tissues

A *tissue* is a group of similar cells that works together to perform specific functions. Tissues represent the next larger unit of study after the cellular level. The body is composed of four different types of tissues: epithelial, connective, muscle, and nerve.

Epithelial tissue is composed of closely packed cells that cover the surface of the body or line the inside of various tube systems within the body. Glandular epithelium forms glands, both exocrine (e.g., sweat glands) and endocrine (e.g., thyroid gland).

Connective tissue is perhaps the most confusing of the four tissue types. It serves to "connect" things, but connection here must be interpreted loosely. Connective tissue includes tendons and ligaments that connect muscle to bone and bone to bone. But connective tissue also includes such varied structures as bone, blood, and loose connective tissue. The common theme among these varied structures is that they contain few cells scattered among abundant intercellular substance.

Muscle tissue possesses the unique capability to produce tension that often results in movement. However, some muscle contraction does not result in observable movement, but only causes a change in the tonal quality of the muscle. Three types of muscle are included in this category: skeletal muscle (voluntary), cardiac muscle (involuntary), and smooth muscle (involuntary).

The fourth type of tissue, *nerve tissue*, transmits an electrical impulse in a rapid and efficient manner. Both the voluntary (skeletal) and involuntary (smooth, cardiac) divisions of the nervous system belong to this category of tissue.

Each of the chapters that follow will close with a short section on practical applications that are useful in day-to-day recreation programming for persons with disabilities. General suggestions for wheelchair safety and lifting patients are presented here.

Term	Definition
Anterior (ventral)	Front of a structure; used to indicate when one structure is in front of another structure
Deep (internal)	Structure positioned close to the center or core of the body
Distal	Further from the attachment of a limb to the trunk than a second structure (e.g., further from the shoulder or hip)
Inferior (caudal)	Structure in a position lower than a second structure; more toward the tailbone
Intermediate	Position between superficial and deep; often used when three structures are discussed
Lateral	Structure positioned more toward the periphery of the body than a second structure
Medial	Structure positioned closer to the midline of the body than a second structure
Posterior (dorsal)	Back of a structure; used to indicate when one structure is behind a second structure
Proximal	Closer to the attachment of a limb to the trunk than a second structure (e.g., closer to the shoulder or hip)
Superficial (external)	Structure that is closer to the surface of the body than a second structure
Superior (cranial)	Structure in a higher position than a second structure; more toward the head

Table 9.5 Summary of directional terms

Practical Applications

Wheelchair Safety

The ability to handle a wheelchair is crucial to the quality of life of the person requiring its use. Wheelchairs are commonly used to access and participate in many recreational activities. Therefore, the chances that a TRS will encounter a person in a wheelchair during his or her career are quite high. Accordingly, the TRS must be knowledgeable of proper wheelchair use, storage, and safety. Most wheelchairs include seat belts, which should be used at all times. Turns should be taken slowly and rapid changes in direction should be avoided. Brakes should be set if the person is transferring to or from the chair, or if the person is working in a stationary position. Wheelchairs are intended for use by one person; do not tow anything or ride tandem with someone. Push wheelchairs up ramps, but back down ramps. When negotiating a curb, slowly tilt the chair backward by stepping on the tilt bar and pulling back on the handles. Pull the back wheels of the chair up to a curb so that the front wheels are in the air and the person is tilted back toward you. When descending a curb, the front wheels should be tipped up in the air and the back wheels brought slowly to the edge of the curb. Lower the chair slowly down the curb by bending your knees.

Lifting Patients

Good posture is essential to lift properly and to avoid injury to yourself or the client. The trunk should be kept in an upright position throughout the length of the spine. The feet should be about shoulder width apart. Use your legs as much as possible while executing the lift. Only bend at the knees and hips. Synchronize your lift with the patient's assist or that of a helper by counting off (e.g., one, two, three, lift). Know your limitations and use help when it is available. If the client has a functional upper extremity, then the client may place one hand behind the head of the lifter to assist in the transfer.

Chapter Summary

This chapter examined the psychomotor domain and addressed the following key concepts:

- Although some behaviors may be characterized as primarily motor for purposes of programming, physical activities include cognitive and affective components.

- Chronic conditions have increased in prevalence and incidence over the last half century with better health care and longer life expectancy.

- Chronic conditions cannot be cured, but only managed.

- Directional terminology used in the health professions refers to an area, a structure, or a relative position.

References

Adams, P. F. and Marano, M. A. (1995). Current estimates from the National Health Interview Survey, 1994. *National Center for Health Statistics. Vital Health Stats, 10,* 81–82.

Anderson, R. N., Kochanek, K. D., and Murphy, S. L. (1997). Report of final mortality statistics, 1995. *Monthly Vital Statistics, 45,* 28–33.

Austin, D. R. (1998). The health protection/health promotion model. *Therapeutic Recreation Journal, 32,* 109–117.

Beaudouin, N. M. and Keller, M. J. (1994). Aquatics solutions: A continuum of services for individuals with physical disabilities in the community. *Therapeutic Recreation Journal, 28,* 193–202.

Berryman, D., James, A., and Trader, B. (1991). The benefits of therapeutic recreation in physical medicine. In C. P. Coyle, W. B. Kinney, B. Riley, and J. W. Shank (Eds.), *Benefits of therapeutic recreation: A consensus view.* Ravensdale, WA: Idyll Arbor.

Caldwell, L. L. and Lee, Y. (1994/95). Perceptions of therapeutic recreation among people with spinal cord injury. *ATRA Annual, 5,* 13–26.

Connolly, P. and Keough-Hoss, M. A. (1991). The development and use of intervention protocols in therapeutic recreation: Documentation of field-based practices. In B. Riley (Ed.), *Quality management: Applications for therapeutic recreation* (pp. 117–136). State College, PA: Venture Publishing, Inc.

Coyle, C. P. and Kinney, W. B. (1990). Leisure characteristics of adults with physical disabilities. *Therapeutic Recreation Journal, 24,* 64–73.

Harrow, A. J. (1972). *A taxonomy of the psychomotor domain.* New York, NY: McKay.

Haywood, K. M. (1993). *Life span motor development* (2nd ed.). Champaign, IL: Human Kinetics.

Kleiber, D. A., Brock, S., Lee, Y., Dattilo, J., and Caldwell, L. (1995). The relevance of leisure in an illness experience: Realities of spinal cord injury. *Journal of Leisure Research, 27,* 283–299.

Lyons, R. F. (1987). Leisure adjustment to chronic illness and disability. *Leisurability, 14,* 4–10.

Malina, R. W. and Bouchard, C. (1991). *Growth, maturation, and physical activity.* Champaign, IL: Human Kinetics.

National Safety Council. (1991). *Accident facts.* Chicago, IL: National Safety Council.

Perry, T. L. (1995). The experience of leisure constraints by families with children with physical disabilities. *Symposium on Leisure Research Abstracts, 11.*

Van Andel, G. E. (1998). TR service delivery and TR outcome models. *Therapeutic Recreation Journal, 32,* 180–193.

Van De Graaf, K. (1998). *Human anatomy* (5th ed.). Boston, MA: McGraw-Hill.

CHAPTER 10
SKELETAL SYSTEM
AND JOINT SYSTEM

This chapter presents the skeletal system first, followed by the system of joints that collectively allow for observable movement and other vital human activities. Muscles are attached to skeletal components and contract movement is produced where different bones meet—at joints. Functions and typical structures of the skeletal and joint systems are followed by a specific presentation of representative structures in each system. For example, you will learn to identify and name specific bones and bones that form selected joints. Following presentation of each system in normal health, relevant disabilities are explained. The next section focuses on therapeutic recreation (TR) interventions and techniques germane to specific disabilities.

Skeletal System

Functions

Along with the joints and muscles, the 206 bones of the normal, adult skeleton produce movement and perform several other important functions that are not as immediately apparent. Bone serves as a reservoir for certain vital trace minerals, such as calcium and phosphorous. The internal regulating systems in the body can tap these mineral reservoirs to maintain health (e.g., adequate blood calcium is essential to normal muscle function). Bone tissue is also involved in the production of blood cells (hemopoiesis). Red blood cells (erythrocytes) and many white blood cells (leukocytes) are produced in red bone marrow. The skeleton also supports and protects vital and susceptible structures.

Prototype Bone

Figure 10.1 illustrates a typical bone. It has been sectioned in the frontal plane to reveal inner structures. As you may observe, bone is not solid through and through. Many bones are hollow, with a central marrow cavity in the shaft section (diaphysis) and porous, spongy

bone located in either end (epiphysis). The end result is a mobile but strong system for the diverse functions of movement and protection that the skeletal system must perform.

Solid, compact bone makes up only a small portion of the total bone mass. It is found mostly in the diaphysis. On either epiphysis, the end of the bone designed to form a joint is covered with *articular cartilage*. The articular cartilage functions to present a smooth surface that facilitates movement. Most types of arthritis involve pathological changes in the articular cartilage.

Bone is also covered on the outside by a fibrous layer called the *periosteum*. Tendons from muscles and ligaments that connect bones anchor to the periosteum.

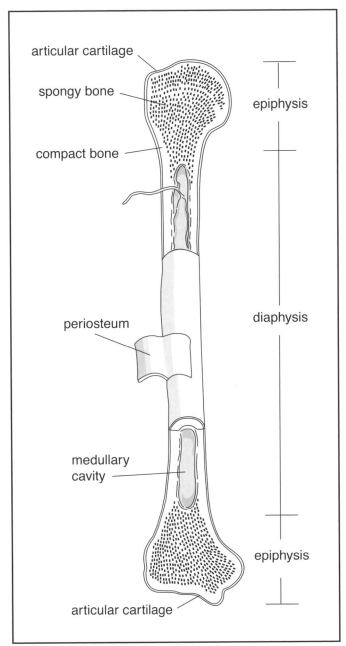

Figure 10.1 Typical bone

The medullary cavity, the hollow, central portion of a long bone, is likewise lined in the area of the diaphysis with a layer of connective tissue called the *endosteum*. Together the periosteum and endosteum maintain bones throughout life by producing new bone tissue on the outside of the bone (periosteum) and breaking down old bone tissue on the inside (endosteum).

Gross Anatomy of the Skeleton

The skeleton can be divided into two parts (see **Figure 10.2**). The *axial skeleton* supports and protects structures along the midline or central axis of the body. It consists of the bones of the skull, middle ear ossicles, vertebral column, rib cage, and the hyoid bone. The second subdivision of the skeleton, the *appendicular skeleton*, consists of the bones of the upper and lower extremities and the bones that comprise the shoulder and hip girdles.

The vertebral column consists of 33 individual vertebrae stacked on top of one another to form a single foundation for posture and body positioning. Between each vertebra lies a disk of fibrocartilage known as an intervertebral disk. Vertebrae are labeled according to region:

- 7 cervical vertebrae in the neck
- 12 thoracic vertebrae in the trunk region
- 5 lumbar vertebrae in the lower back
- 5 fused vertebrae comprise the sacrum
- 4 small vertebrae fuse to form the coccyx (tailbone)

Twenty-two individual bones comprise the skull and form immovable joints with one another called sutures. Suture joints (suture lines) may be seen on the skull in Figure 10.2. The larger of the bones of the skull include the zygomatic, mandible, maxilla, frontal, parietal, and occipital bones.

The rib cage is comprised of 12 ribs, 10 of which articulate directly or indirectly with the sternum anteriorly; all 12 form joints with thoracic vertebrae posteriorly. These joints are slightly movable to allow for subtle posture adjustments. The capacity for limited movement in the thoracic region is consistent with the fact that most of the viscera (organ systems) are housed within the ventral body cavity, and excessive movement would compromise the safety of these soft tissues.

The hyoid bone and the three bones (ossicles) of the middle ear are not pictured in Figure 10.2. The hyoid bone serves as an attachment for many of the muscles of speech. It is located behind (deep to) the mandible, anterior to the cervical portion of the vertebral column, and rests atop the trachea (windpipe). The middle ear

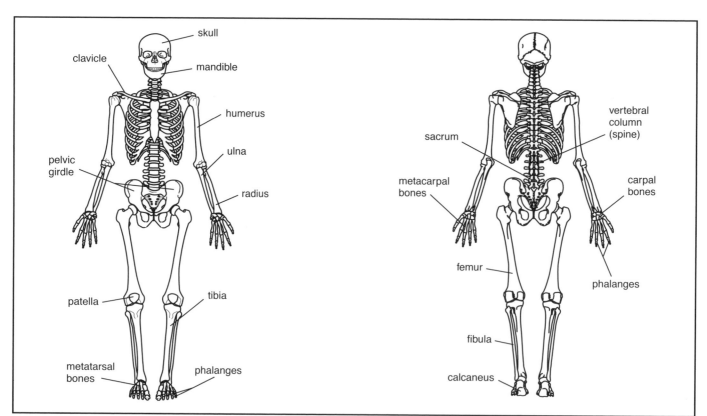

Figure 10.2 Anterior and posterior skeleton

ossicles (malleus, incus, stapes) are embedded within the temporal bone and serve to transmit the vibrations of the tympanic membrane (ear drum) at the end of the external auditory canal to the inner ear where the spiral organ detects the vibrations as sound.

The shoulder girdle is comprised of two bones—the scapula (shoulder blade) and the clavicle (collarbone). The clavicle forms joints with the sternum medially and the scapula laterally. Both of these joints are slightly movable and aid in the proper positioning of the upper extremity. The joint between the clavicle and the scapula is frequently injured in sports and leads to a condition called a separated shoulder.

The scapula is largely a "muscle hanger"—a bone that serves as an origin for many of the muscles that act on the arm and/or the forearm. Hence, it is imperative that the scapula be held rather steady when one of the muscles that takes origin off the scapula is contracting. The scapula also forms the very mobile shoulder joint along with the proximal end of the humerus—called the *head* of the humerus. The shoulder is frequently injured in competitive sports, especially those involving collisions, resulting in a dislocated shoulder (a separation or disarticulation between the humerus and the scapula). Those sports involving throwing projectiles may result in rotator cuff injuries (damage to one or more of the tendons of muscles that insert near the head of the humerus).

The arm lies between the shoulder and the elbow and consists of only one bone—the humerus. The humerus forms the shoulder joint with the scapula. Distally, the humerus forms the elbow joint with the two bones of the forearm.

The forearm lies between the elbow and the wrist. Its skeletal components include two bones—the radius laterally and the ulna medially. The radius and ulna form the elbow joint with the humerus proximally. Distally, the radius only forms the wrist joint with two of the carpals. Unlike the radius, the ulna is not involved in the formation of the wrist joint.

The 8 short bones of the wrist, *carpals*, articulate with one another as well as the radius at the wrist joint. Articulations between the carpals allow for slight movement and make the wrist more pliable. The remaining bones of the hand are the 5 metacarpals that end as the "knuckles," and the 14 phalanges. The thumb is made up of 2 phalanges, while the remaining 4 digits are comprised of 3 phalanges each. The total number of bones in the hand (carpals, metacarpals, and phalanges) is 27.

Many parallels exist in the relationships between the bones of the upper extremity and those of the lower extremity. For instance, the relationship between the bone that forms the pelvic girdle and the femur is similar to that of the scapula and the humerus of the upper extremity. But in the case of the lower extremity, the joint formed is the hip. Unlike the scapula, however, the bone of the pelvic girdle, the os coxa, is the result of the fusing of three bones in the normal adult. Hence, there is no bone comparable to the clavicle in the pelvic girdle.

The thigh lies between the hip and the knee. As with the arm, only one bone is found in the thigh—the femur. It forms the hip joint with the os coxa proximally and the knee with the tibia and patella distally. The patella (kneecap) develops within a tendon (called a *sesamoid* bone) and enhances the effectiveness of the muscles of the anterior surface of the thigh. The patella accomplishes this by improving the angle of pull of these muscles when they contract and produce extension of the leg.

The leg is the area between the knee and the ankle, and like the forearm is comprised of two bones. The tibia is the medial, weightbearing bone of the leg. The fibula is the lateral, nonweightbearing bone of the leg. The fibula does *not* enter into the formation of the knee joint. Like the scapula, it serves largely as a "muscle hanger" for muscles taking all or part of their origin off the fibula and acting on the ankle or foot. Both the tibia and the fibula do enter into the formation of the ankle joint.

The most superior of the bones of the ankle, the *talus*, forms the ankle joint with the fibula and the tibia. There are seven total tarsals, which form slightly movable joints with one another and allow the ankle and foot to be somewhat pliable. The remainder of the foot is arranged similarly to the hand, with five metatarsals (instead of metacarpals) and fourteen phalanges. The great toe, like the thumb, has only two phalanges; the remaining digits have three phalanges each. Note that the great toe is medial in the anatomical position, whereas the thumb is lateral in the anatomical position.

Joints

Types of Joints

A joint is defined as the place where two or more bones meet, or where bone and cartilage meet. Based on this definition, humans have a considerable number of joints. However, most of these joints are either immovable or slightly movable. The presentation on joints here will focus on freely movable joints for the most part because freely movable joints are the most interesting and, unfortunately, the most susceptible to injury and pathology. Joints stabilize and allow for movement between the articulating surfaces. A reciprocal relationship exists between stability and mobility: The more stable a joint the less movement allowed, and vice versa.

Joints can be divided in a number of different ways, based on the amount of movement they allow, the shape of the articulating bones, or the type of connective tissue that holds the bones together. The discussion here will focus on the type of connective tissue as a method for classifying joints, with the amount of movement allowed and the shapes of the articulating bones integrated into the discussion.

Joints that capitalize on the shapes of the articulating surfaces to lend stability to the joint and a strong ligament to hold the bones together are referred to as *fibrous joints*. The sutures of the skull, the distal articulation between the fibula and tibia, and the distal articulation between the radius and ulna qualify as fibrous joints. Fibrous joints are generally immovable or slightly moveable.

Likewise, joints held together by cartilaginous connective tissue are immovable to slightly moveable. Vertebrae stacked one atop the other are held together, in part, by a cartilaginous intervertebral disk. Many back difficulties in later life can be traced to injury or deterioration of the intervertebral disks. The cartilage between the ribs and sternum make this articulation a cartilaginous joint, too.

Synovial joints are freely moveable, a capability resulting from specific structures that characterize a typical synovial joint (see **Figure 10.3**). The structures necessary for a synovial joint include a joint capsule and articular cartilage. The joint capsule encloses the articulating bones and is not found in either fibrous or cartilaginous joint types. A synovial membrane lines the inside of the joint capsule and secretes synovial fluid that acts as a lubricant. Articular cartilage is coated with the synovial fluid to present a smooth, lubricated surface that facilitates movement of the bones within the joint capsule.

Synovial joints have some additional structures, usually designed to improve the stability of the joint. Mobile joints typically have an elaborate system of accessory structures called ligaments. *Ligaments* are strong bands of connective tissue designed to prohibit movement in unwanted directions at the joint. For instance, *hinge joints* allow flexion and extension only in the saggital plane. Hinge joints usually have collateral ligaments placed on medial and lateral borders of the joint to prevent movement in the coronal plane (i.e., abduction, adduction). Ligaments are often injured when a joint is forcibly moved in a direction it is not designed to move in (e.g., as in an ankle sprain).

Synovial joints may also have accessory disks of cartilage within the joint capsule. The knee, for example has two cartilaginous disks called *menisci* that improve the fit between the femur and the tibia. Like ligaments, cartilaginous disks may be damaged when a joint is distorted in an unwanted direction.

Synovial joints are further divided based on the shape of the articulating surfaces of the bones that form the joint (see **Table 10.1**). The surfaces range from two flat bones that simply slide back and forth across one another (e.g., joints between the carpal bone of the wrist) to the very mobile ball and socket joint that allows the most latitude in movement (e.g., shoulder joint between the humerus and the scapula). The types of movements allowed by each type of synovial joint are listed in Table 10.1, along with examples of where each type of joint may be found.

Specific Synovial Joints

Figure 10.4 (p. 178) illustrates some of the synovial joints most often affected by a variety of disabling conditions. The *intervertebral joint* (not shown) is formed between two adjacent vertebrae and includes up to 10 separate joints if articulations with the ribs are included. Osteoporosis, fractures, and disk trauma may affect intervertebral joints.

The *hand* is really a complex of joints between the radius and carpals, the carpals and the metacarpals, metacarpals and phalanges, and between phalanges. The wrist and joints between metacarpals and phalanges, and between phalanges are especially mobile and

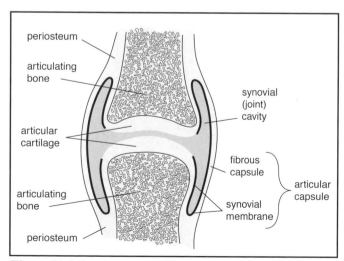

Figure 10.3 Typical synovial joint

therefore most susceptible to injury (e.g., carpal tunnel syndrome, arthritis, fractures).

The *hip* is often injured later in life as a result of a fall. Falls cause 87% of the fractures in the elderly population, initiating a series of health problems that often culminate in death (Baker, O'Neill, Ginsburg & Goohua, 1992). A hip fracture is not usually at the hip joint at all. Rather, what is commonly called a hip fracture is really a fracture of the neck of the femur (just distal to the where the head of the femur articulates at the os coxa).

The *knee* is the frequent site of traumatic, sport-related injuries in teenagers and young adults. Later in life the knee is especially susceptible to disorders of wear and tear. An example of a wear and tear disability is arthritis, which may be secondary to an injury earlier in life or the result of the cumulative wear and tear of a long life. In some cases the knee, as well as the hip, must be replaced in whole or part with an artificial joint or skeletal component. Needless to say, the impact on lifestyle is substantial.

Normal Development

The skeletal system is formed mostly from cartilage. The ossification (bone formation) process begins within the human embryo about the fourth week of gestation. Throughout the developmental years, the skeleton continues to grow. Growth during this period especially accounts for the individual's final adult stature, which is attained somewhere between 18 and 20 years of age.

Bones remain dynamic tissue throughout life. They are not static or inert. Rather, bone is constantly being replenished to accommodate the bone tissue that "wears out" because of the gradual aging process. Furthermore, because bone serves as a mineral reservoir throughout life, it is constantly being modified to meet metabolic demands for calcium and phosphorus.

Joints form where bones articulate with one another. However, joints are not as well supplied with blood and, therefore, do not tend to be as dynamic. In

Type of Joint	Movements possible	Example
Gliding	Two flat surfaces sliding over one another	Between carpal bones of wrist Between vertebrae
Hinge	Convex surface fits into concave surface; movement limited to one axis flexion and extension in the saggital plane	Between humerus and radius/ulna at the elbow Between femur and tibia at the knee Between phalanges in hand and foot
Pivot	Body part rotates around a longitudinal axis	Between first and second cervical vertebrae—C1 (atlas) rotates around the C2 (axis) vertebrae
Ellipsoidal	Convex surface fits into concave surface; movement in two axes—flexion/extension and abduction and adduction in the coronal plane	Between the distal end of the radius and scaphoid/lunate (carpals) to form the wrist joint
Saddle	Two biconcave/convex surfaces fit together; movements are similar to those possible in an ellipsoidal joint	Unique to the articulation between the trapezium of the carpus and the first metacarpal in the hand
Ball and socket	Prominent head fits into a depression on a second bone; most mobile of joints; capable of flexion/extension, abuction/adduction, rotation, and circumduction	Between head of humerus and glenoid fossa of scapula Between the head of femur and and acetabulum of bony pelvis

Table 10.1 Types of synovial joints

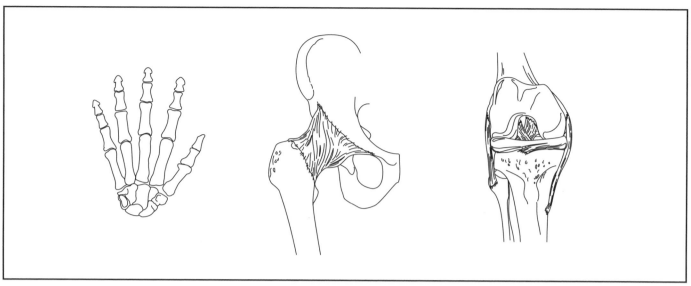

Figure 10.4 Specific synovial joints: hand, hip, and knee

the adult, the poor blood supply to joints also contributes to the slow healing of joints following injury. The articular cartilage that caps the ends of bones that enter into synovial joints is particularly susceptible to wear and tear attributable to the normal aging process, as well as various other inflammatory afflictions (e.g., rheumatoid arthritis).

Primary Disorders of Skeletal and Joint Systems

As in the preceding chapters, the disabilities described here are limited to those most commonly encountered in TR practice. The focus will be on disorders that are serious, chronic, and suitable to TR interventions and techniques. Hence, the disorders and TR specifications that follow should be regarded as representative of the kinds of impairments that therapeutic recreation specialists (TRS) encounter related to the skeletal and joint systems. Disorders affecting skeleton and joints can be developmental, traumatic, or attributable to the aging process.

Developmental Disorders

Cleft palate and spina bifida are examples of congenital disorders. Both relate to failure of the skeleton to develop completely. *Cleft palate* refers to a malformation of the anterior part of the upper jaw and is characterized by a failure of the hard palate to ossify completely. The person with a severe case of cleft palate will present

with a noticeable nasal voice. Together, the tonal qualities of the voice and the cosmetic disfigurement that often correlate with pronounced cleft palate may stigmatize the individual and be the cause of some concern relative to access to normal life experiences and leisure opportunities.

Spina bifida refers to a failure of the vertebral column to develop completely. It is characterized by an opening in the posterior part of the vertebral column, usually in the thoracic and lumbar regions. Spina bifida can range in severity from a mild case that may remain undetected and have very little impact on the person's life, to a severe case where the spinal cord is exposed at the level of the cele (opening in the vertebral column). In the latter case the lesion is referred to as a *myelomeningocele* (both the vertebral column and the spinal cord are involved). In its most severe form (myelomeningocele), the person with spina bifida presents as paraplegic (flaccid-type paralysis of both lower extremities) and unable to control bladder and bowel. Hydrocephalus (fluid accumulation in the brain) secondary to spina bifida is frequent and must be managed surgically by placing a shunt (tube) in the brain to drain excess cerebrospinal fluid into the ventral body cavity. Brain malformations in association with spina bifida are also common.

Adults with spina bifida may have difficulty controlling weight because of inactivity. They are also susceptible to decubiti (skin lesions, pressure sores) caused by a combination of prolonged sitting in one position, minimal ability to change posture, inability to detect places where the skin is rubbed to excess in the lower extremities, and poor circulation. Inability to control the trunk may also lead to the development of scoliosis secondary to spina bifida.

Abnormal curvatures of the vertebral column may present during the developmental years. Four normal curves appear in the vertebral column when it is viewed laterally: cervical, thoracic, lumbar, and sacral (see **Figure 10.5**). However, the same normal curves may be exaggerated and result in a variety of secondary difficulties. When the thoracic curve is excessively concave, the condition is called *kyphosis* (sometimes called Dowager's hump in older adults); an excessive convexity in the lumbar curve is *lordosis*. Both of the conditions are correctable, as they often result from poor posture and muscle weakness. Kyphosis and lordosis respond well to a regimen of corrective exercises and temporary prosthetic bracing.

More severe and sustained is the problem of *scoliosis*—a c-shaped or s-shaped curvature of the vertebral column in the frontal plane. Normal vertebral curves occur only in the saggital plane and can only be seen in a lateral view. Scoliosis can be observed in an anterior or posterior view, where no curves normally exist. Scoliosis is more difficult to correct because it may not be detected early enough and because it often causes permanent changes in the vertebrae affected. Some of the common etiologies that may lead to scoliosis include spina bifida, different leg lengths, and an imbalance of muscle strength on either side of the axial skeleton. In about three fourths of cases, the cause of the scoliosis is idiopathic (unknown). If ossification has advanced well into the developmental years, then the prospects for correction of scoliosis are diminished, though bracing, surgical intervention, and exercise are still used.

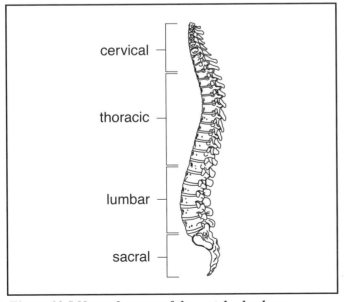

cervical

thoracic

lumbar

sacral

Figure 10.5 Normal curves of the vertebral column

Traumatic Disorders

Traumatic injuries, including amputations and serious fractures, can have a pronounced effect on the skeleton or joints, resulting in a significant impairment. Absence of a limb may be congenital or a result of injury, diabetes mellitus (and associated circulation difficulties), disease (e.g., cancer), or infection. Regardless of the etiology, some general characteristics are common among most persons with amputations.

Amputations distal to a joint are preferable to those proximal to a joint because the disability will be less if another joint is preserved. Prosthetic limbs and devices are frequently employed so long as the individual can tolerate them without developing a skin lesion. The TRS should be vigilant for skin lesions or redness and irritation to avoid development of a decubitus ulceration. Hence, skin care and cosmetic appearance are frequent lifestyle issues for persons with amputations that the TRS may be involved with during recreational programs.

A fracture may be considered serious if the causal event is particularly traumatic (e.g., a crushing injury from a motor vehicle accident), if the fracture involves the growth plate of cartilage in a youth or teen, or if the fracture occurs in late adulthood (past age 70). In the former case, repair may involve surgical intervention and the use of supportive devices (e.g., screws, stainless steel prosthetics). Fractures in general among older adults may be regarded as more serious because of the slower and often incomplete healing process in the vicinity of the injury. The most dramatic example of a serious fracture among older adults is the classic hip fracture—usually the fracture occurs at the neck of the femur. Remediation involves the replacement of the proximal end of the femur with an artificial prosthesis.

In all cases of serious fracture, the involvement of the TRS depends on the extent of incapacitation. Recovery may be complete, albeit prolonged, in cases of serious fracture at all ages. But if the recovery is less than complete the effect of the fracture on the person's leisure lifestyle may be significant. Inability to continue in a favorite sport as a child or teen and mobility restrictions in older adults often lead to lifestyle changes that may call for TR intervention.

Age-Related Disorders

Besides hip fractures, older adults are at risk for two other disorders that affect the skeletal system or joints: osteoporosis and arthritis. In the case of osteoporosis the mineral content in bone experiences a net loss that accumulates over a number of years to weaken bones and make them particularly susceptible to fractures of various types. For example, vertebrae that have lost too much mineral content may start to collapse and compress as a result of a series of minute hairline fractures. The neck of the femur is another site that is especially susceptible to fracture secondary to the loss of excess mineral content resulting from osteoporosis.

Recalling that bone serves as a mineral reservoir, osteoporosis can be thought of as an exaggeration of a normal process—the reallocation of mineral content in bone. The primary cause of osteoporosis is acceleration of the normal bone resorption process, especially in women after menopause. The hormone estrogen seems to preserve bone integrity in women. But as the secretion of estrogen falls during menopause, the loss of the mineral content in bone accelerates to the extent that about 85% of women will experience some degree of osteoporosis. Clinical presentation usually is evidenced by pain and fractures.

Arthritis is a general term that refers to a number of afflictions that cause inflammation of one or more joints. It can occur at any age, but the older adult is more at risk for the form of arthritis related to wear and tear of the joint—osteoarthritis. *Osteoarthritis* (also known as degenerative joint disease) is specific to the articular cartilage that caps the ends of bones that enter into joints. The aging process is associated with the deterioration of cartilage in some individuals, exposing underlying bone tissue. Thinning and pitting of the articular cartilage causes pain and stiffness in the joint. Other symptoms include restricted movement of the affected joint, instability of the joint, and inflammation. Osteoarthritis is more likely at joints that have been injured at some time earlier in life (e.g., a shoulder that has been dislocated).

Although more than one joint may be affected by osteoarthritis, it is not necessarily progressive—moving from one joint to another. In contrast, rheumatoid arthritis is systematic and highly inflammatory, often involving more than one joint. Changes in the synovial membrane lining the inside of the joint cause inflammation and swelling that lead to deterioration of the articular cartilage, irreversible joint instability, and disuse atrophy of the muscle system. As with osteoarthritis, bone tissue then is exposed, resulting in pain. Because of the earlier average age of onset (middle adulthood) and the progressive nature of the disorder, rheumatoid arthritis is frequently more debilitating than osteoarthritis. The individual may suffer intervals of exacerbation of the disease and intermittent periods of remission. Both primary types of arthritis need a balance of rest and exercise, especially exercise that involves range of motion.

Another joint disorder affects the intervertebral disks of the spine. Although anyone can injure an intervertebral disk, older adults are most at risk for deterioration of a disk. The fibrocartilage that comprises the outer portion of the disk may weaken, causing the disk to rupture. The herniated disk often presses on spinal nerves as they exit the vertebral column, causing pain. A precipitating event, such as improper lifting of a heavy object, usually causes the weakened disk to herniate. Because the trauma is most often in the lumbar region, areas supplied by lumbar spinal nerves evidence symptoms (e.g., pain in the back or on the posterior surface of the lower extremity).

Therapeutic Recreation and Orthopedic Impairments

Several themes become evident when examining TR for persons with skeletal and joint impairments, including interrelated chronic conditions, common symptoms, impact on quality of life, and the effect of secondary disabilities. Each of these will be discussed here, along with several research studies. Readers should be aware, however, that many of the research reports cited here had either a small number of subjects, or had a mix of disabilities that included only some persons with skeletal and joint impairments, or had both few subjects and a few persons with skeletal and joint impairments. Hence, the findings reported and recommendations based on the findings should be considered suggestive rather than final, and should be used as a stimulus for further research on these topics.

Interrelated Chronic Conditions

The first theme is the interrelationship between disorders (Carter, Van Andel & Robb, 1995), especially chronic conditions. This means that a person with one disorder is at risk for developing another disorder of the skeletal or joint systems. The interrelationship between disorders crosses over into other systems as well.

The interrelationship between disorders can be better appreciated by recognizing that bone responds to stress in a manner similar to muscle. Positive stress (in the form of exercise) causes bone to adapt to demands by laying down more bone tissue, thus improving strength. Skeletal responses to exercise are particularly marked for weightbearing and resistance exercise. If the skeletal system is not exposed to an optimal amount of stress in the form of weightbearing exercise (e.g., walking, weight training), then the integrity of the skeletal system will deteriorate, making the individual more susceptible to osteoporosis, fractures of the hip and spine, and other chronic conditions.

Because pain is so often associated with many disorders of the skeletal system, falling into a sedentary pattern of living and passive activities is understandable. But inactivity is the last thing that the skeletal system needs to maintain its vitality. Also consider that many disorders result in mobility impairment (e.g., lower extremity amputee), reduction or absence of ambulation (e.g., spina bifida), or progressive decrease in the use of the muscle system (e.g., multiple sclerosis) and the risk of acquiring a comorbid chronic condition becomes clear.

Some comorbid, chronic conditions tend to be found in association with scoliosis, including scoliosis and cerebral palsy (Shephard, 1990), scoliosis and arthritis (Goldberg, Mayo, Poitras, Scott & Hanley, 1994), and scoliosis and breathing difficulties (Shephard, 1990). Other commonly associated disorders are spina bifida and scoliosis and amputations (especially those involving the lower extremity) and diabetes mellitus.

Symptoms in Common

A second theme that emerges out of the literature on rehabilitation and chronic conditions is the number of shared symptoms among the disabilities of the skeletal and joint systems. Pain has already been noted as a common problem—one that has perhaps the most impact on quality of life for those with arthritis, osteoporosis, and other disorders. Pain can interfere with quality of life in a number of ways, from simply causing the person to lead a more passive lifestyle to affecting other psychological states. For example, Varni and colleagues (1996) found that among 160 youth with chronic pain, reports of high levels of perceived pain were associated with higher instances of behavioral problems, depressive symptoms, anxiety, and lower self-esteem.

The work of Varni et al. (1996) underscores the fact that several disorders of the skeleton and joints are associated with psychological symptoms. Depression is a frequently reported problem among individuals with arthritis. Recent studies (Pincus, Griffith, Pearce & Isenberg, 1996; Smedstad, Maum, Vaglum & Kvien, 1996; Taal, Rasker & Timmers, 1997) reveal a consistent relationship between arthritis and reports of depressive symptoms. Kraus and Shank (1992) add persons with amputations to the list of those at risk for developing depressive symptoms in conjunction with their primary disability.

Deterioration of self-concept and self-esteem have logically been associated with orthopedic impairments for some time (Austin, 1987). More recent empirical studies have verified this. The relationship between low self-esteem and some conditions may be attributable to cosmetic differences, as in children with cleft palate (Strauss & Broder, 1990). It may be the salience of the presenting condition (e.g., distorted extremities of the person with severe rheumatoid arthritis). It may also be the restricted mobility associated with pain or progressive disuse (e.g., osteoporosis, arthritis).

Impact on Quality of Life

The third theme shared by many persons with skeletal or joint problems is the marked impact the disability has on the individual's lifestyle and leisure lifestyle. Berryman, James, and Trader (1991) outlined the mechanism for the development of reactive depression based on the inability of a person to regulate his or her own lifestyle because of a chronic disability. The sequence of events leading to reactive depression begins with stress and anxiety resulting from the disability and the perceptions of helplessness on the part of the affected individual. Perceptions of lack of control can then lead to reactive depression as the person generalizes the lack of control over the course of the disability or the pain that results from the affliction.

The salience of the disability may also affect the impact of the impairment on the person's lifestyle. More salient conditions tend to be those that stand out cosmetically (e.g., Hoenk & Mobily, 1987). Hence, even though a person with an amputation, a weight problem, or cleft palate is not as physically limited as someone with rheumatoid arthritis, the former may be more affected in terms of lifestyle limitations because of his or her appearance. Obese and cleft palate children are more anxious, more depressed (Ramstad, Otten & Shaw, 1995), and at greater risk for developing social competence problems (Tobiasen & Hiebert, 1993), such as forming friendships and making satisfactory progress in school.

Specific to leisure lifestyle, skeletal and joint conditions relate to more than the usual limitations. Smith and Yoshioka (1992) investigated the leisure lifestyles of 59 subjects with rheumatoid arthritis. Like other researchers they found that their subjects were more likely than usual to exhibit depressive symptoms. However, Smith and Yoshioka also found that the greater the change in recreation activity from premorbid condition to onset of the arthritis, the higher the report of depressive symptoms. Over 75% of the subjects said that their favorite recreational activity had changed because of rheumatoid arthritis. They offered two possible explanations for the results. The lack of control over lifestyle, as noted earlier in Berryman et al. (1991), may have been associated with reactive depression; or the depression may have been fostered by unpredictable pain and unexpected functional limitations.

Secondary Disabilities

The final theme revealed in the literature relates to a program goal for persons with skeletal or joint impairments—prevention of secondary impairments. For example, those with arthritis are at risk for many chronic conditions (Minor & Lane, 1996) that result from the sedentary lifestyle they often lead ("Prevalence of leisure-time physical activity," 1997). In contrast Helmes et al. (1995) reported that persons with osteoporosis who participated in an exercise program were in significantly better shape with respect to activities of daily living and socialization.

Carter et al. (1995) add prevention of secondary disability to the objectives for persons with arthritis, with potential complications including conditions such as contractures, joint aggravation, posture anomalies, and skin lesions. Furthermore, Shephard (1990) observed that persons with disabilities are not immune from secondary disorders associated with an inactive lifestyle, including obesity, heart disease, and hypertension.

On a positive note, we consider a few reasons why persons with disabilities should participate in exercise. Coutts, McKenzie, Loock, Beauchamp, and Armstrong (1993) tentatively concluded that the exercise capacity of youth with spina bifida was within normal limits. Their subjects possessed the potential to perform at levels comparable to nondisabled peers on several markers of physical performance. Similarly, exercise has been associated with a reduced risk of hip fracture (Grisso et al., 1997) and reduced risk for the development of scoliosis in children (Juskeliene, Magnus, Bakketeig, Darlidiene & Jurkavenas, 1996).

Most authorities recommend mild to moderate exercise to prevent secondary disabilities. For instance, Vuori (1995) concluded that moderate intensity physical activity would benefit almost all musculoskeletal disorders at all ages. Furthermore, Panush and Holtz (1994) maintained that reasonable leisure time exercise can be performed safely by persons with arthritis, if

exercises were limited to the normal range of motion at joints, and were continued within the margins of the individual's comfort. In almost every report the research community is recommending *leisure time* exercise and physical activity, not the calculated therapy so characteristic of physical medicine and exercise prescriptions.

Therapy

The problem with conditions such as osteoporosis, arthritis, and the like is that the disabilities do not go away. Curing in the traditional sense is unlikely, so the focus of conventional rehabilitation tends to be on management of symptoms and prevention of secondary disabilities. Accordingly, therapeutic recreation specialists should seek to intervene with orthopedic impairments by managing pain, decreasing depression while increasing self-esteem, and preventing secondary disabilities.

Pain Management

Research-based techniques that address pain include relaxation, aquatics, and exercise. The active mechanisms for the effectiveness of these techniques are often poorly understood. However, cross-sectional and correlational studies and small sample projects have demonstrated encouraging results.

Various relaxation methods, biofeedback, massage, acupuncture, and guided imagery may relieve pain in two ways. Relaxation and related methods may augment the person's conviction that pain can be controlled, thus supporting perceptions of control and psychological health in spite of the presenting pathology. In contrast to the psychological explanation, a physiological mechanism that operates by stimulating nervous pathways interrupting the pain pathway may be in effect. This pathway may be as simple as the stimulation of touch receptors and nerves by massage or biofeedback that block the course of the pain information to the brain, or it may be more obscure, such as the pathway in operation during acupuncture.

Like relaxation, the effectiveness of exercise in the relief of pain is not well understood, but nevertheless potent. One possible mechanism for the management of pain through exercise includes the well-known stimulation of the brain's natural analgesics (e.g., endorphins) through some types of exercise.

Another mechanism that explains the effectiveness of exercise relates to progressive muscle weakness that tends to correlate with disorders that have a high incidence of pain as a comorbid symptom. Dekker, Tola, Aufdemkampe, and Winckers (1993) argued that muscle weakness is the key variable in a sequence of events that includes exercise and pain and ends in disability. They maintain that negative affect (e.g., depressive symptoms, perceptions of loss of control and helplessness) fosters a disposition to avoid pain. To avoid pain the individual avoids pain-related activities. As an example, for the arthritic patient, gross motor activities such as ambulation, chores around the home, and weightbearing recreational activities are likely to be avoided. The marked decrease in gross motor activity induces progressive muscle weakness because of disuse and thereby advances disability.

Decreasing Depression and Increasing Self-Esteem

The role of exercise in the management of pain underscores negative affect as another focal point of therapy. Exercise is also effective in the management of depressive symptoms, particularly in groups most at risk for the development of pain in relation to chronic conditions of the skeletal and joint systems. For example, Mobily, Rubenstein, Lemke, O'Hara, and Wallace (1996) reported a longitudinal study of community-dwelling older adults. They found that subjects with high depressive symptoms at baseline were significantly less likely to report high depressive symptoms three years later if they walked every day.

If a decrease in activity also decreases self-esteem, then continued physical activity may be the treatment of choice. Involvement in an array of activities is apt to promote self-concept and self-esteem, and may encourage perceptions of control and choice. Perceived control may have been the mediating variable in a study (Sherrill, Hinson, Gench, O'Kennedy & Low, 1990) that demonstrated that young athletes with disabilities (including amputations and other conditions) scored within normal subscale ranges for self-concept.

Preventing Secondary Disabilities

Prevention of secondary disabilities represents the third initiative for therapeutic efforts with individuals experiencing skeletal and joint disabilities. Given the extensive scientific and popular literature on the usefulness of exercise in preventing many chronic conditions and pathologies, one can conclude that the same benefits would apply to those with disabilities if they were able

to maintain a program of regular exercise. Of course, the preventable secondary disabilities depend upon the chronic conditions already present in the client.

For example, persons with osteoporosis are at risk for vertebral or hip fractures because of the susceptibility of their skeletal systems. Regular exercise may help them avoid a hip fracture. Stevens, Powell, Smith, Wingo, and Sattin (1997) learned that older adult subjects with no limitations in activities of daily living who participated in vigorous exercise (i.e., heavy physical activity at least three times per week) were half as likely to suffer a hip fracture as their inactive peers. Although Stevens et al.'s subjects did not report manifest osteoporosis, the results do point toward an initiative that may help avoid a secondary complication often associated with osteoporosis.

An earlier study reported by Jaglal, Kreiger, and Darlington (1993) supports the findings of Stevens and associates. Women between the ages of 55 and 84 were asked about past and present exercise habits. Those reporting either frequent physical activity in the past or recent moderate intensity physical activity lowered their risk for a hip fracture by almost one half. An important aspect of the Jaglal et al. finding is that the effects of past and recent physical activity were independent of one another. Their findings imply that even if a person is sedentary for an extended period of time, beginning a program of regular, moderate exercise still holds the promise of reducing the risk of developing one secondary disability (hip fracture in this case).

To the specific example of the osteoporosis–hip fracture relationship, we can add other more subtle aggravations associated with skeletal and joint problems. These include restrictions in range of motion, contractures, disuse atrophy, wasting of the muscle system, skin lesions, and infections. An array of emotional disorders (e.g., anxiety, stress, psychosomatic disorders), and substance abuse (particularly in cases where pain is persistent and/or the person is limited in his or her leisure choices or bored) are also included. Any number of recreational programs that motivate the client to engage life and not acquiesce in disability may prove to be beneficial.

If the person uses a wheelchair, then spending some time out of the chair will remove pressure from at risk areas of the skin that bear the stress of seated or recumbent positioning. Music may be used to engage the person in rhythmic movements that serve to enhance range of motion at affected joints. Such a program would also reduce the probability of contractures. Likewise, mat-based, recumbent exercises would put the individual in a new position and temporarily remove pressure from at risk areas for skin lesions (e.g., buttocks, heel, posterior surface of the leg and thigh).

Most epidemiological studies show that only 10% to 20% of the U. S. population participates in a program of regular exercise, with the lower percentage typical if the qualifier "of adequate intensity" is added. Persons with disabilities, especially ones accompanied by pain during movement, are probably participating at an even lower rate than the samples reported in the literature (i.e., even more sedentary than the typical adult). Hence, the amount of exercise-induced stimulus necessary to derive benefit is likely less in persons with disabilities than for an asymptomatic peer. This means that low intensity physical activity may provide significant benefits among persons with skeletal and joint disorders. Recreational-based exercise programs, therefore, do not have to be risky.

Specific Programs and Protocols in Therapy

Exercise Programs

Shephard (1990) outlined some general goals for exercise programs for persons with disabilities, including physiological gain, metabolic control (weight control), flexibility and range of motion, anaerobic power (strength), and habituation (learning). However, Shephard's goals may be too ambitious for some conditions (e.g., osteoporosis). Ambulation may present too great a risk for persons with advanced osteoporosis—the obvious stress of weightbearing and the increased risk of a fall. Fortunately, Swezey's (1996) review of the literature corroborated earlier observations of Marcus et al. (1992): resistance exercise (e.g., resistance bands, lightweight training) result in benefits to the skeletal system and muscle system equal to those derived from weightbearing activities (e.g., walking). Hence, the patient with severe osteoporosis can improve the integrity of the skeleton by participation in a resistance exercise program, avoiding some of the risks inherent in ambulatory programs of exercise.

In 1988 Buettner described a moderate intensity exercise program for older adults with chronic conditions, including kyphosis, contractures at some joints, and hip fracture. She used therabands and light weights to provide resistance. In addition, a beach ball and vestibular "donut" were used to train joint sense. Sensory stimulation was provided through an air flow mat and varied visual, tactile, and auditory stimuli. The

22 participants in the program demonstrated significant improvements in flexibility, strength, and ambulation following participation twice a week for one year. Buettner concluded that such programs held considerable promise for cutting costs in long-term care.

One existing protocol for persons with arthritis takes a more conservative approach. Murphy (1998) describes a three-phase treatment plan that includes the following goals:

- Express past and new leisure skills
- Develop leisure problem-solving skills
- Improve social interaction
- Explore leisure attitudes
- Increase in physical and/or intellectual activity level
- Provide information about leisure resources
- Reintegrate into the community
- Provide leisure opportunities

Most of the modalities are less physically active than the literature seems to support. Understandably, however, a cautious approach may be indicated in this case because if the person is hospitalized for arthritis, either surgery or aggravation of the arthritis is likely the cause. Nevertheless, Murphy's protocol does share the use of sensory stimulation as a modality in common with Buettner's program.

Exercise, physical activity, and sport have been frequently identified as activities with the potential to reverse or prevent the development of some physiological and psychological comorbid conditions. But caution needs to be used with individuals who manifest skeletal and joint problems, making consultation with a physician or other qualified health professional a necessity. For example, a person with advanced osteoporosis may benefit from a moderate program of weightbearing activity (e.g., walking) and resistance exercises (e.g., resistance bands), but that same person may be at risk for a fracture because weightbearing may stress a bone to excess. Likewise, a person with arthritis may benefit from an increase in physical activity in general, but if a joint is fused or excessively painful, then adaptations may be necessary for participation.

When customary precautions are taken, a mild to moderate program of recreational exercise is feasible for persons experiencing pain accompanied by depressive symptoms or either symptom in isolation. Both the TRS and the physical therapist use exercise as a modality, but in a very different manner. The TRS is concerned with coverage of symptoms through the *patient-driven* choice of exercise, rather than a *prescriptive* regimen of exercises used in physical therapy. This means that programs as simple as walking, using resistance bands, using light weights, or water-based exercise can have a high probability of success in the management of pain and depressive symptoms characteristic of skeletal and joint disabilities.

Aquatic Therapy

Programming challenges for persons with skeletal and joint difficulties may explain Levine's (1996) general recommendation of water-based activity programs. Water offers three very desirable programming features that offset the risks of land-based activities. Water's buoyancy minimizes the stress of the weight of the limb on the joint. Water offers natural resistance to movement, causing muscles to work harder and placing positive stress on the skeletal system. Finally, a water environment affords protection of skeletal parts from excessive jarring and other potential trauma in the activity environment. Weighing the desirable features of a water-based activity program against those of a conservative, land-based activity program (e.g., weightbearing activities) is necessary in the program planning phase of the TR process.

Two notable water-based TR interventions have been described in the recent literature. Beaudouin and Keller (1994) reported on a project titled Aquatic-Solutions. The authors described assessments, evaluations, and goals for chronic pain specific to skeletal-related and joint-related disabilities. Physical goals for chronic pain included increasing flexibility and endurance. Psychosocial goals included decreasing depression, increasing locus of control, and improving self-concept—all comorbid, psychological concomitants of pain and skeletal and joint impairment.

Beaudouin and Keller (1994) described the program plan for Aquatic-Solutions as "a combination of water exercises and adapted aquatics to alleviate specific physical and psychosocial conditions, and increase functional abilities" (p. 195). Implementation consisted of stretching and range of motion exercises, muscle toning exercises, and strength and endurance exercises. The program was initially delivered on a one-to-one basis to account for individual fitness levels and to allow for adjustment to the water-based exercises. The transition phase of the program was small group based, with the groups organized around shared disabilities and symptoms. The maintenance portion of the program usually took place after 6 to 8 weeks. In the maintenance phase the individual was referred to an integrated, community-based aquatics program.

Several years before Beaudouin and Keller described their program, Weiss and Jamieson (1988) explained an aquatic exercise program (the Hydro-Cal-Aerobics program) based in the community with the purpose of bringing exercise programs to underserved "hidden disability" groups (e.g., those with orthopedic conditions or chronic pain). Like Beaudouin and Keller, Weiss and Jamieson were also concerned about the concomitant emotional problems that frequently accompanied these disorders—depression, anxiety, insomnia, disturbed eating patterns, and abuse of medication.

The Hydro-Cal-Aerobics program appeared to be similar in content to that of Beaudouin and Keller's, with stretching and flexibility exercises followed by strength and endurance exercises. The main program difference was the 30 minutes of cardiovascular training embedded within Weiss and Jamieson's 1-hour program. Another difference between the two aquatic exercise programs was that Weiss and Jamieson's program was less explicitly outcome based and the evaluations were more informal. The authors surveyed participants to evaluate the program and found that most of the clients said that their medical condition had improved as a result of the program. Of those who reported depression at the beginning of the program, all said they "felt better" after the program. In addition, Weiss and Jamieson evaluated leisure and social outcomes in their post hoc survey of participants. Over 75% of the subjects reported that they made new friends, over 20% resumed an old leisure activity, and about 18% tried a new leisure activity.

Although no specific aquatics program is described by Jansma and French (1994), they do give a general recommendation to involve persons with spina bifida in aquatics programs. They note that the person with spina bifida can experience motor control in the water that he or she may not be able to experience when in a wheelchair. Goals for the client with spina bifida in a water-based program are familiar enough: weight control (a significant problem for adults with spina bifida), increase endurance, emotional and social outlet, and overcoming fear of the water. So long as the toileting regimen of the client with spina bifida is well-managed, water-based activity programs should be feasible and without unusual difficulties.

Leisure Education

The goals for leisure education for persons with skeletal and joint impairments relate to inclusion in mainstream recreation programs, transition into the community, acquiring new or adapted leisure skills, and adherence to a program of physical activity.

Inclusion

Inclusion in the least restrictive environment is not a new idea. Legislation mandating an appropriate education for persons with disabilities during the developmental years has existed for some time. Inclusion efforts were further encouraged with the implementation of the Americans with Disabilities Act (ADA) in the 1990s. Physical education has been at the forefront of the normalization effort as the only subject explicitly required for persons with disabilities during the developmental period.

Inclusion of youth with disabilities in educational opportunities with their nondisabled peers has met with mixed success. Connor-Kuntz, Dummer, and Paciorek (1995) found that over 90% of persons with spina bifida surveyed were in physical education; however, only a little more the half of the respondents participated in *regular* physical education. Likewise, over 80% of the subjects said they participated in sports, but less than half reported participation in school sports. Those excluded from regular physical education reported that the primary reason for the exclusion was concern over bowel and bladder control.

Results reported by Connor-Kuntz et al. (1995) may have motivated Aufsesser (1991) to add an unusual option for inclusion on his continuum of least restrictive environments for physical education. In Aufsesser's model of integration, community-based physical education is positioned between integrated physical education and split placement (in adapted physical education and regular physical education). Aufsesser's model points to the important role of community-based programs, such as those coordinated by a TRS working for a municipal recreation department. Aufsesser reasoned that because youth with disabilities would eventually become adults with disabilities who reside in the community, orienting them to community-based programs made perfect sense.

An illustration of Aufsesser's ideas at work is represented in a case study published by Green and DeCoux (1994). The researchers worked with parents and program directors to integrate an 8-year-old with spina bifida into a youth basketball program. Their findings revealed that with properly configured conditions, inclusion and participation in regular recreational sport programs within the community is feasible and attainable. Their results indicated that integration was

successful with respect to participation indicators (e.g., how many times the client handled the ball per game) and social indicators (e.g., who subjects would invite to a party at their house).

Unfortunately, as with the specific findings on the integration of youth with spina bifida into regular physical education in public schools, disabled populations in general are still rejected in the community (Austin, 1987; Kraus & Shank, 1992). Cleft palate and obesity may provide an acid test for progress in attitudes toward persons with disabilities because both conditions involve cosmetic differences but no functional disabilities. Strauss and Broder (1990) maintained that cosmetic appearance still made a significant difference in attitude formation. Tobiasen (1990) reasoned that people impute psychological characteristics based on physical characteristics (e.g., persons with cleft palate are less smart, less friendly, less popular).

Transition

Transition initiatives are vitally important if the aspirations represented by the ADA will ever be realized. Attitudes of persons without disabilities are not the only barrier—sometimes the person with the disability may present a self-imposed mental barrier. For example, over 75% of Smith and Yoshioka's (1992) subjects with arthritis reported that they had made significant changes in their leisure lifestyles following development of the impairment. Smith and Yoshioka concluded that persons with arthritis should increase their activity repertoire to neutralize the impact of the disease on leisure lifestyle. If persons with arthritis are representative of other disability groups, then we may expect many persons with disabilities to succumb to societal expectations of how persons with disabilities should behave (e.g., persons with pain should not be exercising).

New or Adapted Skills

Instead of acquiescing in the disability, persons with impairments must work to overcome internal and external barriers to participating in a satisfying leisure lifestyle, whether that means learning new activities, maintaining premorbid activities (Carter et al., 1995), or both. Indirect evidence for the importance of remaining engaged in life is found in a recent study (Crotty et al., 1994) of 75 young women with rheumatoid arthritis. Over time Crotty and associates discovered that psychosocial variables were as significant as physical variables in predicting function. Social relationships and maintaining leisure interests were as important as pain in determining endpoint functional ability.

A second study corroborates the findings of Crotty et al. Katz and Yelin (1995) discovered that the loss of valued activities (e.g., visiting family, crafts and hobbies, vacations) increased the risk of rheumatoid arthritic subjects developing marked depressive symptoms by almost fourfold. Furthermore, when the loss of valued activities was reported in conjunction with significant functional impairment, the risk of developing depressive symptoms increased more than 10 times. Functional impairment alone, however, did not significantly increase the risk for the development of depressive symptoms. Katz and Yelin (1995) concluded:

> Therapies or programs designed to help persons with RA [rheumatoid arthritis] maintain activities that are important to them, or perhaps find adequate alternative activities, may be very effective in helping them maintain psychological well-being. (p. 55)

Assistance in developing and maintaining recreational activities may be provided through programs aimed at facilitating the transition from school to community or from healthcare setting to community. One such program described in the literature is Close Encounters (Maddy, 1988). Close Encounters was given impetus by concerns expressed by teenagers with developmental disabilities during clinic visits. They said they felt socially isolated much of the time—lacking friends and depending on their families for social activities. Many of the youth expressed an interest in entering college, presenting an acute need for a program designed to assist in the transition into a more independent and responsible environment.

Youth between ages 13 and 21 were recruited to participate in Close Encounters for two weeks during the summer months. Inclusion criteria for the program were average intelligence and independence in self-care or in directing self-care. Goals consistent with the ultimate aim of independent, community living included improving social skills, developing satisfying friendships, increasing independence, improving knowledge of community resources, and advancing self-understanding and understanding of others. The program included daily seminars on leisure resources and skills, assertiveness, college life, sexuality, self-defense, apartment living, social skill development, and meal preparation, among others. Evenings and weekends were set aside for activities which the participants planned and implemented themselves. Formative and summative evalua-

tions were used to improve the Close Encounters experience. Participant evaluations were based on attainment of individualized objectives related to responsibility, self-care, use of community resources, cooperation, and group participation.

Another method of empowering clients through leisure education is based on the premise that knowledge and competence are self-reinforcing. Through acquiring new skills in leisure experiences and activities, persons with disabilities advance the breadth of their leisure repertoire and augment perceptions of competence. Perceptions of competence and adequacy may support perceptions of control on the part of the person with the disability. Perceived control and competence have long been hallmarks of the therapeutic effect of recreation (Iso-Ahola, 1980; Shary & Iso-Ahola, 1989) and have been included in some more contemporary models of therapeutic recreation service delivery (e.g., Datillo & Kleiber, 1993).

Although little research exists linking acquiring leisure skills and competencies and perceived control, the logic supporting the association is compelling. Reason suggests that perceptions of control will be likely if the person can execute an activity with some acceptable degree of competence. Further, acquisition of a broad and varied repertoire of leisure skills enhances the probability of long-lasting perceptions of control because it insulates the person against the loss of leisure activities because of a disability (e.g., Smith and Yoshioka's (1992) subjects who changed leisure activities after being diagnosed with rheumatoid arthritis). The person with a larger repertoire of leisure skills to choose from is more adaptable and less likely to fall victim to perceptions of helplessness and hopelessness (see Mobily, Lemke & Gisin, 1991).

Crawford (1989) used individualized reinforcers and instruction to enhance the leisure skills on playground apparatus of five subjects with severe mental retardation and accompanying physical disabilities (two subjects had spina bifida). Three of the five subjects acquired at least one new playground skill (e.g., learned to use a piece of playground equipment) and improved in their social skills. One of the three that showed improvement was a subject with spina bifida. Whether these subjects also enhanced perceptions of control and competence is not known, but the probability of perceived control resulting seems possible.

Adherence

Adherence is the final area addressed by leisure education for persons with skeletal and joint impairments.

Adherence to a well-rounded leisure lifestyle in general and adherence to a regular program of physical activity more specifically are of central interest. Persons with disabilities face the very same difficulties and report the very same barriers to participation in a program of regular exercise as their nondisabled peers (Shephard, 1990). The main obstacles to participation relate to environmental factors—cost, availability of facilities, and transportation. Intrinsic barriers are also evident, and include lack of interest, lack of time, and secondary health and medical problems.

Minor and Brown (1993) reported on a study of exercise adherence among 120 patients with arthritis and concluded that the reasons for not maintaining a self-directed exercise program were similar to those in the general population. However, more of the reasons pertained to internal factors (anxiety about exercise, depression, aerobic capacity, and pain), compared to external factors—support of friends. Nevertheless, most of the barriers to adherence to a recreational exercise program appear to be subject to modification, whether the obstacle exists in the environment or within the individual's own psyche. The TRS focusing on improving adherence should direct efforts toward modifying one or more of the significant obstacles reported by the client.

Recreation Participation

Growth in wheelchair sports and adventure experiences for persons with orthopedic impairments has been apparent over the last decade (Austin, 1987). These activities are examples of the benefits of programs designed to include persons with disabilities in a broad diversity of leisure experiences available to the general public. The following studies detail some of the inclusion initiatives for persons with skeletal or joint problems.

Burns (1995) evaluated a camping experience of four subjects with spina bifida. Two of the subjects improved self-esteem. Perhaps equally important, the same campers were observed to interact progressively more with other campers than with counselors as the camping experience continued. These outcomes might well be anticipated in light of the commonly known finding from inclusion studies that indicates that mere physical integration is not enough to change attitudes. The sustained camping experience may have provided sufficient time for the able-bodied campers to overcome reluctance to interact with their peers with spina bifida and advance the genuine quality of the camping experience for all members of the party.

Subjects in a study by McAvoy, Schatz, Stutz, Schleien, and Lais (1989) included persons with osteoporosis and amputations. The researchers examined anxiety levels of campers with disabilities following wilderness experiences of variable lengths (1 day, 3–5 days, 7–12 days). Compared to a control group that received a nonwilderness recreational activity, those who participated in the wilderness experience tended to be less anxious. The reduction in anxiety was statistically significant when subjects participating in the one-day trips were dropped from the analysis. The latter result is in keeping with the common finding mentioned earlier—sustained experiences are more likely to result in sufficient exposure to allow for meaningful interactions which are more apt to produce genuine attitude change. The net benefit in the case of the McAvoy et al. (1989) study was that anxiety levels also declined as a result.

McAvoy et al. (1989) also debriefed campers with disabilities using a qualitative interview. Subjects frequently reported positive lifestyle changes. Beneficial changes in relationships, recreation skills, attitudes toward persons with disabilities, tolerance of others, tolerance of stress, and skills in approaching new situations were all noted in the findings.

Subjects with arthritis were among those involved in a horseback riding experience provided by Brock (1988). Student riders participated in classes two times a week for eight weeks. As a result of the experience, Brock hoped to find improvement in medical criteria (posture, coordination, spasticity, and hypotonia), sport and recreation skills (balance, skill, coordination, and strength), and educational and psychological variables (vocabulary, behavior, self-confidence, motivation, and locus of control). Significant improvements were noted in arm and leg coordination following completion of the program; however, none of the other variables improved significantly.

The results of the Brock study point to an important concern for TRS delivering services for the purpose of recreation participation instead of for therapy or education. When the objective of the program is to enhance the quality of the participant's recreation experience (e.g., enjoyment, intrinsic motivation, friendships), then the markers used to evaluate the effectiveness of the program ought to focus on the recreational experience, not the concomitants (e.g., low self-esteem, anxiety, depression) of chronic conditions. The efforts of the TRS can be misguided if he or she focuses on "side effects" in preference to the quality of the experience. Focusing on the quality of the recreation experience when the main program intent is recreation participation amounts to doing what you profess to be doing.

Others (Haun, 1966; Hunnicutt, 1980; Lee, 1987) have cautioned the profession about the trap of side effects. To be certain, the TRS hopes that the softball game that integrates peers with and without disabilities will help decrease anxiety and depression. But when recreation participation is the focus of the service delivery effort, the other aspects of therapy—goals and objectives that relate to symptoms or preventing secondary disabilities, assessments of relevant variables, and evaluation of client progress toward attaining clinical goals—are less evident.

This does not mean that community-based TR cannot or should not address clinical goals. Rather, whenever the program (clinical or community) intent is stated to be recreation participation, then the TRS is obliged to remain faithful to that purpose. Focusing on side effects or clinical outcomes under the conditions that prevail when the intent of service delivery is recreation participation also marginalizes the quality of the recreation experience as an important outcome of the comprehensive TR effort.

Practical Applications

Medical Screening for Exercise Programs

Simple preliminary screening devices are abundant; one of the best is the revised Physical Activity Readiness Questionnaire (rPAR-Q) by Shephard, Thomas, and Weller (1991). Following preliminary screening the questionnaire should be reviewed by a consulting physician. Further examination may be warranted if the cooperating physician believes consultation with the family doctor is indicated. In most cases, with the conservative approach and mild to moderate exercise programs recommended here, the physician will approve and even encourage participation.

Pain as a Marker

The obvious precautions mentioned in the literature remind TRS that pain, limited range of motion, and functional limitations are common to many skeletal and joint problems. Hence, *reasonable* and *moderate* are often used as qualifiers for leisure time exercise programs for persons with disabilities, including those with skeletal and joint disabilities. The calls for caution and a conservative approach to leisure time exercise in the literature may have prompted some authorities (e.g., Carter et al., 1995) to recommend an even safer approach to recreation-based physical activity—the use of water as an environment for exercise. In either event, pain should be used as a marker for the upper limits of safe participation. Reports of pain by participants should not be ignored or treated lightly; pain should prompt the program leader to adjust the exercise according to the person's capacity to tolerate.

A Conservative Approach

In some cases, pain may not be evident, even when the risk of provoking secondary problems exists. For example, participants with advanced osteoporosis should be kept within appropriate margins of safety, because the very activity designed to improve skeletal integrity also puts the individual at risk for injury (e.g., hip fracture). Bone customarily responds favorably to the stress of exercise, but when the integrity of the skeleton is compromised, as is the case in osteoporosis, proceeding cautiously is advised. Translated into practical application, this means that nonweightbearing exercise should be the first recourse with osteoporotic clients. Examples presented in the earlier section on TR interventions—aquatic programs and weight training— are considered more conservative than weightbearing activities and may yield similar results. High impact activities and contact sports are, therefore, contraindicated.

Watch for Skin Lesions

The TRS must remain vigilant for early signs of skin breakdown, including irritations, red or inflamed segments of the skin, or indications of pain from the client. Early precaution can prevent significant problems in the future. A brief cessation of activity or a simple change of posture may be all that is required to avoid development of troublesome and occasionally lethal ulcerations of the skin.

Use Clean Procedures When Toileting

Competence in toileting is a cultural concern and clearly a potential obstacle to inclusive recreation experiences. (Recall the report by Connor-Kuntz et al. [1995] of reasons articulated for not allowing students with spina bifida to participate in regular physical education.) Beyond basic self-care or self-directed competence in toileting, the TRS may often be required to assist in toileting of clients (e.g., empty a leg bag). Appropriate precautions should be followed at all times to protect the client from urinary tract, bladder, or kidney infections, all of which can be serious or even life-threatening. Most agencies have protocols and procedures for assisted toileting, and for meeting toileting emergencies in the field.

Encourage Tolerance

For the most part, unless secondary conditions are present, clients with skeletal and joint conditions will not present with any cognitive impairments. At times, persons with orthopedic disorders may be less than patient with clients they are grouped with who have some cognitive or psychological involvement. For instance, grouping persons with post hip fracture, osteoporosis, and arthritis with clients who have experienced a stroke or who have Alzheimer's disease is not unusual. (In fact, judging by the TR literature,

grouping mobility impairments into the same programs is the norm.) One possible strategy to counteract intolerance is to establish mentoring relationships or partnerships between persons with and without cognitive impairments, or to have an experienced person without cognitive impairment serve as a peer leader.

Chapter Summary

This chapter examined the skeletal system and joint system and addressed the following key concepts:

- The primary functions of the skeletal and joint systems are support and movement.
- Older adults are most frequently affected by problems with skeletal and joint systems, including osteoporosis, arthritis, fractures, and postural abnormalities.
- Common problems associated with disorders of the skeletal and joint systems present as pain, impaired mobility, depression, and marked constraint to leisure lifestyle.
- Persons with skeletal and joint impairments usually do not have comorbid cognitive deficits.
- Pain management is the most important goal because it is prerequisite to addressing other problems.
- Low impact recreational-level exercise has shown good results with this group.
- Those with developmental disabilities of the skeletal system frequently encounter barriers to inclusion.

References

Aufsesser, P. M. (1991, Winter). Mainstreaming and least restrictive environment: How they differ. *Polestar*, 31–34.

Austin, D. R. (1987). Recreation and persons with physical disabilities. A literature synthesis. *Therapeutic Recreation Journal, 21*(1), 36–44.

Baker, S. D., O'Neill, B., Ginsburg, M. J., and Goohua, L. (1992). *The injury fact book* (2nd ed.). New York, NY: Oxford University Press.

Beaudouin, N. M. and Keller, M. J. (1994). Aquatics solutions: A continuum of services for individuals with physical disabilities in the community. *Therapeutic Recreation Journal, 28*, 193–202.

Berryman, D., James, A., and Trader, B. (1991). The benefits of therapeutic recreation in physical medicine. In C. P. Coyle, W. B. Kinney, B. Riley, and J. W. Shank (Eds.), *The benefits of therapeutic recreation: A consensus view* (pp. 235–288). Ravensdale, WA: Idyll Arbor.

Brock, B. J. (1988). The effects of therapeutic horseback riding on physically disabled adults. *Therapeutic Recreation Journal, 22*(1), 34–43.

Buettner, L. L. (1988). Utilizing developmental theory and adaptive equipment with regressed geriatric patients in therapeutic recreation. *Therapeutic Recreation Journal, 22*(3), 72–79.

Burns, J. L. (1995). The psychosocial effects of a therapeutic camping experience on first time campers with spina bifida. *Symposium on Leisure Research Abstracts*, 34.

Carter, M. J., Van Andel, G. E., and Robb, G. M. (1995). *Therapeutic recreation: A practical approach* (2nd ed.). Prospect Heights, IL: Waveland.

Connor-Kuntz, F. J., Dummer, G. M., and Paciorek, M. J. (1995). Physical education and sport participation of children and youth with spina bifida myelomeningocele. *Adapted Physical Activity Quarterly, 12*, 228–238.

Coutts, K., McKenzie, D., Loock, C., Beauchamp, R., and Armstrong, R. (1993). Upper body exercise capacity in youth with spina bifida. *Adapted Physical Activity Quarterly, 10*, 22–28.

Crawford, M. E. (1989). The development of age appropriate outdoor playground behaviors in severely disabled children. In F. N. Humphrey and J. H. Humphrey (Eds.), *Recreation: Current selected research* (pp. 91–108). New York, NY: AMS Press.

Crotty, M., McFarlane, A. C., Brook, P. M., Hopper, J. L., Bieri, D., and Taylor, S. J. (1994). The psychosocial and clinical status of younger women with early rheumatoid arthritis: A longitudinal study with frequent measures. *British Journal of Rheumatology, 33*(8), 754–760.

Datillo, J. and Kleiber, D. A. (1993). Psychological perspectives for therapeutic recreation research: The psychology of enjoyment. In M. J. Malkin and C. Z. Howe (Eds.), *Research in therapeutic recreation: Concepts and methods* (pp. 57–76). State College, PA: Venture Publishing, Inc.

Dekker, J., Tola, P., Aufdemkampe, G., and Winchers, M. (1993). Negative affect, pain and disability in osteoarthritis patients: The mediating role of muscle weakness. *Behaviour Research & Therapy, 31*(2), 203–206.

Goldberg, M. S., Mayo, N. E., Poitras, B., Scott, S., and Hanley, J. (1994). The Ste-Justine Adolescent Idiopathic Scoliosis Cohort Study: Part II: Perception of health, self and body image, and participation in physical activities. *Spine, 19*(14), 1562–1572.

Green, F. P. and DeCoux, V. (1994). A procedure for evaluating the effectiveness of a community recreation integration program. *Therapeutic Recreation Journal, 28*(1), 41–47.

Grisso, J. A., Kelsey, J. L., O'Brien, L. A., Miles, C. G., Sidney, S., Maislin, G., Lapann, K., Moritz, D., and Peters, B. (1997). Risk factors for hip fracture in men. Hip fracture study group. *American Journal of Epidemiology, 145*(9), 786–793.

Haun, P. (1966). *Recreation: A medical viewpoint.* New York, NY: Teacher's College Press.

Helmes, E., Hodsman, A., Lazowski, D., Bhardwaj, A., Crilly, R., Nichol, P., Drost, D., Vanderburgh, L., and Pederson, L. (1995). A questionnaire to evaluate disability in osteoporotic patients with vertebral compression fractures. *Journal of Gerontology. Series A, Biological Sciences & Medical Sciences, 50*(2), M91–M98.

Hoenk, A. H. and Mobily, K. E. (1987). Mainstreaming the play environment: Effects of previous exposure and salience of disability. *Therapeutic Recreation Journal, 21*(4), 23–31.

Hunnicutt, B. K. (1980). To cope in autonomy: Therapeutic recreation and the limits to professionalization and intervention. *Journal of Expanding Horizons, 7,* 121–134.

Iso-Ahola, S. E. (1980). Perceived control and responsibility as mediators of the effects of therapeutic

recreation on the institutionalized aged. *Therapeutic Recreation Journal, 14*(1), 36–43.

Jaglal, S. B., Kreiger, N., and Darlington, G. (1993). Past and recent physical activity and risk of hip fracture. *American Journal of Epidemiology, 138*(2), 107–118.

Jansma, P. and French, R. (1994). *Special physical education: Physical activity, sports, and recreation.* Englewood Cliffs, NJ: Prentice-Hall.

Juskeliene, V., Magnus, P., Bakketeig, L. S., Dailidiene, N., and Jurkuvenas, V. (1996), Prevalence and risk factors for asymmetric posture in preschool children aged 6–7 years. *International Journal of Epidemiology, 25*(5), 1053–1059.

Katz, P. P. and Yelin, E. H. (1995). The development of depressive symptoms among women with rheumatoid arthritis. The role of function. *Arthritis & Rheumatism, 38*(1), 49–56.

Kraus, R. and Shank, J. (1992). *Therapeutic recreation service: Principles and practices* (4th ed.). Dubuque, IA: Brown.

Lee, L. L. (1987). A panic attack over therapeutic recreation being considered therapeutic. *Therapeutic Recreation Journal, 21*(2), 71–78.

Levine, G. R. (1996). Neuromuscular disorders. In D. R. Austin and M. E. Crawford (Eds.), *Therapeutic recreation: An introduction* (2nd ed., pp. 184–212). Boston, MA: Allyn & Bacon.

Maddy, B. J. (1988). Close encounters: Promoting social independence in adolescents with physical disabilities. *Therapeutic Recreation Journal, 22*(4), 49–55.

Marcus, R., Drinkwater, B., Dalsky, G., Dufek, J., Raab, D., Slemenda, C., and Snowharter, C. (1992). Osteoporosis and exercise in women. *Medicine & Science in Sports & Exercise, 24*(6), S301–S307.

McAvoy, L. H., Schatz, E. C., Stutz, M. F., Schleien, S. J., and Lais, G. (1989). Integrated wilderness adventure: Effects of personal and lifestyle traits of persons with and without disabilities. *Therapeutic Recreation Journal, 22*(3), 50–64.

Minor, M. A. and Brown, J. D. (1993). Exercise maintenance of persons with arthritis after participation in a class experience. *Health Education Quarterly, 20*(1), 83–95.

Minor, M. A. and Lane, N. E. (1996). Recreational exercise in arthritis. *Rheumatic Diseases Clinics of North America, 22*(3), 563–577.

Mobily, K. E., Lemke, J. H., and Gisin, G. J. (1991). The idea of leisure repertoire. *Journal of Applied Gerontology, 10*, 208–223.

Mobily, K. E., Rubenstein, L. M., Lemke, J. H., O'Hara, M. W. and Wallace, R. B. (1996). Walking and depression in a cohort of older adults: The Iowa 65+ rural health study. *Journal of Aging and Physical Activity, 4*, 119–135.

Murphy, C. (1989). Protocol for arthritis service. In C. Land, A. Marmer, S. Mayfield, M. K. Gerski, and C. Murphy (Eds.), *Protocols in therapeutic recreation* (pp. 12–17). Alexandria, VA: National Recreation and Park Association.

Panush, R. S. and Holtz, H. A. (1994). Is exercise good or bad for arthritis in the elderly? *Southern Medical Journal, 87*(5), S74–S78.

Pincus, T., Griffith, J., Pearce, S., and Isenberg, D. (1996). Prevalence of self-reported depression in patients with rheumatic arthritis. *British Journal of Rheumatology, 35*(9), 879–893.

Prevalence of leisure-time physical activity among persons with arthritis and other rheumatic conditions. United States, 1990–1991. (1997). *Morbidity & Mortality Weekly Report, 46*(18), 389–393.

Ramstad, T., Ottem, E., and Shaw, W. C. (1995). Psychosocial adjustment in Norwegian adults who had undergone standardized treatment of complete cleft lip and palate, II. Self-reported problems and concerns with appearance. *Scandinavian Journal of Plastic & Reconstructive Surgery & Hand Surgery, 29*(4), 329–336.

Shary J. M. and Iso-Ahola, S. E. (1989). Effect of a control-relevant intervention on nursing home residents' perceived competence and self-esteem. *Therapeutic Recreation Journal, 23*(1), 7–16.

Shephard, R. J. (1990). *Fitness in special populations.* Champaign, IL: Human Kinetics.

Shephard, R. J., Thomas, S. and Weller, I. (1991). The Canadian home fitness test: 1991 update. *Sports Medicine, 1*, 359.

Sherrill, C., Hinson, M., Gench, B., Kennedy, S. O., and Low, L. (1990). Self-concepts of disabled youth athletes. *Perceptual and Motor Skills, 70*, 1093–1098.

Smedstad, L. M., Moum, T., Vaglum, P., and Kvien, T. K. (1996). The impact of early rheumatoid arthritis on psychological distress. A comparison between 238 patients with RA and 116 matched controls. *Scandinavian Journal of Rheumatology, 25*(6), 377–382.

Smith, S. A. and Yoshioka, C. F. (1992). Recreation functioning and depression in people with arthritis. *Therapeutic Recreation Journal, 26*(4), 21–30.

Stevens, J. A., Powell, K. E., Smith, S. M., Wings, P. A., and Sattin, R. W. (1997). Physical activity, functional limitations, and the risk of fall-related fractures in community-dwelling elderly. *Annals of Epidemiology, 7*(1), 54–61.

Strauss, R. P. and Broder, H. (1990). Psychological and sociocultural aspects of cleft lip and palate. In J. Bardach and H. L. Morris (Eds.), *Multidisciplinary management of cleft lip and palate* (pp. 831–837). Philadelphia, PA: W. B. Sanders.

Swezey, R. L. (1996). Exercise for osteoporosis: Is walking enough? The case for site specificity and resistive exercise. *Spine, 21*(23), 2809–2813.

Taal, E., Rasker, J. J., and Timmers, C. J. (1997). Measures of physical function and emotional well-being for young adults with arthritis. *Journal of Rheumatology, 24*(5), 994–997.

Tobiasen, J. M. (1990). Psychosocial adjustment to cleft lip and palate. In J. B. Bardach and H. L. Morris (Eds.), *Multidisciplinary management of cleft lip and palate* (pp. 820–825). Philadelphia, PA: W. B. Saunders.

Tobiasen, J. M. and Hiebert, J. M. (1993). Clefting and psychosocial adjustment. Influence of facial aesthetics. *Clinics in Plastic Surgery, 20*(4), 623–631.

Varni, J. W., Rapoff, M. A., Waldron, S. A., Gragg, R. A., Bernstein, B. H., and Lindsley, C. B. (1996). Chronic pain and emotional distress in children and adolescents. *Journal of Developmental & Behavioral Pediatrics, 17*(3), 154–161.

Vuori, I. (1995). Exercise and physical health: musculoskeletal health and functional capabilities. *Research Quarterly for Exercise & Sport, 66*(4), 276–285.

Weiss, C. R. and Jamieson, N. (1988). Hidden disabilities: A new enterprise for therapeutic recreation. *Therapeutic Recreation Journal, 22*(3), 9–17.

CHAPTER 11 MUSCULAR SYSTEM

Muscles attach to the skeleton. When muscles contract they produce movement at joints. Although movement is the primary function of the muscle system, it performs other important tasks. An explanation of the functions of the muscle system will be followed by a presentation of the three different types of muscle: skeletal muscle, cardiac muscle, and smooth muscle. This will lead to a brief discussion of how muscles work (contract) to produce movement and the role of the nervous system in muscle contraction. As with the skeletal system, the chapter will then move to a presentation of the gross anatomy of the system. This section will include the names of some of the more important muscles that produce familiar movements, the primary actions of the major muscle groups, and the peripheral nerves that innervate the same muscles. Next, normal development of the muscle system will be discussed briefly. The most common disorders specific to skeletal muscles will be described after normal development. The final section of the chapter addresses therapeutic recreation (TR) interventions and techniques focused on the specific disabilities that preferentially affect the muscle system.

Muscle Tissue

Functions of Muscle

The major function of muscle is to produce movement. Because the movement function of the muscle system figures in many of the activities programmed by the TR Specialist, and because many of the more conspicuous disabilities directly or indirectly involve the muscle tissue and mobility, this text emphasizes the movement function of the muscle system.

Nevertheless, the muscle system has other important roles. The shivering observed in conditions of low temperature is a function of the muscle system. The general activity of the muscle system in physical work and exercise produces a significant amount of heat that can increase body temperature in low thermal conditions, or must be dissipated in conditions of excess heat. The posture function of the muscle system is largely performed by muscles that act on the axial portion of the skeleton.

Muscles that regulate posture often contract in only very slight increments to put the body in a better working position. The muscles of posture sustain submaximal contractions over prolonged periods of time, and are adept in "sharing the work" of maintaining a specific posture over a long time.

Types of Muscle

Most of the discussion of muscle in the present chapter pertains to skeletal muscle. *Skeletal muscle* moves the skeleton. In contrast to smooth and cardiac muscle, skeletal muscle is under voluntary control. Skeletal muscle cells also have more than one nucleus, whereas cardiac and smooth muscle cells have the more usual one nucleus per cell. *Cardiac muscle* is found in only one location: the heart. *Smooth muscle* is found lining the walls of many tube systems (e.g., digestive system, urinary system, vascular system) found in the ventral body cavity. Cardiac and smooth muscle are not under voluntary control. A person cannot choose for the muscle of the heart to contract or not; nor can he or she choose to relax the smooth muscle lining the walls of an artery to allow more blood to flow to an area of high demand. Even though cardiac and skeletal muscles differ in function, they look remarkably similar under a light microscope. (Further discussion of cardiac and smooth muscle may be found in the chapters on the cardiopulmonary systems and the visceral systems.)

Muscle Contraction

Gross muscle (visible to the unaided eye) contains many *muscle cells* (also called muscle fibers). *Muscle contraction* literally means that a muscle cell shortens. If enough muscle cells within a gross muscle are stimulated to contract to overcome a specific resistance, then observable movement occurs.

Muscles attach to bones by means of a strong band of connective tissue called a *tendon*. Because muscles have at least two (sometimes more) attachments to bones, the shortening muscle usually produces movement at a joint by pulling one bone closer to the other. The attachment of a muscle that usually stays stationary during contraction is known as the *origin*; the attachment that moves is called the *insertion*. The muscle proper is located between the origin and the insertion and is known as the "gaster" or muscle belly (see **Figure 11.1**, p. 196).

Muscles shorten because of contractile proteins (myofilaments) contained within muscle cells. When

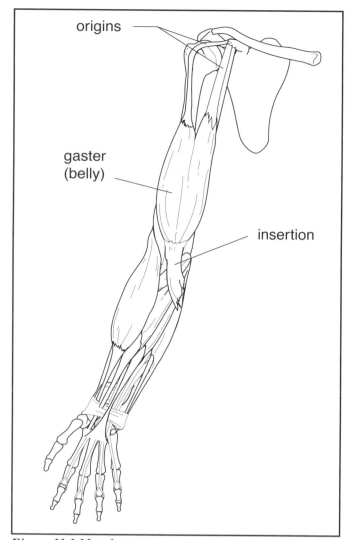

Figure 11.1 Muscle components

stimulated by a nervous impulse, two types of myofilaments—thick and thin—will shorten the individual muscle cell. When the number of muscle cells stimulated within a specific muscle is sufficient to overcome the resistance, then movement results. Some very important contractions, however, produce no movement (see "Muscle Tone").

Neuromuscular Junction

A muscle cell needs stimulation from a *neuron* (nerve cell) to contract. This nervous stimulation occurs at the *neuromuscular junction*. One is located on every muscle fiber within a gross muscle (see **Figure 11.2**). Analysis of a neuromuscular junction reveals several important anatomical structures. The muscle cell at a neuromuscular junction has a depression in the cell membrane where the neuron stimulates it called the motor end plate. The part of the neuron that stimulates

the muscle cell is known as the axon. The *axon* extends from the central area of the neuron into the periphery to stimulate muscles. The close-up of the neuromuscular junction in Figure 11.2 shows that the axon is swollen at its termination (end bulb) and contains many small bodies (vesicles). The *vesicles* contain the transmitter substance—a chemical messenger that passes from the neuron to attach to the cell membrane of the skeletal muscle cell. The transmitter substance causes the muscle cell to be stimulated and begin a sequence of events that eventually leads to contraction of the muscle cell.

The anatomy of the human nervous system is most efficient. The axon portion of one neuron forms neuromuscular junctions with more than one muscle cell. The association of one neuron to a number of muscle cells is called a motor unit. Some motor units are "gross," with one neuron innervating several hundred to thousands of muscle cells within any given muscle. Other motor units are known as "fine" because the neuron innervates only a few muscle cells. Generally, *fine motor units* are typical of muscles that are required to execute intricate and complex tasks. Therefore, the muscles that control the digits of the hand and foot are examples of muscles organized into fine motor units. *Gross motor units* are found in muscles that are responsible for movements that do not require a great deal of precision, such as the muscles of posture (erector spinae group) and muscles of ambulation (most of the muscles of the lower extremity).

The implication of the concept of a motor unit for rehabilitation efforts should not be overlooked. For example, if a pathology affects a muscle organized into fine motor units, then restoration of the capabilities of that muscle will take longer than for a muscle organized into gross motor units. This means it takes longer for a person to use the hand again than it does to learn to walk again. Rehabilitation here assumes complete recovery from the lesion, which is almost never the case.

Muscle Tone

Stimulation of a single muscle cell advances the state of contraction of the entire gross muscle. The more muscle cells stimulated the more the tone of any given muscle. Muscle tone means that in every skeletal muscle, some muscle cells are contracting at any given moment in time. If you palpate your biceps brachii muscle you may confirm that it exhibits a certain level of resilience even when you are not producing an observable contraction. The reason is muscle tone—a few of the muscle cells within the biceps brachii are contracting, but not enough to produce movement.

Tone is especially important for maintaining good posture, because an upright (standing) posture is largely a function of the muscle tone among the deep back muscles responsible for extending the vertebral column. Some of the muscle cells within the gross muscles that comprise the erector spinae group (see **Figure 11.3**, p. 198) are contracting just enough to resist the forces of gravity and weight of the body that are acting to draw the person into a recumbent position. Yet, if a person maintains good posture, movement is not customarily seen.

Muscle tone is also a significant concern in working with several disabilities that have origin in the nervous system, but manifest as muscle dysfunction. Some pathologies of the nervous system (e.g., a peripheral nerve injury) lead to *hypotonia*—the lack of or complete absence of sufficient muscle tone. Other disorders of the nervous system may result in hypertonia or an excess amount of muscle tone. The most severe presentation of hypertonia is exhibited in spasticity, a condition often associated with spinal cord injury.

Gross Anatomy of the Muscle System

This section will name and identify the function of the significant muscles acting on the axial skeleton and appendicular skeleton. The general pattern of nervous innervation of the muscle system will also be described. **Figure 11.4** (p. 199) presents an overview of many of the more superficial gross muscles. In some regions muscles are found in multiple layers—superficial, intermediate, and deep. Knowing the level or layer presented is essential.

Muscles Acting on the Axial Skeleton

Muscles of the *axial skeleton* produce subtle movements that help maintain posture and place the body in a better working position. Axial muscles include the muscles of facial expression, muscles of the tongue, muscles of mastication, neck muscles, abdominal muscles, muscles that act on the vertebral column, and muscles of respiration.

Muscles of the Neck

Most of the muscles found in the posterior neck region are either continuations of deep back muscles, such as the semispinalis capitis and longissimus capitis (see Figure 11.3), or superficial muscles such as the trapezius and sternocliedomastoid (see Figure 11.4). The trapezius, semispinalis capitis, and longissimus capitis extend the head. The sternocliedomastoid flexes the head. All but the trapezius rotate the head.

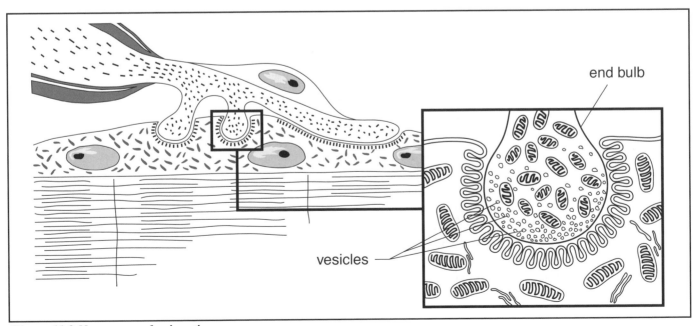

end bulb

vesicles

Figure 11.2 Neuromuscular junction

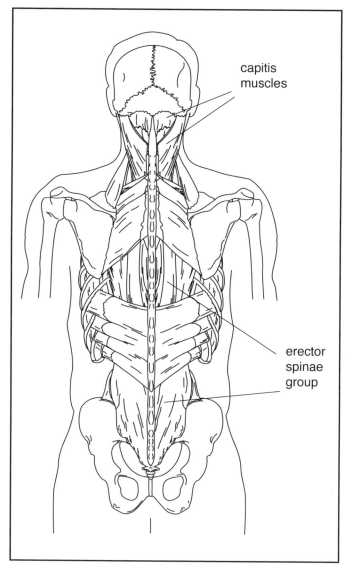

Figure 11.3 Erector spinae (deep back muscles)

Muscles Acting on the Vertebral Column

The erector spinae muscle (see Figure 11.3) comprises several groups of short muscles that connect vertebra to vertebra, or vertebrae to ribs. Collectively the erector spinae acts as one long muscle to extend the vertebral column. Its actions are essential to maintaining an upright posture and to lifting objects. The semispinalis capitis and longissimus capitis muscles that extend the head are continuations of the erector spinae group that runs the length of the vertebral column from the sacrum to skull. Another muscle that will produce extension of the vertebral column is the quadratus lumborum, which will produce lateral flexion of the vertebral column if only one side contracts.

Muscles of Respiration

Although not shown, the *muscles of respiration* and their actions in ventilation (breathing) will be discussed briefly. The diaphragm is a dome-shaped muscle that increases the superior to inferior space of the thoracic cavity (i.e., it pulls down to enlarge the thoracic cavity). The external intercostal muscles (the muscles between the ribs) increase the anterior to posterior dimension of the thoracic cavity (i.e., they pull out on the ribs to enlarge the thoracic cavity). Together, the diaphragm and the external intercostals act to create a situation favorable to inspiration because the pressure inside the thoracic cavity is made less than that of atmospheric air. When pressure inside the thoracic cavity is less than atmospheric pressure, inspiration results.

Expiration tends to be a recoil of stretched intercostal muscles and the elastic quality of healthy lung tissue. Internal intercostal muscles (also between the ribs) can draw the ribs closer together slightly in forced expiration. Abdominal muscles may also assist with forced expiration by making pressure inside the thoracic cavity greater than atmospheric pressure.

Muscles Acting on the Appendicular Skeleton

Upper Extremity

A number of muscles take origin on the axial skeleton and act on the shoulder (scapula) or the arm (humerus). Some of these muscles are illustrated in Figure 11.4.

Muscles of the Abdominal Wall

Two of the four abdominal muscles can be observed in whole or part in **Figure 11.5**. The external abdominal oblique and the deeper internal abdominal oblique produce lateral rotation of the trunk. The centrally placed rectus abdominis draws the thorax anteriorly and effectively flexes the vertebral column by pulling its attachments on the ribs and sternum closer to its origin on the pubic bone of the os coxae. A fourth abdominal muscle (not seen in Figure 11.5) is the transversus abdominis. Like the internal abdominal oblique, the transversus abdominis lies deep to the more superficial abdominal muscles. All four of the abdominal muscles act to compress the abdominal wall as in completing a crunch exercise or a sit-up.

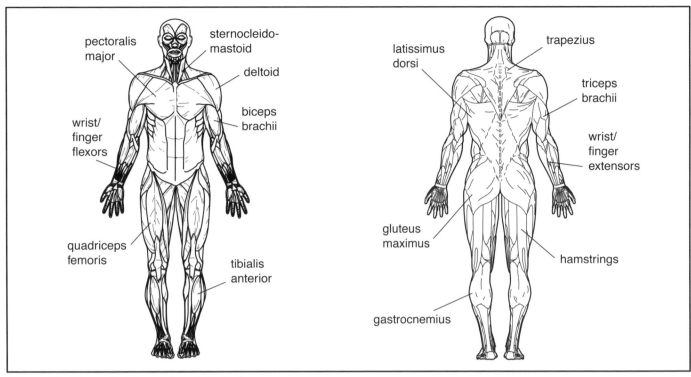

Figure 11.4 Superficial muscles of the body

Trapezius has already been mentioned as a muscle that acts on the head, but it also adducts and elevates the scapula (as in shrugging the shoulders). Adduction and elevation of the scapula is also the primary function of three muscles that take origin on the vertebral column and insert on the medial border of the scapula—the levator scapulae, rhomboid minor, and rhomboid major. The three adductors of the scapula are found in the intermediate layer of the upper back, between the trapezius (superficially) and the deep erector spinae muscles.

Two other muscles that act on the scapula—the pectoralis minor and the serratus anterior—produce only slight movements in the scapula. Both muscles hold the scapula steady while muscles taking origin on the scapula act on the arm and the forearm (e.g., biceps brachii).

Pectoralis major covers serratus anterior and pectoralis minor on the anterior thorax. Pectoralis major converges to insert on the humerus from a broad, expansive origin on the sternum and costal cartilages of the ribs near the sternum. Pectoralis major will adduct, flex and medially rotate the humerus. Another superficial muscle that may be seen in Figure 11.5 on both anterior and posterior views is the deltoid. Its major function is abduction of the upper extremity, but it also assists in flexion and extension of the humerus.

The counterpart of the pectoralis major on the lower back is the latissimus dorsi muscle. It arises from a broad origin like the pectoralis major. Its tendon travels under the axilla (armpit) and inserts on the humerus. The latissimus dorsi will adduct and medially rotate like pectoralis major, but it will extend the humerus instead of flexing it. The actions produced by contraction of the latissimus dorsi muscle are identical to those necessary to produce the crawl stroke in swimming.

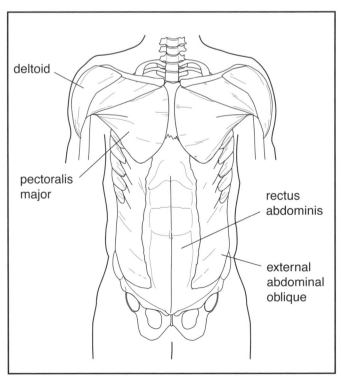

Figure 11.5 Muscles of the anterior trunk

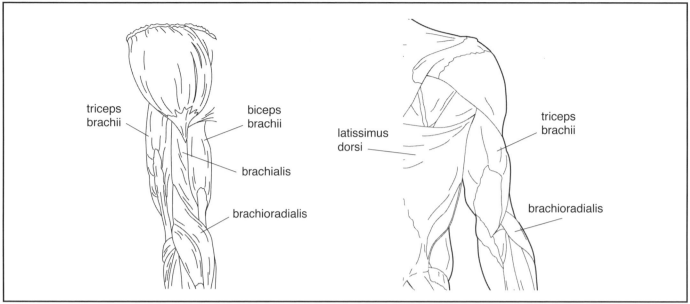

Figure 11.6 Muscles acting on the forearm (antebrachium)

In the intermediate, posterior layer of the upper back (deep to trapezius) are four muscles that take their origin off the scapula and insert on the humerus. Superior to inferior, the muscles are the supraspinatus, infraspinatus, teres minor, and teres major. These muscles act largely as adductors and lateral rotators of the humerus. Besides the latissimus dorsi and pectoralis major, another medial rotator of the humerus is the subscapularis, found on the anterior surface of the scapula (in the subscapular fossa). Because of its deep position, the subscapularis is only slightly visible in Figure 11.5.

Muscles that act on the forearm (radius and ulna) generally take origin off either the scapula or the humerus. Those on the anterior surface of the humerus flex the forearm and those on the posterior surface extend the forearm. **Figure 11.6** shows three anterior muscles: the superficial biceps brachii, the deep brachialis (only partially seen), and the antero-lateral brachioradialis. There are two posterior muscles: pervasive, three-headed triceps brachii and a second small muscle called the anconeus.

Seventeen muscles take origin in the forearm and the humerus and act on the wrist or digits. Most of these muscles are named after the primary action each produces. For instance, the pronator teres pronates the hand (turns the palm down), the flexor digitorum superficialis flexes the fingers, the flexor carpi radialis flexes the wrist (the carpus), and the flexor pollicis longus flexes the great digit (the thumb) of the hand. Only the more superficial of the muscles that act on the wrist or digits are seen in **Figure 11.7**. The palmaris longus flexes the wrist, but otherwise the name of each muscle gives its action.

Figure 11.7 also illustrates some of the intrinsic muscles of the hand—muscles that act on the digits that are located in the hand. Intrinsic muscles of the hand are not enumerated specifically, but for the most part these muscles are also named for the primary actions (e.g., the adductor pollicis adducts the thumb).

Lower Extremity

Muscles that act on the lower extremity are for the most part larger and easier to identify, and they tend to work in groups that share common actions. Those that move the thigh, for instance, can be organized into three logical groups: a medial adductor group (groin), a posterior extensor group, and an anterior flexor group. In addition, muscles of the lower extremity are more apt to act on two joints. Muscles act on two joints when their tendons cross two joints.

Muscles acting on the thigh (femur) take origin off the os coxa and/or part of the vertebral column. **Figure 11.8** (p. 202) shows the mass of muscle on the anterior surface of the thigh. However, many of these muscles take origin on the femur, cross the knee joint, and act on the leg (tibia and fibula). The superficial sartorious actually acts on two joints—it flexes both the thigh and the knee. Likewise the rectus femoris of the quadriceps femoris muscle group flexes the thigh and extends the leg. The remaining muscles that comprise the quadriceps femoris act only on the knee. Two deep muscles are also responsible for flexing the thigh—the iliacus and the psoas major. Sometimes the latter two muscles are referred to as one muscle—the iliopsoas.

Muscles on the medial surface of the thigh also take origin off the os coxa and insert on the femur, with adduction of the lower extremity as their primary action. Many of the muscles that adduct the lower extremity have adductor in their names—adductor longus, adductor brevis, and adductor magnus. The gracilis and the pectineus are also adductors of the lower extremity. Because the gracilis crosses the knee as well it will also flex the leg.

The posterior surface of the hip (the buttocks or gluteal region) is dominated by a large superficial muscle—the gluteus maximus. It is the primary extensor of the thigh. Two muscles deep to gluteus maximus, the gluteus medias and gluteus minimis (not seen completely in Figure 11.8), are medial rotators of the thigh. The hamstring group represents three muscles—biceps femoris, semitendinosus, and semimembranosus—that cross two joints like the rectus femoris on the anterior surface of the thigh. Therefore, the hamstrings will help the gluteus maximus extend the thigh and produce flexion of the leg at the knee joint. Only one muscle is found on the lateral surface of the os coxae and abducts on the lower extremity. The tensor fasciae latae can be partially seen in Figure 11.8.

Figure 11.8 also includes most of the muscles that act on the leg. All four of the muscles that comprise the quadriceps femoris (rectus femoris, vastus medialis, vastus lateralis, vastus intermedius) converge on a common tendon that inserts on the anterior surface of the tibia to produce extension of the leg at the knee (as in kicking a football).

The three muscles of the hamstring group represent the counterparts of the quadriceps femoris on the posterior surface. The hamstrings act to flex the leg at the knee. The hamstrings are assisted in flexing the leg by two other muscles that act on two joints: the sartorious and the gracilis.

Tendons of muscles that take origin on the fibula and the tibia cross the ankle joint to act on the foot at the ankle or on the digits. Some parallels can be drawn between the muscles acting on the hand and those acting on the foot. First, many of the muscles are named after their primary actions. Second, some of the muscles have names that are almost identical to those in the forearm. Third, the foot contains some intrinsic muscles that act on the digits, just like the hand.

Figure 11.9 (p. 202) illustrates the muscles of the leg that act on the foot. An anterior group of muscles act to dorsiflex the foot at the ankle, with some of the deeper muscles (not seen in Figure 11.9) also acting on the digits or great toe (e.g., extensor digitorum longus, extensor hallucis longus). The tibialis anterior muscle is the most discernible of the anterior muscle group, and it is a significant dorsiflexor of the foot. A smaller peroneus tertias muscle also assists with dorsiflexion of the foot.

The tendons of two muscles on the lateral surface of the leg pass posterior to the laterally positioned fibula thereby causing plantar flexion of the foot at the ankle. The two lateral muscles are the peroneus longus and peroneus brevis. The posterior surface of the leg is dominated by the substantial gastrocnemius (calf)

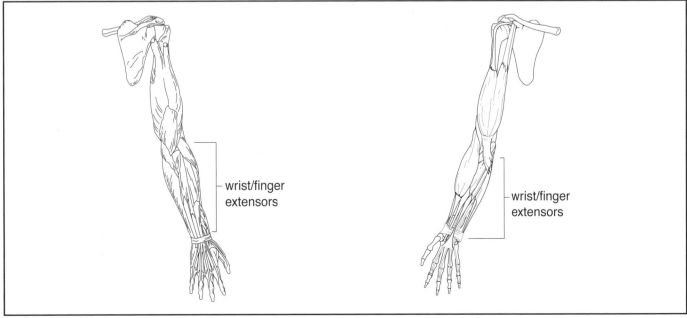

Figure 11.7 Muscles acting on the wrist (carpas) and fingers (phalanges)

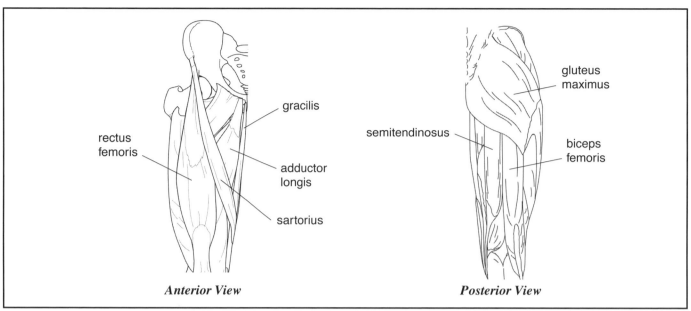

Figure 11.8 Muscles of the hip and thigh

muscle; it is a powerful plantar flexor of the foot at the ankle. Only slightly visible in Figure 11.9 is the deeper soleus muscle; its primary action is plantar flexion of the foot. Two muscles are not seen in on the posterior view of the leg, but their names reveal their primary functions—flexor digitorum longus and flexor hallucis longus (hallux refers to the big toe). Finally, the deep tibialis posterior also plantar flexes the foot.

Nervous innervations for the muscles discussed above are summarized in **Table 11.1**. The nerves listed form neuromuscular junctions with muscle cells that comprise the muscles listed. The table is intentionally general and organized according to the area or muscle group innervated in all but a few cases.

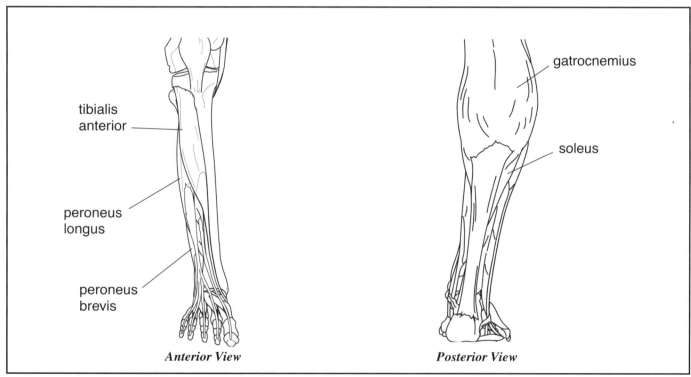

Figure 11.9 Muscles of the leg that act on the ankle and the foot

Normal Development

Muscle cells begin forming about the fourth week of fetal life and are functional after about four months. Shortly before birth precursor cells to muscle cells stop forming. Therefore, an individual is born with all of the muscle cells he or she will ever have. This has important implications for future potential with respect to muscular fitness and future conditioning and rehabilitation. To some extent, muscle strength and capability are genetically determined. The number of muscle cells one is born with predetermines the upper limits of muscle fitness. The fact that all muscle cells are present at birth for any given individual also urges a search for an explanation for how muscles increase in strength.

The strength of any muscle is a function of the cross-sectional area of the muscle (i.e., how big the muscle is). The number of muscle cells that make up a muscle determines its size. As a rule, larger muscles are comprised of more muscle cells and are stronger muscles. However, a person who exercises will condition a muscle and improve its strength. How do muscles get stronger if genetically limited to the number of muscle cells present at birth? The simple answer is that strengthening exercises cause the cells that comprise any given muscle to get larger. The more complicated answer pertains to the effect exercise has on individual muscle cells. As a general rule, muscle cells will adapt to higher than usual demands of exercise by synthesizing more contractile units. This means that more thick and thin myofilaments are produced and packed inside the well-conditioned muscle cell than the unfit muscle cell. The net result is larger muscle cells and a larger gross muscle.

After birth, the mastery of muscle control in humans is a protracted process when compared to that of other animals. The ambulation that takes a horse only hours to learn takes the human about a year. Besides the acquisition of strength and endurance capabilities throughout the developmental period, humans also occupy extensive time perfecting the control of the muscle system by the nervous system. This latter process, known as *motor learning*, really never stops and is in effect at any time in life when we try to learn a new task, including learning many recreational activities.

Peripheral Nerve	Area Innervated
Dorsal rami	Muscles of the deep back
Accessory	Sternocliedomastoid, trapezius
Phrenic	Diaphragm
Intercostals	Intercostal muscles, muscles of the abdominal wall
Pectoral nerves	Pectoral muscles
Dorsal scapular	Rhomboids and levator scapulae
Suprascapular	Supraspinatus, infraspinatus
Thoracodorsal	Latissimus dorsi
Long thoracic	Serratus anterior
Axillary	Deltoid, teres minor
Ulnar	1 1/2 muscles of the anterior forearm and intrinsic muscles of the hand
Upper and lower subscapular	Subscapularis, teres major
Radial (superficial and deep)	Muscles of the posterior arm and forearm, brachialis
Musculocutaneous	Biceps, coracobrachialis, brachialis
Median	Muscles of the anterior forearm and intrinsic muscles of the hand
Iliohypogastric	Muscles of the abdominal wall
Ilioinguinal	Muscles of the abdominal wall
Femoral	Muscles of the anterior thigh
Obturator	Muscles of the medial thigh
Inferior gluteal	Gluteus maximus
Superior gluteal	Gluteus medias and minimis, tensor fascia lata
Tibial	Muscles of the posterior thigh and leg
Peroneal (common, deep, superficial)	Muscles of the lateral and anterior leg

Table 11.1 Summary of nervous innervations

Primary Disorders of the Muscle System

Muscular Dystrophy

Muscular dystrophy refers to a group of disorders with the common symptom of progressive muscle weakness that leads to atrophy (decrease in muscle size and strength). Healthy muscle tissue is replaced by connective tissue and fat, which are not capable of contraction.

One curious symptom of the most frequent type of muscular dystrophy (Duchenne type) is pseudohypertrophy. Because fat and connective tissue replace healthy muscle tissue, the muscle's external presentation lends an appearance of sound conditioning, even of hypertrophy. In reality, the disease is only a facade for health, the muscles involved are not functional and experience necrosis (tissue death).

Postural complications secondary to muscular dystrophy are not unusual. As the client loses muscle function he or she moves from slightly impaired ambulation to a waddling gait (Jansma & French, 1994) which results when muscles acting on the vertebral column become involved (e.g., erector spinae, abdominal). To compensate the subject may carry the arms more posteriorly and protrude the abdomen. Hence, lordosis is not uncommon among children with muscular dystrophy who are still ambulatory. Inevitably, the ability to ambulate is lost. As more muscles are affected and the disease progresses, control of the trunk is compromised; scoliosis may then develop.

Contractures (shortening of muscles and connective tissue) may preferentially develop in muscles and tendons immediately affected by the disease. Contractures effectively reduce range of motion and flexibility in the affected joints. Loss of range of motion, in turn, significantly affects functional ability and may pose a health risk because pronounced contractures make skin care around the affected joints difficult. Skin lesions are a possibility.

Later, muscles of respiration, such as the intercostals and the diaphragm, experience loss of contractile units. Respiratory capacity is then affected, and the adolescent in more advanced stages of the disease may only have 25% of the normal ventilatory capacity of an able-bodied peer (Wanke et al., 1994). If scoliosis develops, then respiratory movements and ventilatory capacity may be further inhibited (Bar-Or, 1996).

The childhood (*Duchenne*) type of muscular dystrophy is the most severe and most common. It typically manifests during the preschool years and culminates in death, usually in late adolescence or young adulthood. The disease is genetic (carried by a recessive gene) and usually passed from mother to male infant. Mortality is associated with involvement of cardiac muscles and muscles of respiration and opportunistic infections.

Especially in children and adolescents with muscular dystrophy, the TR Specialist may expect to confront an array of psychological complications secondary to the primary diagnosis. The typical teen with muscular dystrophy is immature and difficult to motivate, perhaps as a result of intuition into the dismal long-term prognosis of his disability. He may be somewhat withdrawn as well because of frequent hospitalization, overprotection by parents, or because of lack of sufficient opportunity to interact with peers in a normal manner.

An adult form of muscular dystrophy is known as *facio-scapulo-humeral*, named after the areas preferentially affected. As the name indicates, muscles of the face, shoulder girdle, and arm are most affected. The facio-scapulo-humeral version of the disorder does not advance as quickly as the Duchenne type, and it occurs with about the same frequency in women as in men. Unlike the Duchenne form of the disease, the prognosis for the facio-scapulo-humeral type is reasonably good—progression of impairment is slower and a near normal life span may be anticipated. The patient with facio-scapulo-humeral muscular dystrophy may even experience periods of remission.

Myasthenia Gravis

Myasthenia gravis is sometimes included with muscular dystrophy because of the common symptom of muscle weakness. However, its focal point of dysfunction is at the neuromuscular junction instead of the muscle cell proper. The transmission of an impulse from the neuron to the muscle cell is incomplete. Receptor sites on the muscle cell normally occupied by transmitter substance molecules from the neuron are blocked, probably by an antibody produced by the individual.

Symptoms of myasthenia gravis include muscle weakness, often pronounced in ocular muscles (dropping eyelid) and muscles of mastication (difficulty chewing). Weakened respiratory movements and difficulties with speech may also be evident. Muscles of the extremities, especially at the proximal extent, may exhibit progressive weakness.

Ambulation and movements against more than the usual amount of resistance may be labored as a result of myasthenia gravis. Fatigue progressively develops during a routine day. Movement against resistance or holding one position against gravity is a technique for assessing muscle weakness in patients with myasthenia gravis.

Drug treatment can help manage the impact of myasthenia gravis. The drugs may suppress the autoimmune response or facilitate the transmission of the nerve impulse. For example, some pharmacological agents inhibit an enzyme responsible for clearing the transmitter substance from the neuromuscular junction. In some severe cases, the thymus gland may be removed to suppress the autoimmune response (Busch, Machen, Pichlmeier, Emskotter & Izbicki, 1996).

Guillain-Barre Syndrome

Guillain-Barre syndrome results in a flaccid type of paralysis and a diminished muscle tone in the affected regions of the body. It results from a demyelination process (destruction of the protective covering of the nerve fiber). Some research suggests the disease may be an autoimmune disorder, similar to myasthenia gravis. Facial muscles and muscle of respiration are preferentially affected. Muscles atrophy because of the absence or below normal amount of stimulation from the affected peripheral nerves. If the muscles of respiration are affected the patient may have to spend some time on a respirator for breathing support. The disorder is self-limiting and most patients experience complete recovery.

Frailty

Only about 20% of the U. S. population exercises on any regular basis. The rate of exercise decreases for older segments of the population, although exercise is more important for middle-aged and older adults that for younger people. Exercise is known to retard a host of age-related impairments, chronic conditions, and diseases. Exercise now appears to be so vital that its absence predisposes an identifiable syndrome of low muscle fitness: *frailty*.

Frailty puts the individual at risk for a number of chronic conditions, including osteoporosis, hip fracture, and serious falls. Indirectly, significant muscle weakness resulting from disuse and sedentary lifestyle may lead to heart disease, high blood pressure, and diabetes mellitus.

Progressive deterioration in the ability to perform activities of daily living is especially apparent among older adults (Cutler, 1994). As a result of subpar muscle fitness, the capacity of an individual to meet personal needs and address activities of daily living is severely limited. Frailty can predispose seniors to falls and institutionalization. Muscle weakness has been associated with impaired balance, sit-to-stand movement, and the risk of falls (Kauffmann, 1994).

Frailty and subsequent falls threaten the independence and well-being of elderly persons. In noninstitutionalized elderly adults, between one fourth and one third fall in a year (Tideiksaar, 1994). The situation is even more critical in nursing homes; falls among elderly patients in nursing homes exceeds 60% (Tinetti, 1987). Frail older persons fall more frequently than active ones, about three times more often (Speechley & Tinetti, 1987). Another danger of falls is that they frequently lead to morbidity and even death of older adults (Sattin, 1992; Tideiksaar, 1994). Falls are the cause of 87% of the fractures in the older adults and often begin a sequence of health difficulties that end in death (Baker, O'Neill, Ginsburg & Goohua, 1992).

Research has shown that a leading cause of falls is weakness in the lower extremities (Rosado, Rubenstein, Robbins, Heng, Shulman & Josephson, 1989). Robbins et al. (1989) compared elderly fallers to nonfallers residing in the community and in residential care settings. Older adults with weakness of the lower extremities had three to eight times the risk of falling than those without lower extremity weakness. Therefore, the data suggest that muscle weakness or frailty is a risk factor in subsequent falls.

TR Intervention

General Observations

Considerable controversy exists over how to treat young people with muscular dystrophy. For the most part, disagreement surrounds the usefulness of exercise in cases where progressive muscle weakness is inevitable, and the fear that exercise may even exacerbate the progression of the disease process. Scant research is available on this topic. Those advocating for exercise with muscular dystrophy are generally conservative in their approach, emphasizing maintenance of range of motion, prevention of contractures, and possible enhancement of breathing mechanics as goals.

Although ultimately quality of life should be the focus of any intervention—especially among individuals with muscular dystrophy—a clear interface exists between physical capacity and quality of life. For example, decrements in breathing mechanics and abnormal fatigue seem to be related to perceived quality of life among young people with muscular dystrophy (Ahlstrom, Gunnarsson, Kihlgren, Arvill & Sjoden, 1994). Therefore, improvement in breathing mechanics may logically be expected to be associated with improved quality of life.

Improvement in quality of life is even the objective of some invasive surgical procedures designed to improve breathing. For instance, spinal fusion improved the breathing ability (forced vital capacity) in three of eight subjects with muscular dystrophy, and seven of the subjects improved use of their upper extremities and sitting balance as a result of the procedure (Matsumara, Kang, Nozaki & Takahashi, 1997). Likewise, Bunch and Siegel (1993) reported on the quality of life of subjects subsequent to a surgical procedure that fixed the scapula. They followed up with their patients with facio-scapulo-humeral type muscular dystrophy to learn the effects on quality of life. All but one of the 12 subjects were "pleased" with the impact the procedure had on the quality of life. The improvement in quality of life may have been a function of gains in strength and lifting ability reported by subjects.

Therapy

Therapeutic recreation professionals (e.g., Carter, Van Andel & Robb, 1995; Kraus & Shank, 1992) and adapted physical educators (e.g., Jansma & French, 1994; Sherrill, 1986) recommend exercise for persons with progressive muscular diseases, with qualifications. Typical parameters limit goals for exercise for persons with progressive muscular disorders to the following: improve range of motion, decrease contractures, prevent obesity, improve respiration, prevent posture problems (e.g., lordosis), and improve muscle strength (Carter et al., 1995; Jansma & French, 1994; Levine, 1996; Sherrill, 1986).

However, Bar-Or (1996) maintained that no systematic evidence supports the contention that exercise can improve muscle strength in individuals with Duchenne type muscular dystrophy. The TR practitioner must ask: Do I implement a program of exercise without knowing whether it has reasonable prospects for improving the person's condition? The answer depends on the goal.

A study by Wanke et al. (1994) may provide a measure of guidance. The researchers randomly assigned subjects with Duchenne type muscular dystrophy to treatment and control groups. Subjects in the treatment group completed breathing exercises against resistance for six months. Ten of the subjects in the

treatment group showed significant improvement in respiratory function. Five subjects were dropped from the treatment because they showed no improvement after one month of exercise. The five who were dropped *did not* suffer any adverse effects from exercise. Wanke et al. concluded that respiratory muscle training is beneficial for persons in the early stages of Duchenne type muscular dystrophy.

Consistent with the Wanke et al. (1994) findings, Levine (1996) encouraged mild to moderate exercise for clients with Duchenne type muscular dystrophy to tolerance. Exercise programs designed to accomplish goals other than improvement of muscle strength (e.g., improve respiratory muscle function, improve range of motion, prevent obesity, prevent contractures) seem to hold promise of advancing the person's quality of life through improved function.

Vilonzi and colleagues (1994) discovered that 15 patients with muscular dystrophy and moderate impairment of lung function improved respiratory function following a training program for respiratory muscles. Wanke et al. (1994) motivated subjects by using video games as a reward for proper training. Likely, researchers were encountering some of the psychosocial concomitants of the disease process (e.g., immaturity, lack of motivation) and recreation activities were salient enough to encourage compliance with an unpleasant but beneficial intervention—breathing exercises.

An aquatics-based exercise program may produce good results in the young person with muscular dystrophy, similar to those with skeletal and joint impairments. Jansma and French (1994) and others (Carter et al., 1995; Sherrill, 1986) endorse exercise in the water designed to improve body mechanics (posture) for persons with muscular dystrophy. Water offers a protective and buoyant environment that provides enough resistance for exercise. The TR Specialist should be aware, however, of the possibility of hypothermia among persons with progressive muscular impairments.

Exercise programs for persons with myasthenia gravis hold more potential to improve muscle strength than for clients with muscular dystrophy. Lohi, Lindberg, and Andersen (1993) exposed 11 subjects with mild to moderate myasthenia gravis to a strength training program for muscles acting on the knee and elbow. Subjects demonstrated significant improvement in knee extensor strength following training. Only minimal gains in muscle strength were noted in muscles at the elbow. The researchers attributed the uneven increments in strength to insufficient length of training and workload. Subjects did not complain of pain or discomfort during the exercise protocol. Two subjects reported that they increased their walking distance.

General rules governing physical activity for persons with myasthenia gravis primarily concern fatigue. Persons with myasthenia gravis experience fatigue during a day of routine activity. Therefore, frequent rest periods should be built into therapeutic recreation programs—physically active or sedentary (Carter et al., 1995). Aquatic-based physical activity should include frequent rest because water's buoyancy supports the weight of the body and may help delay the onset of fatigue.

TR Specialists have reason to be optimistic for the prospects of improving the quality of life of the frail older adult. Research on the improvement of strength in older adult subjects has been hopeful. Evans' (1995) review of literature lead him to conclude that progressive resistance training (weight training) is effective in reversing the muscle wasting in the lower extremities of elderly subjects. Fiatarone and associates (1994) used a program of progressive resistance training with frail older adults. Leg strength, walking speed, and stair climbing capability improved markedly. The improvements were most noticeable in the most at-risk (for falls) elderly adults (Fiatarone et al., 1994). Research has demonstrated that older adults are physically trainable (i.e., they can show improvement in muscle function and strength).

Improvements in strength may translate into improvement in quality of life. Researchers have maintained that adequate perceptual-motor ability and muscular strength are essential for functional independence. For instance, one study (Sonn, Frandin & Grimby, 1995) reported that older subjects who were dependent in instrumental activities of daily living were more likely to have slower gait speed, lower grip strength, less knee extensor strength, and disruptions in stair climbing ability.

Lower extremities are not the only muscle groups to benefit from progressive resistance training. Although upper extremity strength has not been as well-studied, the implications of preliminary functional disability studies in this area are clear. For example, some researchers (Ostwald, Snowdon, Rysavy, Keenen & Kane, 1989) have found that loss of manual ability effectively categorized elderly women into different living conditions (nursing home, retirement home, or living in community). Their findings underscored the results of two earlier studies (Williams & Hornberger, 1984; Williams, Hadler & Earp, 1982) showing that independence or dependence in living condition among older adults was associated with manual capability. Balance,

lower extremity strength, and falls all intercorrelate. Balance is a function of lower extremity strength and endurance. Difficulty with balance and equilibrium are risk factors for falls among older adults (Graafmans et al., 1996; Lord & Clark, 1996; Tinetti, Williams & Mayewski, 1986).

The negative side of the encouraging research on progressive resistance training with older adults is that many of the studies have been completed in highly controlled settings, using sophisticated weight training equipment. These conditions are far from customary in practical, field settings encountered by the TR practitioner. Fortunately, recent studies have moved the progressive resistance methodology of the laboratory into the field. For example, Mobily, Mobily, Lane, and Semerjian (1998) found that older adult subjects were able to significantly improve flexibility, coordination, strength, endurance, and agility following an 8-week program of progressive resistance training in a field setting (a senior center). Pending replication studies, TR Specialists should be able to plan and implement progressive resistance training programs for at risk older adults as well as for those interested in preventing deterioration of the muscle system.

Specific Programs and Protocols in Therapy

Mobily and Mobily (1997) have developed a protocol for progressive resistance training for at-risk community-dwelling older adults. To meet field requirements for TR Specialists in the community, the protocol satisfies several essential criteria:

- Capable of improving strength and functional fitness while being low risk (see Mobily, Mobily, Lane & Semerjian, 1998)

- Practical—low cost, simple, and easy to implement

- Systematically administers dosage (i.e., overload or enough resistance to produce an improvement in strength)

- Progressive (i.e., enough latitude for the addition of more resistance as the person becomes stronger)

- Delivered in a nonthreatening manner to make the program enjoyable and accessible

- Provides for assessment and evaluation of participants through the use of a simple and quantifiable battery of functional fitness tests (see Osness et al., 1990) that measure flexibility, coordination, strength, endurance, and agility

Given these criteria, free weights (hand weights) offer a logical alternative to the expensive equipment characteristic of more controlled settings (e.g., exercise testing laboratories, rehabilitation facilities, residential care centers).

The protocol was designed to serve small groups (no more than 8). Participants completed 40-minute exercise sessions 2–3 times per week for a minimum of 8 weeks. Participants began with a 5-minute warm-up, which included a series of stretching exercises, controlled breathing, relaxation techniques, and tai chi separately or in combination. The muscle-conditioning portion of the program ran about 30 minutes. The exercises, specifically selected to improve muscular strength and endurance, employed light weights with resistance ranging from 4 to 15 pounds. The exercises were progressive in nature—older adults moved to increased demand levels on their own, limited by the ability to exercise comfortably with increased resistance. Participants completed the exercises in sets of 3, using 8–10 repetitions per set. Rapid early progression led to completing 3 sets of 15 repetitions each without increasing the resistance. Only after the individual is able to complete three sets of 15 should resistance be increased. Once the weight is increased, the number of repetitions for each of the sets should be dropped down to 8–10. Finally, for five minutes after completion of the muscular conditioning portion of the program, each participant completed cool-down exercises. The cool-down exercises may be identical to those in the warm-up, or the TR Specialist may wish to emphasize relaxation more than flexibility to bring a pleasant closure to the session.

Safety is always a concern when conducting physical interventions with older adults. All such programs carry a small amount of risk; however, the literature suggests that older adults are at risk if they do nothing at all. Piscopo (1979) emphasized safety features such as conducting activities slowly, using light weights, avoiding ballistic movements, warming up, and cooling down. These features were implemented in this program. Careful screening before beginning an exercise program is mandatory. We endorse the use of the revised Physical Activity Readiness Questionnaire (Shephard, Thomas & Weller, 1991). Following preliminary screening, the questionnaire should be reviewed by a consulting physician, who may refer the subject to a family physician for further examination prior to approval. In the implementation of this protocol, and previous

versions of the protocol in the preceding two years, no applicant was told not to participate by a physician.

Leisure Education

Muscular dystrophy syndrome usually does not evidence significant cognitive impairment. Leisure education, therefore, presents some worthwhile possibilities for advancing the quality of life of those with muscular dystrophy. Acquisition of a broad, diversified leisure repertoire through leisure education allows the individual to adapt to the progressive impairment intrinsic to the disease. As the physical capacity to participate in some activities is lost, the person with a large and varied repertoire of leisure activities can accommodate and adapt by drawing on a reservoir of meaningful leisure alternatives.

Muscular dystrophy also tends to advance from proximal to distal in the extremities. This means that the use of the digits and fine motor skill in the hands is preserved early in the disease course. As the disease advances, the person with muscular dystrophy remains a good candidate for activities that capitalize on the fine motor skills that are retained. Accordingly, Levine (1996) suggests that activities such as writing, artistic expression, crafts, journaling, and calligraphy offer potential for educational goals within the leisure education dimension of TR service.

Inevitably, as Carter et al. (1995) remind us, the young adult with muscular dystrophy will become progressively less active because of the loss of effective muscle tissue. Hence, the person will come to rely on less active and perhaps more creative activities for self-expression when transitioning into the late teen years. Unfortunately, because of the relatively rapid progression of the disorder, the typical adolescent with Duchenne type muscular dystrophy is apt to exhibit immaturity in several ways that may obstruct social relationships.

Psychosocial problems are common among persons with Duchenne type muscular dystrophy. Low motivation, withdrawal, and social isolation frequently result from immaturity and lack of confidence (Kraus & Shank, 1992; Sherrill, 1986). Practically speaking, the adolescent with muscular dystrophy may have fewer dates, fewer friends, and greater difficulty leading a meaningful leisure lifestyle as a result (Kraus & Shank, 1992).

Emphasizing the social values of participation (Sherrill, 1986) and interaction with peers (Jansma & French, 1994) appears to be a prudent course to follow. After the physical capacities to participate have eroded, the fortunate teen will still have the meaningful friendships built through leisure socialization. Goals for leisure education should therefore be focused on developing social relationships and acquiring social skills, instead of the technical aspects of the activity at hand. Specific activities become less significant, only serving as a format for the development of social skills and the maturation of the client.

Nevertheless, leisure education efforts may also focus on acquisition of skills and competencies that can carry over for several years of deteriorating muscle function. The dual goals for leisure education for persons with muscular dystrophy suggested here (developing social skills and teaching carry-over leisure skills) urge the use of social-leisure activities or group activities. This may be a challenge given the probable immaturity and lack of self-esteem of the client. These secondary characteristics may discourage interaction and predispose many attempts to plan and implement social interaction programs to failure.

In response, leisure education for persons with muscular dystrophy may need to be more structured because of the immaturity of the participants. The structure may provide just enough regulation to encourage more mature behaviors. For instance, use of a positive reinforcement schedule may minimize socially inappropriate behavior early in leisure socialization, while peer modeling of acceptable behavior may prove to be productive in building social skills later.

Loovis (1985) found some evidence for the use of structure in leisure education. Loovis studied toy preferences in 15 orthopedically impaired children. Among the 15 was a 4-and-a-half-year-old with muscular dystrophy. The findings indicated that the children were able to express clear toy preferences through their actions and play behaviors. However, the researcher also observed that a large percentage of play intervals constituted use of the toys in nondesigned ways. Loovis (1985) concluded that children with orthopedic disabilities needed structured settings for toy play—they need to be taught how to play.

Because the findings are *not* restricted to subjects with muscular dystrophy, applications to leisure education must be regarded as suggestive. Nevertheless, by recommending that positive reinforcement and cueing should be used to help structure leisure education experiences of clients with muscular dystrophy, Loovis has provided some guidance for synthesizing effective educational strategies for children with muscular dystrophy.

Leisure skill instruction is also of use for the *frail older adult* for many of the same reasons noted for the individual with muscular dystrophy. Progressive reduction of muscle size (atrophy) is common to both conditions. But the atrophy experienced by frail older adults (disuse atrophy) is not as predictable in its progression.

The frail client may wish to augment physical capacities and reduce the risk of developing a chronic condition secondary to frailty (e.g., hip fracture). If the person is medically cleared for a program of exercise, the TR Specialist will often learn that the subject evidences considerable apprehension about the program. Much of the anxiety is based on a lack of knowledge about safety, how vigorous the exercise needs to be, and resources available for exercise for elderly citizens. Through leisure education, the older adult learns correct exercise techniques, acquires skills, improves confidence, and decreases apprehension. Apart from the exertion commonly associated with work, formal programs of exercise and physical activity are foreign concepts to many elderly adults. Hence, in the case of exercise for older adults, leisure education may have to precede the use of exercise as a therapeutic modality.

Recreation Participation

The lessons learned through leisure education are expressed in recreation participation. Recreation participation serves as a forum for access to intrinsically valuable activities. Kraus and Shank (1992) maintain that leisure activities allow an accessible means for creative expression when other active outlets erode with the loss of physical capacity. Accordingly, TR Specialists are advised to enrich the present leisure experiences of clients with intrinsically valuable activities. The emphasis should be placed on living for the present and near future (Sherrill, 1986).

Adaptations and accommodations in activities should be delayed as long as possible for persons with muscular dystrophy. Normal and near normal levels of activity should be expected early in the course of muscular dystrophy (Sherrill, 1986). Encouraging the child with muscular dystrophy to participate with nondisabled peers may support perceptions of control, build the foundation for sustained social relationships, and facilitate integrated activities when adaptations become necessary.

Focusing on intrinsically valued leisure activities feeds directly into a second goal of recreation participation for clients with muscular dystrophy: perceived control. Perceived control is a function of intrinsic motivation and perceived freedom. Levine (1996) recommends that the child with muscular dystrophy be encouraged to do as much as possible independently, or with minimal assistance. The TR Specialist can augment perceptions of control by configuring the leisure environment for success and social validation.

As the disease progresses, children know they are no longer able to control as many aspects of their lives as they did in the recent past. Configuring an environment for success assists in directing the child's perceptions in an accurate manner. Participation in freely chosen leisure activities underscores perception of control so long as the TR Specialist reinforces to the client that the choice was his and no one else's. Perception of control is furthered by directing the child's attention toward the cause of the success in the activity—the child himself or herself. Hence, recreation participation becomes a subtle but potent milieu for internal causal attributions and cultivation of perceptions of personal control in circumstances where lack of control over one's life often exists. Other opportunities for success and social validation provided by Levine (1996) include volunteering, advocacy, and participation in support groups, although immaturity may again be an obstacle here.

The situation is somewhat different for adults with the facio-scapulo-humeral type of muscular dystrophy, although personal control remains an issue. Many adults with muscular dystrophy cannot continue to work indefinitely. Insofar as work is a significant source of self-esteem, substitute activities for the support of self-esteem must be found, including recreation and avocational activities and community service through volunteering. Similar recommendations are given for clients with myasthenia gravis (Carter et al., 1995).

Practical Applications

Capitalize on Abilities

Clearly, the prognosis for early onset muscular dystrophy is not optimistic and progressive deterioration is predictable. Nevertheless, the TR Specialist should not overlook the capabilities preserved in the young person with muscular dystrophy: unaffected cognitive ability and preserved use of distal extremities.

Anticipate Adaptations and Accommodations

Adjustments to activities are inevitable because of the progression of Duchenne type muscular dystrophy. Sometimes simple adjustments in rules facilitate participation during early stages of muscular dystrophy. Later, adaptations may be more extensive, including not only rules but also equipment (e.g., Nerf balls), assistive devices (e.g., wheelchairs), and social support.

Focus on Quality of Life

Different methods for improving quality of life may enhance perceptions of control through recreation activities. Augmenting functional abilities through progressive resistance training and other exercise programs also supports quality of life among frail older adults and clients with myasthenia gravis. Building social support and meaningful friendships is also accomplished through recreation activities.

Emphasize Prevention

For frail older adults, persons with myasthenia gravis, and clients with the facioscapulohumeral type of muscular dystrophy, exercise programs translate into prevention of secondary conditions. Hip fracture, deterioration of functional abilities, and loss of independence may be prevented by a vigorous program of recreationally based exercise. Of course, consultation with the person's attending physician is not only a reasonable precaution, but also necessary to determine whether the client is below a threshold of impairment that may respond to exercise.

Chapter Summary

This chapter examined the muscular system and addressed the following key concepts:

- Muscle is a tissue, organ, and system with primary responsibility for movement.

- A muscle produces movement by shortening (contracting) and drawing one bone closer to another.

- Although pathology is often manifested as muscle dysfunction, there are few disorders intrinsic to the muscle system.

- Cautious use of respiratory exercises with recreational reinforcers may improve quality of life among children and adolescents with muscular dystrophy.

- Strength training with light weights has proven to be very effective with frail older adults.

- Psychosocial outcomes should be emphasized among children and adolescents with muscular dystrophy.

References

Ahlstrom, G., Gunnarsson, L. G., Kihlgren, A., Arvill, A., and Sjoden, P. O. (1994). Respiratory function, electrocardiography and quality of life in individuals with muscular dystrophy. *Chest, 106,* 173–179.

Baker, S. D., O'Neill, B., Ginsburg, M. J., and Goohua, L. (1992). *The injury fact book* (2nd ed.). New York, NY: Oxford University Press.

Bar-Or, O. (1996). Role of exercise in the assessment and management of neuromuscular disease in children. *Medicine and Science in Sports and Exercise, 28,* 421–427.

Bunch, W. H. and Siegel, I. M. (1993). Scapulothoracic arthrodesis in facioscapulohumeral muscular dystrophy. Review of seventeen procedures with three to twenty-one-year follow-up. *Journal of Bone & Joint Surgery—American Volume, 75,* 372–376.

Busch, C., Machen, A., Pichlmeier, U., Emskotter, T., and Izbicki, J. R. (1996). Long-term outcome and quality of life after thymectomy for myasthenia gravis. *Annals of Surgery, 224,* 225–232.

Carter, M. J., Van Andel, G. E., and Robb, G. M. (1995). *Therapeutic Recreation: A practical approach* (2nd ed.). Prospect Heights, IL: Waveland.

Cutler, N. E. (1994). Functional limitations and the need for personal care. In B. R. Bonder and M. B. Wagner (Eds.), *Functional performance in older adults* (pp. 210–222). Philadelphia, PA: F. A. Davis Co.

Evans, W. J. (1995). Exercise, nutrition, and aging. *Clinics in Geriatric Medicine. 11,* 725–734.

Fiatarone, M. A., O'Neill, E. F., Ryan, N. D., Clements, K. M., Solares, G. R., Nelson, M. E., Roberts, S. B., Kehayias, J. J., Lipsitz, L. A., and Evans, W. J. (1994). Exercise training and nutritional supplementation for physical frailty in very elderly people. *New England Journal of Medicine, 330,* 1769–1775.

Graafmans, W. C., Ooms, M. E., Hofstee, H. M., Bezemer, P. D., Bouter, L. M., and Lips, P. (1996). Falls in the elderly: A prospective study of risk factor and risk profiles. *American Journal of Epidemiology, 143,* 1129–1136.

Jansma, P. and French, R. (1994). *Special Physical Education: Physical activity, sports, and recreation.* Englewood Cliffs, NJ: Prentice-Hall.

Kauffmann, T. (1994). Functional performance in older adults. In B. R. Bonder and M. B. Wagner (Eds.), *Functional performance in older adults* (pp. 42–61). Philadelphia, PA: F. A. Davis, Co.

Kraus, R. and Shank, J. (1992). *Therapeutic Recreation Service: Principles and practices* (4th ed.). Dubuque, IA: Brown.

Levine, G. R. (1996). Neuromuscular disorders. In D. R. Austin and M. E. Crawford (Eds.), *Therapeutic Recreation: An introduction* (2nd ed., pp. 184–212). Boston, MA: Allyn & Bacon.

Lohi, E., Lindberg, C., and Andersen, O. (1993). Physical training effects in myasthenia gravis. *Archives of Physical Medicine & Rehabilitation, 74*, 1178–1180.

Loovis, E. M. (1985). Evaluation of toy preference and associated movement behaviors of preschool orthopedically handicapped children. *Adapted Physical Quarterly, 2*, 117–126.

Lord S. R. and Clark, R. D. (1996). Simple physiological and clinical tests for accurate prediction of falling in older people. *Gerontology, 42*, 199–203.

Matsumara, T., Kang, J., Nozaki, S., and Takahashi, M. P. (1997). The effects of spinal fusion on respiratory function and quality of life in Duchenne muscular dystrophy. *Rinsho Shinkeigaku—Clinical Neurology, 37*, 87–92.

Mobily, K. E. and Mobily, P. R. (1997). Reliability of the 60+ functional fitness test battery for older adults. *Journal of Aging an Physical Activity, 5*, 150–162.

Mobily, K. E., Mobily, P. R., Lane, B. K., and Semerjian, T. Z. (1998). Using progressive resistance training as an intervention with older adults. *Therapeutic Recreation Journal, 32*, 42–53.

Osness, W. H., Adrian, M., Clark, B., Hoeger, W., Raab, D., and Wiswell, R. (1990). *Functional fitness assessment for adults over 60 years* (2nd ed.). Dubuque, IA: Kendall/Hunt.

Ostwald, S. K., Snowdon, D. A., Rysavy, S., Keenen, N. L., and Kane, R. L. (1989). Manual dexterity as a correlate of dependency in the elderly. *Journal of the American Geriatrics Society, 37*, 963–969.

Piscopo, J. (1979). Indications and contraindications of exercise and activity for older persons. *Journal of Physical Education and Recreation, 50*, 31–34.

Robbins, A. S., Rubenstein, L. Z., Josephson, K. R., Shulman, B. L., Osterweil, D., and Fine, G. (1989). Predictors of falls among elderly people. *Archives of Internal Medicine, 149*, 1628–1633.

Rosado, S. A., Rubenstein, L. Z., Robbins, A. S., Heng, M. K., Shulman, R. L., and Josephson, K. R. (1989). The value of halter monitoring in evaluating the elderly patient who falls. *Journal of the American Geriatric Society, 37*, 430–434.

Sattin, R. W. (1992). Falls among older persons: A public health perspective. *Annual Review of Public Health, 13*, 489-508.

Shephard, R. J., Thomas, S., and Weller, I. (1991). The Canadian Home Fitness Test: 1991 update. *Sports Medicine, 1*, 359.

Sherrill, C. (1986). *Adapted physical education and recreation: A multidisciplinary approach*. Dubuque, IA: Brown.

Sonn, U., Frandin, K., and Grimby, G. (1995).Instrumental activities of daily living related to impairments and functional limitations in 70-year-olds and changes between 70 and 76 years of age. *Scandinavian Journal of Rehabilitation Medicine, 27*, 119–128.

Speechley, M. and Tinetti, M. (1987). Falls and injury in frail and vigorous community elderly persons. *Journal of the American Geriatric Society, 39*, 46–52.

Tideiksaar, R. (1994). Falls. In B. R. Bonder and M. B. Wagner (Eds.), *Functional performance in older adults* (pp. 224–239). Philadelphia, PA: F. A. Davis, Co.

Tinetti, M. E. (1987). Factors associated with serious injury during falls by ambulatory nursing home residents. *Journal of the American Geriatric Society, 35*, 644–648.

Tinetti, M. E., Williams, T. F., and Mayewski, R. (1986). Fall risk index for elderly patients based on number of chronic disabilities. *American Journal of Medicine, 80*, 429–434.

Tseng, B. S., Marsh, D. R., Hamilton, M. T., and Booth, F. W. (1995). Strength and aerobic training attenuate muscle wasting and improve resistance to the development of disability with aging. *Journals of Gerontology*. Series A, Biological Sciences & Medical Sciences, *50*, 113–119.

Vilonzi, D., Bar-Yishay, E., Gur, I., Shapira, Y., Meyer, S., and Godfrey, S. (1994). Computerized respiratory muscle training in children with Duchenne muscular dystrophy. *Neuromuscular Disorders*, *4*, 249–255.

Wanke, T., Toifl, K., Merkle, M., Formanek, D., Lahrmann, H., and Zwick, H. (1994). Inspiratory muscle training in patients with Duchenne muscular dystrophy. *Chest*, *105*, 475–482.

Williams, M. E., Hadler, N. M., and Earp, J. L. (1982). Manual ability as a marker of dependency in geriatric women. *Journal of Chronic Diseases*, *35*, 115–122.

Williams, M. E. and Hornberger, J. C. (1984). A quantitative method of identifying older persons at risk for increasing long term care services. *Journal of Chronic Diseases*, *37*, 705–711.

CHAPTER 12
NERVOUS SYSTEM

Nervous impulses communicate information about two things: *sensory information* to the spinal cord and brain about the internal or external environment or *motor information* that directs muscles to contract. Sensory information and motor information are integrated in the brain. We think about whether we want to make a response relative to changes in our environment. Some motor responses, however, occur at a subconscious or reflex level as well.

A *pathway* is the route followed by a nerve impulse from origin to its final destination. Scientists have discovered that neurological pathways are organized according to specific modalities. Hence, we can speak of pathways for pain, temperature, touch, voluntary motor activity, and posture adjustments. Knowledge of pathways is useful for diagnostic purposes, for prediction and explanation of symptoms, and for planning rehabilitation efforts when people experience trauma that interrupts one or more of the pathways. Sensory pathways begin with a specific kind of receptor and end either in the cerebrum or the cerebellum. Motor pathways begin in the cerebral cortex or the brainstem and end at the neuromuscular junction, where the muscle is stimulated by a peripheral nerve.

Nervous tissue is specialized to transmit an electrical impulse determined by the concentration of sodium and potassium ions on either side of a nerve cell membrane. The exchange of ions causes a reversal in the polarity (electrical charge) of the nerve cell membrane—this is known as a nerve impulse. While this brief and simplified physiological description of nervous activity is technically correct, it is more useful to think of a nerve impulse as information traveling from one point or structure to another. The primary unit in this communication network is the nerve cell, or neuron.

Many neurological impairments result from an interruption in the communication pathway (e.g., spinal cord injury). Most of the limitations that result from severing the spinal cord by way of a traumatic lesion are not because nerve cells are destroyed. Rather, the paraplegia or quadriplegia that often result are attributable to the interrupted communication between the brain and the spinal cord. The brain can no longer tell the spinal cord what to do.

This chapter describes the composition of nervous tissue and the organization of the nervous system. Basic anatomy of the nervous system and primary disorders that affect nerves follow. Specific protocols for head injuries and spinal cord injuries are next. Finally, the chapter examines leisure education and recreation participation with a focus on persons with head injuries, spinal cord injuries, and cerebral palsy.

Nervous Tissue Composition

All neurons share several features. A central area containing the nucleus and other organelles (e.g., mitochondria) is called the perikaryon or cell body. Processes (projections) extend from the cell body and can be labeled according to whether they bring the nerve impulse toward the cell body (*dendrite*) or take the nerve impulse away from the cell body (*axon*). One common type of neuron is illustrated in **Figure 12.1**, the *multipolar neuron*. Many processes are labeled as dendrites, and only one is labeled as an axon. All neurons have at least one dendrite and one axon; some have more.

The processes that extend out from the cell body allow the neuron to communicate with muscle cells

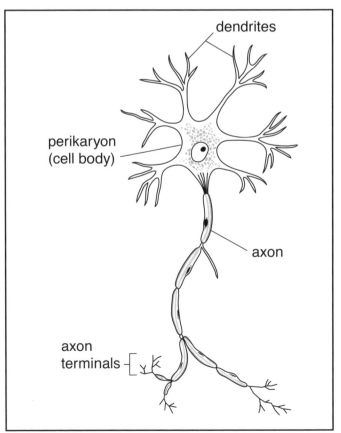

Figure 12.1 Multipolar neuron

through the neuromuscular junction. Nerve cells also communicate with one another by way of a synapse, a structure similar to a neuromuscular junction. A *synapse* may be understood in the same way as the neuromuscular junction, as the location where a chemical message is sent from one neuron to a second neuron. Like the neuromuscular junction, a transmitter substance conveys the chemical message. Although the actual transmitter substance may vary, the idea is the same: transmission of an impulse from one structure to another.

Also apparent in Figure 12.1 is a fatty substance that coats the axon at regular intervals. This substance (*myelin*) significantly increases the conduction velocity of a myelinated nerve cell process. Either an axon or a dendrite may be myelinated, although only the axon is myelinated in Figure 12.1. The pattern of myelination lends a distinct pattern of coloration to nervous tissue that can be distinguished with the naked eye. White matter consists of myelinated nerve cell processes—axons and dendrites. Gray matter is made up of unmyelinated axons and dendrites and cell bodies of neurons that are also unmyelinated. A particular language is then used to talk about gray matter and white matter in nervous tissue, depending on where it is located.

Organization of the Nervous System

Central Nervous System and Peripheral Nervous System

The gray and white matter of the nervous system is organized according to location. All nervous tissue housed inside of the vertebral column and skull is considered part of *the central nervous system* (CNS) and all nervous tissue outside of the vertebral column and skull is considered part of the *peripheral nervous system* (PNS). White matter is named according to its location in the CNS or PNS. White matter in the PNS is called a *nerve* and in the CNS it is known as a *tract*. Likewise, gray matter is known as a *ganglion* in the PNS and called a *nucleus* in the CNS.

Sensory and Motor Portions of the Nervous System

The nervous system can also be understood from another point of view: whether the information is

sensory or motor. **Figure 12.2** illustrates the four functional divisions of the nervous system. The division of the nervous system according to function depends on where the sensory information is coming from or where the motor information is going. Sensory information can arrive at the CNS from one of two areas—the external environment or the internal environment. Sensory information about the external environment (e.g., pain in the fingertip from a burn) is classified as *somatic sensory*, whereas information about the internal environment (e.g., pain in the small intestines from an ulcer) is categorized as *visceral sensory*. (In some texts the term "afferent" may be used in place of "sensory.") Similarly, motor information can be classified according to its destination—either to voluntary (skeletal) muscle or involuntary (smooth or cardiac) muscle. If the motor impulse travels to skeletal muscle, it is classified as *somatic motor*. (In some texts the term "efferent" may be used in place of "motor.") If the information is going to involuntary muscle, it belongs to the *visceral motor* classification.

As mentioned previously, somatic motors are specific to skeletal muscle and visceral motors are specific to involuntary muscle. One of the distinguishing features of the visceral motor classification is that it uses two neurons. The visceral motor group also includes *ganglia*, clusters of nerve cell bodies that aggregate together. Ganglia of the visceral motor portion of the nervous system form from aggregations of the second cell bodies in the two-neuron sequence of innervation.

Somatic motors and visceral motors also have different effects on muscle. In the somatic motors, the effect is always excitation—moving the skeletal muscle toward contraction. In the visceral motors, the effect may be either excitatory or inhibitory. For example, some visceral motors can stimulate the heart to beat faster, while innervation from other visceral motors can cause the heart to beat more slowly.

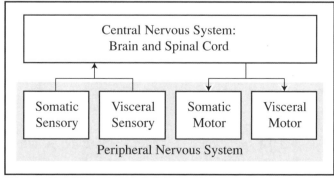

Figure 12.2 Functional divisions of the nervous system

Autonomic Nervous System

Visceral motors *only* are also given another name: the *autonomic nervous system* (ANS). The ANS is divided according to the location of the first cell body in the two-neuron sequence and the effect produced. The *sympathetic division* of the ANS is located in the thoracic and lumbar regions of the spinal cord; it is sometimes called the *thoraco-lumbar division* of the ANS. The *parasympathetic division* of the ANS is found as part of some cranial nerves in the brain and the sacral portion of the spinal cord; it is sometimes called the *cranio-sacral division* of the ANS.

Function is another way to distinguish the sympathetic and parasympathetic divisions of the ANS. The sympathetic serves to mobilize the body's resources to meet emergency situations (sometimes called the "fight or flight" response). The parasympathetic division is responsible for more routine, day-to-day activities and acts to conserve energy. An example of a sympathetic effect is to increase the heart rate; the parasympathetic effect would be to slow down the heart rate. Likewise, the parasympathetic division helps digest food, whereas the sympathetic effect would slow digestion.

The ANS accomplishes its reciprocal effects by means of dual innervation. As a rule, organs containing smooth or cardiac muscle receive fibers (axons) from both divisions that allow for the response that best suits the particular circumstances. The functions of the ANS are automated, not subject to voluntary control and not usually attended to by conscious thought. This is a remarkable adaptive quality of the human nervous system and frees the brain to concentrate on solving problems rather than worrying about, for example, the moment-to-moment adjustments necessary for the digestion of food.

Functions of the Nervous System

Neurons are very specialized in the propagation of impulses. If this capacity for transmitting impulses is broken into finer parts, then nervous tissue has four important functions:

1. Provide information about the internal and external environments—everything from temperature to vision.
2. Control and regulate internal body functions, such as ventilation (breathing), blood pressure, and acid-base balance. These vital activities operate within a narrow range of acceptability and allow little margin for error. This particular function is taken care of for us at a largely subconscious level.
3. Think. Although no one knows with certainty what this means at a physiological level, we all count on the results and depend upon predictable, logical, and rational human activity predicated on thoughtfulness. We are surprised and offended by thoughtless behavior. At the psychological level thought means that new, sensory information must be integrated with old, remembered information and learned data to decide on whether a motor response is required.
4. Regulate instinctual behaviors—everything from thirst and hunger to survival emotions and sex drive. These behaviors are not a distinguishing feature of the human nervous system, but necessary to life. It is the function the human nervous system shares with the nervous systems of lower species.

Normal Development

The nervous system begins to form within 3 weeks of conception. It begins as a neural plate derived from one of the three basic layers of the embryo—the *ectoderm*. The plate soon deepens into a neural fold and eventually becomes a tube, deep to the outer layer of skin—the *epidermis*. The neural tube develops into the central nervous system. The caudal (inferior) portion becomes the spinal cord. If the neural tube fails to close completely at its caudal extent, then the myelomeningocele form of spina bifida is present at birth. The central canal seen in a cross section of the spinal cord in the normal adult (see **Figure 12.3**, p. 218) is all that remains of the space in the middle of the neural tube of the embryo and fetus.

The brain is a result of the swelling of different portions of the cranial (superior) part of the neural tube. The peripheral nervous system (nerves and ganglia) forms from the neural crest, a smaller, separate portion of the neural tube. Most cranial and peripheral nerves are formed from the cells that comprise the neural crest.

The nervous system is fully differentiated at the time of birth. As with the muscle system, a person is born with all the nerve cells he or she will ever have. However, nerve tissue will continue to grow in size (i.e., the brain gets larger) and integrate functions during the developmental years.

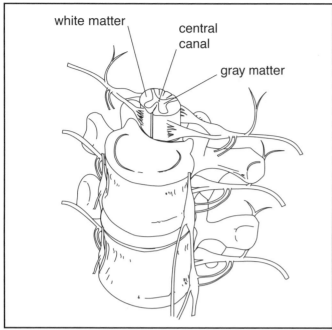
Figure 12.3 Cross-section of the spinal cord

Gross Anatomy of the Nervous System

Brain

The brain is divided into four different parts: brainstem, diencephalon, cerebrum, and cerebellum. The brainstem, diencephalon, and cerebellum operate at the subconscious level, whereas the cerebrum operates as the conscious part of the brain. The majority of the activities of the brain occur at a subconscious level. This frees the cerebrum to concentrate on more complex cognitive operations, such as solving problems, learning, and complex motor activities. The subconscious parts of the brain take care of a lot of the tedious details, from regulation of blood pressure to coordination of motor activities such as speaking, writing, and typing. All of these activities are complex, serial tasks (witness the difficulty a child has learning to walk, talk, or write for the first time), but are quite automated in the normal human adult.

Brainstem

The brainstem is the continuation of the spinal cord as it enters the skull (see **Figures 12.4** and **12.5**). It is composed of the three parts: the inferior medulla oblongata, the intermediate pons, and the superior cephalic midbrain. Each part of the brainstem shares several subconscious tasks and contains centers for vital functions, including regulation of blood pressure, ventilation, and heart rate. All parts of the brainstem contain the same tracts that are found in the spinal cord. This continuation of tracts allows for communication between the spinal cord and different parts of the brain.

The brainstem also contains nuclei (clusters of gray matter in the CNS) that give rise to a number of cranial nerves. (The functions and locations of the cranial nerves are presented as part of the spinal cord because they function as spinal nerves for the most part.) Other nuclei in the brainstem give rise to motor tracts that control neurons in the anterior gray horns of the spinal cord. Motor tracts that originate in the brainstem nuclei operate at the subconscious level. For instance, one important tract is the rubro-spinal tract, responsible for posture and muscle tone in skeletal muscles. The red nuclei of the midbrain give off axons that coalesce to form this tract in the brainstem and eventually in the lateral funiculi of the spinal cord.

Diencephalon

At the superior extent of the brainstem lies the diencephalon. The diencephalon is comprised of two parts: the thalamus and the hypothalamus (see **Figure 12.5**). The *thalamus* is a cluster of nuclei that serve as a sensory relay station. The sensory tracts that have traversed the spinal cord and the brainstem synapse on

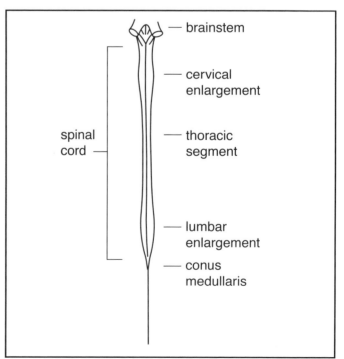
Figure 12.4 Spinal cord and brainstem

the nuclei of the thalamus. Thalamic nuclei send axons to the cerebrum where the sensory impulses can be perceived at a conscious level. Like the tracts and the brainstem, the thalamus is part of an information pathway for sensory modalities (e.g., pressure, touch, pain, temperature, joint sense).

The *hypothalamus* controls the ANS, the system that stimulates involuntary muscle and glands. The hypothalamus also controls several aspects of automated activities, including feeding cycles, sleep cycles, thirst cycles, and temperature regulation. By way of a stalk of tissue known as the pituitary stalk (infundibulum) the hypothalamus controls many of activities of the endocrine system through connection with the master endocrine gland—the pituitary gland. (The relationship between the hypothalamus and the pituitary gland is discussed further in Chapter 15, Visceral Systems.)

Cerebrum

By way of analogy, the cerebrum represents the cap of a mushroom whose stalk is composed of the brainstem and the diencephalon. The cerebrum is the most advanced part of the brain—the anatomical feature that most distinguishes the human mind from that of lower species. Like other parts of the nervous system, the cerebrum is made up of gray matter and white matter. The difference between the arrangement of white and gray matter in the cerebrum is that the gray matter is located in the outer shell of the cerebrum—the cerebral cortex. The white matter is in an intermediate position and another aggregation of gray matter (the basal nuclei) is found in the deepest layer of the cerebrum.

(Neither the white matter nor the deep gray matter of the cerebrum is shown in Figure 12.5.)

The cortex is divided into four lobes: temporal, parietal, occipital, and frontal (see Figure 12.5). Temporal, parietal, and occipital lobes receive and interpret sensory impulses. The frontal lobe initiates voluntary motor commands. Axons from the cortex of the frontal lobe become motor tracts that descend through the brainstem and spinal cord to transmit volitional motor commands to the anterior horn of the spinal cord. The anterior horn then sends axons into the periphery through spinal nerves that innervate muscles and cause willful movement. The neurons of the anterior horn of the spinal cord are subject to the control of the tracts that carry motor commands from the frontal lobe of the cerebral cortex, as well as other areas of the brain that operate at the subconscious level (e.g., brainstem).

As with the balance of the CNS, the cerebrum is anatomically symmetrical, with two identical cerebral hemispheres (right and left). The lobes of the cerebral cortex have different functions. The frontal lobe controls most voluntary, conscious, motor activity through its descending motor tracts. The occipital lobe receives light information from the specialized receptor for light, the retina at the posterior extent of the eye. The parietal lobe receives and interprets information for all other sensory modalities (e.g., pain, temperature, taste) except hearing. The temporal lobe is dedicated to audition; however, the closely related function of language is found only on the left hemisphere. This has important implications for the symptoms associated with lesions to the left versus right temporal lobe. For example, a person who suffers a stroke to the left temporal lobe will likely have difficulty with language.

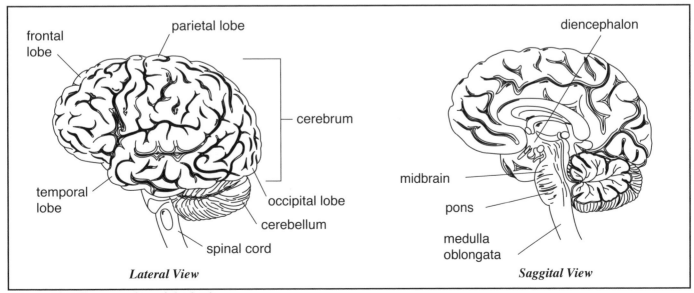

Figure 12.5 Cross-section of the brain

The neuron cell bodies that comprise the cortex process information, including reception of sensations, perceptions and understanding of sensations, and decisions about whether to respond to the stimuli and how to respond to the stimuli. Each lobe of the cortex may connect with the opposite cerebral hemisphere, another part of the brain altogether, or another lobe on the same cerebral hemisphere by way of myelinated axons that comprise the intermediate white matter of the cerebrum.

For instance, the temporal lobe receives the sound information associated with a question asked in the classroom from the specialized receptor for sound in the inner ear. Auditory information is sent to the temporal lobe where we hear the sound and understand the sound information (language). If one particular student wishes to verbalize an answer to the question, then the temporal lobe must communicate with the frontal lobe where the motor commands necessary for a verbal response are organized. Axons carrying motor commands from the frontal lobe travel by way of tracts to synapse on neurons in the anterior gray horns in the cervical levels of the spinal cord. Axons from these neurons exit the spinal cord by way of spinal nerves and eventually stimulate the muscles of speech. An answer to the question is then articulated.

Although the cerebral hemispheres are anatomically symmetrical, functional distinctions exist between the two hemispheres. The left hemisphere, the so-called dominant hemisphere, controls language. Analytical ability tends to reside on the dominant hemisphere too. Creativity, aesthetic ability, perceptual ability, and spatial understanding are located on the right hemisphere, the nondominant hemisphere. Cerebral control of the body is contralateral. Therefore, when the cerebrum is damaged by trauma of some kind, symptoms tend to manifest on the opposite side of the body.

Deep to the superficial cortex and the intermediate white matter is another aggregation of gray matter known as the basal nuclei (not shown in Figure 12.6). The *basal nuclei* operate at a subconscious level and control automated movements of the trunk (posture), hip and shoulder girdles, and proximal limb muscle groups. The basal nuclei also appear to play a role in the adjustment of muscle tone necessary for intentional movements. More generally, the basal nuclei regulate involuntary, stereotyped (well-learned and automated) movements (e.g., alternately swinging the arms during walking).

Cerebellum

Motor coordination is an automated neurological activity. We do not have to occupy conscious thought with the order in which to contract muscles, the force of the each contraction, and its duration. These tasks are performed at the subconscious level by the cerebellum (see Figure 12.5). Initiation of motor actions begin elsewhere (e.g., cerebral cortex, nuclei in the brainstem), but are coordinated by the cerebellum.

Through its connections with the brainstem, the cerebellum receives moment to moment joint sense information (proprioception) so that contractions may be adjusted accordingly. The proprioceptive information also allows the cerebellum to make subtle posture adjustments by influencing muscle tone through its connections with the brainstem. *Proprioception* maintains balance and correct posture. Accordingly, the cerebellum also plays a role in balance and posture adjustments.

The cerebellum is organized in a manner similar to the cerebrum, with a thinner cortex of gray matter superficial to white matter. The neurons found in the cerebellum are not the same as those found in the cerebral cortex. Cerebellar control of the body is ipsilateral (same-sided) in contrast to the contralateral control exerted by the cerebrum.

Spinal Cord

The *spinal cord* transmits information to and from the brain and controls spinal reflexes. The spinal cord neither thinks nor controls volitional activity on its own. The brain regulates most of the activities of the spinal cord with the exception of spinal reflexes.

The gross anatomy of the spinal cord is illustrated in Figure 12.4. The spinal cord is shaped like a long hourglass with a tapered tail (the *conus medullaris*). Closer to the brain is an area of greater width called the *cervical enlargement*. Likewise, there is another wider portion in the lower back region called the *lumbar enlargement*. The enlargements are explained by the presence of the extra neurons necessary for innervation of the muscles of the upper and lower extremities. Less muscle mass occupies the trunk region, and hence the spinal cord is narrower in the thoracic segment.

A typical cross section of the spinal cord is presented in Figure 12.3. Although each level of the spinal cord may vary from this pattern somewhat, the fundamental structure of the spinal cord is the same throughout its entire length. A characteristic H-shaped pattern of gray matter is found in the central portion of the spinal cord. In the middle of the gray matter is a central canal. The gray matter has four horns or extensions from the crossbar of the H-shape. The two posterior horns are generally thought to be sensory in function, whereas the two anterior horns are primarily motor. Cell bodies and unmyelinated nerve fibers dominate the infrastructure of the gray matter of the spinal cord.

Large areas of white matter surround the central gray matter of the spinal cord. As with all white matter, that of the spinal cord contains myelinated axons and dendrites. The white matter of the spinal cord is organized into three distinct areas (*funiculi*): anterior funiculus, posterior funiculus, and lateral funiculus. The funiculi contain *tracts*, columns of axons traveling to the brain or coming down from the brain. The tracts represent the functional connection between the brain and the spinal cord. When the tracts are interrupted through injury, the communication between the spinal cord and the brain is interrupted. Therefore, tracts are absolutely essential for normal, voluntary control of the body.

Spinal Nerves

Spinal nerves form peripheral nerves. They represent access for sensory impulses from receptors back to the spinal cord and exit for motor impulses from the spinal cord to muscles. Each level of the spinal cord gives off a variable number of spinal nerves. A total of 31 pairs of spinal nerves can be identified: 8 cervical, 12 thoracic, 5 lumbar, 5 sacral, and 1 coccygeal.

Cranial Nerves

Cranial nerves are similar to spinal nerves in function but not in location. Although not as uniform in function as spinal nerves, the 12 pairs of cranial nerves bring sensory impulses back to the CNS and take motor commands to muscles. Cranial nerves are associated with different parts of the brain and brainstem and the structures they innervate are usually in and around the face. Cranial nerves I and II are associated with the cerebrum. Numbers III and IV originate in the midbrain part of the brainstem. Numbers V–VIII arise in the pons, the second part of the brainstem. Finally, cranial nerves VIII through XII belong to the part of the brainstem closet to the spinal cord, the medulla oblongata. A summary of the names and functions for each of the cranial nerves is found in **Table 12.1** (p. 222). Note that cranial nerve number VIII is listed for both the medulla oblongata and the pons because

portions of the nerve are found in both portions of the brainstem.

Spinal Reflexes

Reflexes are automated responses to specific stimuli. Spinal reflexes do not require involvement of the brain; no conscious thought is necessary. The components of a spinal reflex are always the same, regardless of the specific stimulus or response. The five components necessary for any spinal reflex include a receptor, a sensory neuron, an association neuron, a motor neuron, and an effector (see **Figure 12.6**, p. 223). In the case of the withdrawal reflex, the receptor is a pain receptor. The sensory neuron transmits the pain information back to the spinal cord where the association neuron passes the impulse on to the motor neuron. The motor neuron is stimulated to send an impulse to the effector, in this case a skeletal muscle. The net effect is contraction of the muscle to remove the hand from the painful stimulus (e.g., a flame). That is why this particular spinal reflex is called a "withdrawal" reflex.

Although the five components are always the same, subtle variations in reflexes are specific to the receptor and the effector. The receptor may change according to the stimulus (e.g., a pain receptor does not respond to cold), and the effector may be different (e.g., a gland, smooth muscle, or cardiac muscle). The spinal cord will execute reflexes as long as the stimulus is sufficient to provoke the response, with or without involvement of the brain. This fact has vital implications for the symptoms associated with spinal cord and injury and some injuries to the brain. For example, spinal reflexes continue even after the spinal cord is severed. Below the level of damage, this can lead to spacisity.

In sum, the spinal cord represents the interface between the periphery and the brain. Sensory axons bring information from receptors through peripheral nerves to the spinal cord. Motor axons take impulses from the spinal cord to muscles to stimulate contraction. By way of sensory tracts, the spinal cord informs the brain of important environmental events. Through motor tracts the brain exerts control over the spinal cord, especially neurons in the anterior gray horn, the motor portion of the gray matter of the spinal cord. Through the motor tracts, the brain can preferentially control motor impulses from the spinal cord to muscles. The tracts of the spinal cord then form a crucial part of a pathway for voluntary motor activity from the brain to the muscles. In the normal human the brain is in control of the spinal cord through the tracts found in the white matter of the spinal cord.

Peripheral Nerves

Peripheral nerves (or simply "nerves") are formed from axons and dendrites. Nerves supply motor innervation to muscles for contraction and transmit sensory information back to the CNS for processing by the spinal cord and brain. Nerves are derived from spinal nerves associated with each level of the spinal cord. Peripheral nerves are considered mixed nerves in the sense that most contain axons from both sensory and motor portions of the nervous system. This means that when nerves are injured, usually the person experiences both sensory and motor losses, though to a lesser extent than with an injury to the CNS.

Examples of peripheral nerves include all of the nerves that supply motor innervation to the muscles. All of these nerves contain both sensory and motor components, even though the muscle system chapter addressed only the motor component.

Primary Disorders of the Nervous System

Overview of Primary Disorders

Figure 12.7 (p. 224) represents some of the primary disorders of the nervous system, demonstrating the relationships between muscles, receptors, peripheral nerves, the spinal cord, and the brain. The model illustrates the principles of communication and control in the neuromuscular systems. Control is exerted by communication between structures. Communication is attained by axons within nerves and tracts. The principles of control are as follows:

- Brain controls the spinal cord by way of motor tracts
- Spinal cord controls the muscle system by way of nerves

Origin	Cranial Nerve	Function
Cerebrum	I. Olfactory	Smell
	II. Optic	Vision
Midbrain	III. Oculomotor	Motor innervation to eye muscles
	IV. Trochlear	Motor innervation to eye muscles
Pons	V. Trigeminal	Motor muscles for chewing; sensory to front of head
	VI. Abducens	Motor innervation to eye muscles
	VII. Facial	Motor to facial muscles of expression (e.g., smiling); sense of taste; stimulates salivation and crying
Pons and Medulla Oblongata	VIII. Vestibulo-cochlear	Hearing and balance
Medulla Oblongata	IX. Glosso-pharyngeal	Swallowing, taste, and salivation; monitors blood pressure
	X. Vagus	Swallowing, taste, and speech; provides autonomic innervation to most of the viscera in the ventral body cavity
	XI. Accessory	Motor innervation to the trapezius and sternocliedo-mastoid muscles
	XII. Hypoglossal	Motor innervation to the tongue

Table 12.1 Summary of cranial nerves

- Receptors transmit sensory information to the spinal cord by way of nerves
- Spinal cord communicates the sensory information to the brain by way of sensory tracts

Understanding this schematic should assist the student in appreciating the implications of various lesions placed between any two structures. The disorders used to demonstrate resulting symptoms are not exhaustive, but representative of lesions that produce predictable patterns of symptoms.

Muscular dystrophy (#1 in Figure 12.7) produces muscle weakness without neurological involvement. Damage to the nervous system does not cause muscular dystrophy. The focal point of *myasthenia gravis* (#2 in Figure 12.7) is the neuromuscular junction. The action of the transmitter substance is blocked and the result is again muscular weakness, but no nerve structures are involved. Frequently the result of a traumatic lesion, such as a gunshot, knife wound, or an accident that causes a significant laceration, *peripheral nerve injury* (#3 in Figure 12.7) is the first of the disorders that involves nervous tissue. When the axons in the nerve are severed, a very specific pattern of symptoms (known as the signs of a lower motor neuron lesion) manifests: flaccid paralysis, absent tendon reflex, and progressive atrophy.

Flaccid paralysis is caused by depriving the muscle or muscles innervated of motor stimulation. A *tendon reflex* (also known as a stretch reflex) occurs when a physician taps on your patellar tendon (at the knee) and you exhibit a slight knee jerk. Physicians try to elicit

tendon reflexes during physical assessment to determine the integrity of the pathway from muscle to spinal cord and back. If a slight knee jerk is not elicited, then the physician has reason to suspect damage to one or more of the structures involved in a spinal reflex. When a peripheral nerve is severed, both sensory and motor axons are cut. This means that the stretch information does not reach the spinal cord, nor are cut motor axons capable of responding to the stretch stimulus. If dennervation is prolonged, then the muscle(s) affected will decrease in size and strength. *Atrophy* is the term we introduced in the muscle system chapter, and *progressive* may be added here because the longer the muscle is deprived of nerve stimulation, the more the loss of effective muscle tissue. *Guillain Barre Syndrome* results in symptoms comparable to those described above for a peripheral nerve injury (see Chapter 11, Muscular System).

Fortunately, two aspects of peripheral nerve injury make it less grim than it may seem otherwise. First, peripheral nerves have considerable ability for repair. The severed axons regenerate and prognosis is good because the cell body of the affected neurons sustains no damage. Second, peripheral nerve injuries result in localized and limited impairment. For example, if the femoral nerve is damaged, muscles of the anterior thigh would exhibit the characteristic symptoms—flaccid paralysis, absent tendon reflexes, and progressive atrophy—but the symptoms would be limited to the anterior thigh.

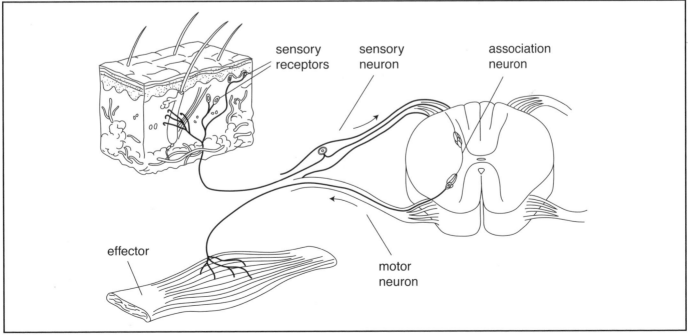

Figure 12.6 Spinal reflex

A disorder that preferentially destroys neurons in the anterior gray horn of the spinal cord would cause flaccid paralysis because of the motor neurons can no longer transmit an impulse. Tendon reflexes would be absent, again because the motor neurons of the anterior gray horn could not respond to the "stretch" stimulus. And progressive atrophy would result if the damage to the motor neurons of the anterior horn was sustained or permanent. *Poliomyelitis* (or simply *polio*; #4 in Figure 12.7) is just such a disorder. It is a virus (parasite) that invades neurons in the anterior gray horns and destroys them. The damage is permanent in this case, unlike that of a peripheral nerve injury. The extent of involvement depends upon how far the disease process spreads. Polio is generally controlled through immunization and therefore not frequently encountered in the modern world; however, its clinical description remains valuable for instructional purposes.

Spinal cord injury between cervical and lumbar enlargements (#5 in Figure 12.7) will predictably result in paraplegia, paralysis of both lower extremities. If the lesion occurs closer to the cervical enlargement, at the T1 or T2 level for example, then the person will have less capability to control the trunk. If the damage is closer to the lumbar enlargement, at T10 or T11, then most of trunk control will be retained. (The level of lesion has implications for wheelchair sports and will be discussed further in the recreation participation section of this chapter.)

Initially, the patient experiences a period of spinal shock following trauma. Spinal shock may last as long as several weeks and the person is completely unable to control voluntary and involuntary functions. The symptoms of spinal shock resemble those of a lower motor neuron lesion plus the loss of control of some autonomic functions (e.g., bowel and bladder control). After the period of spinal shock, the individual will experience return of function in tissues innervated by the spinal cord above the level of the lesion; below the level of the damage the person will experience the signs of an upper motor neuron lesion. Sensory signs persist after spinal shock as well. Whenever the spinal cord is completely sectioned, the person will be unable to detect sensations in the area of the body innervated by spinal nerves below the level of the lesion.

The amount of recovery below the level of the lesion depends on whether the cord is completely or partially severed. Partial trans-section leaves open the possibility that a variable number of tracts connecting brain and spinal cord remain operational. In general, if the axons in a tract within the CNS are damaged, the prospects for repair are not good when compared to the

return one might expect with a peripheral nerve injury. Neurons do not seem to be very successful in effecting repair within the CNS. Regardless of the level of lesion, so long as the damage is between the enlargements the individual will manifest the signs of an upper motor neuron lesion along with his or her paraplegia: voluntary paralysis, spasticity with hyperreflexia, and a positive Babinski.

Voluntary paralysis results because the person cannot complete transmission of a motor command from the cerebrum to the neurons in the anterior horn of the spinal cord. Essentially, the spinal cord below the level of the lesion continues to operate independent of control of the brain. Because one of the two basic functions of the spinal cord does not require input from the brain, spinal reflexes continue to operate below the level of the lesion, even after spinal cord injury. The difference is that the affected person can no longer override spinal reflexes with impulses from the brain. This means that tendon reflexes will be hyperactive and result in spasticity.

Spasticity is conspicuous when the practitioner is attempting to assist with range of motion through manual guidance. For example, pulling on the heel with the client in a seated position will elicit a stretch reflex initially. The reaction of the inexperienced practitioner is to pull even more forcefully. This will likely result in

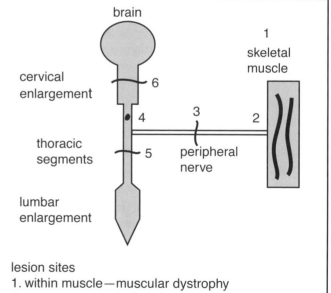

lesion sites
1. within muscle—muscular dystrophy
2. at neuro-muscular junction—myasthenia gravis
3. peripheral nerve injury
4. at spinal segment, anterior gray horn—poliomyelitis
5. sectioned spinal cord between cervical and lumbar enlargements
6. sectioned spinal cord at the level of the cervical enlargement

Figure 12.7 Primary disorders of the nervous system

even more vigorous resistance on the part of the client. Clearly, the person is not capable of voluntarily controlling the lower extremity; the practitioner has set off a stretch reflex with only a slight stretch. A slight stretch would not normally provoke a stretch reflex when tracts that carry motor impulses from the brain remain in tact. But those pathways have been cut as a result of the trans-section of the spinal cord. The key to successfully completing range of motion with a spinal cord injury is to make certain that the stretch is slow and gradual, because the speed of the stretch is a key variable in provoking the reflex. If the person's limb resists range of motion, then pause for a short time until the reflex subsides. The symptom of *hyperreflexia* is why the kind of paralysis experienced by a person with a spinal cord injury is sometimes called spastic paralysis. *Spastic paralysis* (too much muscle tone and excessive tendon reflex) contrasts markedly with flaccid paralysis (no muscle tone and no tendon reflex).

The final symptom associated with a spinal cord lesion is a *positive Babinski*. With a positive Babinski, the toes extend upon stimulation of the sole of the foot (e.g., scrapping a tongue depressor across the bottom of the foot). This response is normal in infants but indicates damage to the CNS after infancy.

The symptoms that result following complete trans-section of the spinal cord at the level of the cervical enlargement (#6 in Figure 12.7) are identical to those observed with trans-section that causes paraplegia—voluntary paralysis, spasticity, and a positive Babinski. The difference between lesions #5 and #6 lies in the extent of impairment, not in the symptoms. Damage that involves the cervical enlargement will result in *quadriplegia*—involvement of all four extremities. *Involvement* is used instead of paralysis because the portion of the spinal cord superior to the trans-section continues to function normally. This means that most quadriplegics are not completely paralyzed in all four extremities; they retain some use of their upper extremities. The higher the site of the lesion, the more the impairment. For instance, trans-section at C8 will not cause as much impairment of the upper extremities as a lesion at C5. While both individuals are considered quadriplegic, the person with a C5 lesion experiences more loss of function. This also explains why a person with quadriplegia may still be a candidate for a manual wheelchair and may still participate in wheelchair basketball.

Disorders of the Brain

Different parts of the brain have different responsibilities and damage to each part will yield different symptoms. Sometimes, the signs of an upper motor neuron lesion will result from trauma of some sort to neurons in the brain, other times not. Symptoms can be predicted with some accuracy from an understanding of what one part of the brain does when healthy. Inferring that these functions will be disturbed when that part of the brain is damaged usually reveals a general pattern of symptoms. The following sections address disorders of the brainstem, cerebrum, and cerebellum, as well as multiple sclerosis, cerebral palsy, and seizure disorders.

Disorders of the Brainstem

Disorders of the brainstem that a therapeutic recreation specialist (TRS) may work with are fairly uncommon. Specific pathologies may preferentially affect one of the cranial nerves (e.g., trigeminal neuralgia). Interruption of the motor or sensory tracts may take place in the brainstem (discussed in the section on cerebral impairments). But disabilities that have an origin in the brainstem are not common. This may well be attributable to the high mortality rate associated with lesions in the brainstem. Damage to brainstem nuclei often involves centers responsible for vital functions (e.g., cardiac centers, respiratory centers). When centers controlling vital functions are involved, little margin for compromise exists and the person is at great risk of death.

Disorders of the Cerebrum

Damage to the cerebrum will often produce some measure of voluntary paralysis. Whether the other symptoms of an upper motor neuron lesion accompany the voluntary paralysis depends on the location of the problem. Some of the motor tracts found in the spinal cord begin in the cerebrum. When these are damaged *anywhere* between the brain and the spinal cord, the predictable signs of an upper motor neuron lesion are evident.

Spinal cord injury results in interruption in this communication near the termination of the motor tract (just before the axons synapse on lower motor neurons in the anterior horn of the spinal cord). The lesion to the motor tracts from the cerebrum to the spinal cord can occur at a much more superior level, in the brainstem or in the cerebrum for instance.

Again, the predictable pattern of upper motor neuron lesion signs occurs. An example of a disorder that often results in the signs of an upper motor neuron lesion is a *cerebrovascular accident* (CVA or stroke). A *stroke* is a vascular lesion to one or more of the arteries that supply blood to the brain. Compromised blood supply will rapidly cause problems because of the brain's critical need for the oxygen carried in the blood stream.

Because cerebral blood supply enters the brain from an inferior route, arterial blood must travel from deep to superficial, in a superior direction to the cerebral cortex. Strokes often occur as the artery makes its way through deep and intermediate structures toward the cortex. Accordingly, strokes often affect the intermediate white matter of the cerebrum.

Many strokes interrupt the communication between the cerebrum and the spinal cord by damaging tracts near their origin in the cerebrum. Likewise, a stroke may damage the tract from the cerebrum through the brainstem to the spinal cord. Regardless, the symptoms are again those associated with upper motor neuron lesions.

The trauma associated with damage to the motor tracts in the brain is customarily limited to one side of the brain. The typical stroke will produce a variable amount of *hemiplegia*, (paralysis to one side of the body) instead of paraplegia or quadriplegia.

The extent of hemiplegia depends on how much of the tract is damaged. Because the tracts are larger in or near the cerebrum, a stroke may not completely interrupt all of the axons in the tract. This is analogous to partially severing a peripheral nerve. Nevertheless, the signs of an upper motor neuron lesion will be present on the affected side with either complete or partial destruction of the tract. (Strokes are discussed further in Chapter 14, Cardiopulmonary Systems.)

In contrast to strokes, head injuries may affect either superficial or deep structures of the brain. Head injuries may be open or closed. An *open head injury* means that a penetrating wound has been introduced into the skull and brain tissue, such as the result of a gunshot wound or a fracture. A *closed head injury* results when the brain is bounced against the skull without sustaining a penetrating trauma. In either case significant brain damage can result.

Immediate symptoms are specific to the area damaged. Because the *cerebral cortex* is the most superficial structure of the cerebrum and the largest structure of the brain, the cortex is often the focal point of the primary injury and resulting symptoms. But additional problems—cerebral edema (brain swelling), infection, or hematomas (blood clots)—may develop secondary to the initial injury.

Hemotomas may develop in the protective coverings surrounding the brain (*meninges*) or in the brain tissue itself. Blood clots are dangerous because they put pressure on brain tissue and compress it. Functional manifestations of the pressure depend on the area involved. Partial paralysis on one side of the body (hemiparesis) fixed and dilated pupils on one side, or impairments in balance or vision are examples of symptoms secondary to head injury. Portions of the brain may even herniate into other areas (e.g., part of the cerebrum may herniate inferiorly) if the pressure is excessive and not relieved.

Meningitis and encephalitis may develop following an open head injury, though other causes of these infections include surgery, viruses (e.g., herpes simplex), and viral infections elsewhere in the body (e.g., influenza). *Meningitis* refers to an infection of the protective coverings of the CNS, the meninges. *Encephalitis* refers to infections of the brain tissue proper. Infections of the meninges or the CNS functional tissue may cause deafness, brain damage, and mental retardation.

Another less common group of disorders may affect the deepest layer of the cerebrum—the basal nuclei. The syndrome of characteristics common to lesions to the basal nuclei includes the presence of involuntary movements, changes in muscle tone, and difficulties with posture. The person with an impairment stemming from damage to the basal nuclei may present with any of the following: involuntary tremor (alternating, rhythmic contractions), choriform movements (rapid, jerky, brisk movements), or athetosis (slow writhing movements, especially in the distal extremities).

Parkinson's disease is one of the more common forms of impairments localized in the basal nuclei. The person presents with an unchanging, masklike (unemotional) facial expression, tremors in the distal extremities, difficulty walking, and slow, monotone speech. Not infrequently, individuals with Parkinson's disease may later develop Alzheimer's disease. Typical onset for Parkinson's disease is past age 50.

Disorders of the Cerebellum

Balance difficulties and problems with coordination are hallmarks of cerebellar lesions. Subtle adjustments in the position of the trunk become more problematic for the person with a cerebellar lesion. The client is unsteady and at great risk for falling.

Uncoordinated movements resulting from cerebellar lesions can manifest in several different ways. Movements may break apart (called *decomposition of movement*) into separate units instead of appearing as one smooth, continuous movement. By way of analogy, if an essay represents a normal, smooth and coordinated movement, then the outline for the essay represents decomposition of movement.

Ataxia is a general term used to refer to uncoordinated movement. Ataxias may be manifested in several ways. Tremors during intentional movement are common with cerebellar lesions. Overshooting or pastpointing when moving an extremity toward a target (as in picking up a small object) is observed as well.

Speech is a complex motor activity that is well-learned and integrated by adulthood. However, with the onset of cerebellar pathology, speech may become uncoordinated, resulting in a slurring of words and a general slowness of speech that suggests uncertainty. Many of the symptoms of a cerebellar lesion may be mimicked if alcohol is used to excess—slurred speech, ataxic gait, uncoordinated movements.

Multiple Sclerosis

Multiple sclerosis (MS) may occur at several different locations in the CNS. Like a stroke, MS will produce different symptoms depending on the area affected.

MS is a disease of unknown etiology that causes deterioration of the myelin (demyelination) that covers many of the nerve fibers in the CNS. Some risk factors for MS include residence in a temperate climate and familial history of MS. Some authorities believe that the immune system may also be implicated.

The demyelinating process causes decreased conduction velocity or blocks the conduction of the nerve impulse altogether. Areas preferentially affected include optic pathways and structures, the cerebellum, motor tracts from the brain to the spinal cord, and some sensory tracts in isolation or combination.

Common impairments include speech disturbance, balance problems, vertigo (dizziness), blurred vision, gait difficulties, and tremors. Experts (e.g., Porth, 1990) maintain that increases in body temperature or ambient temperature worsen symptoms, although others suggest that the evidence for the temperature/symptom relationship is less clear and highly variable (Ponichtera-Mulcare, 1993). The disease is most often progressive, with each episode more severe than the last. The person shows less improvement during each subsequent period of remission. Depression and other mood disorders are common, probably responses to the unpredictability of the disease process.

Manifestation of the disease is phasic. The client experiences intervals with acute symptoms and heightened impairment alternating with periods of remission and normal or near normal health. Four patterns of disease progression are usually described: classical, acute, benign, and progressive (Woods, 1992).

The *classical* pattern is the most common, with episodes of symptom onset alternating with remission over many years. Each episode is usually more severe and each subsequent period of remission less complete. The *acute* form presents with rapid onset and progression with little or no remission. The prognosis for patients with the acute form is very poor. The *progressive* form of MS is similar to the acute type of MS—the patient presents with little or no indication of remission—but the progressive form advances more slowly than the acute form. Symptom onset and exacerbation are more gradual. The *benign* form presents with very attenuated symptoms. Full recovery or infrequent, mild episodes with the benign form of MS are likely.

Cerebral Palsy

Cerebral palsy (CP) is a syndrome of neurological disorders present at birth that affect various parts of the brain. The extent and type of impairment depends upon the area in the brain affected and the amount of damage. Injury during the birth process, insufficient oxygen to the fetus during gestation, and toxins are common causes of CP. Because of the time of onset, CP is considered a developmental disability.

Types of CP are named after symptoms common to the areas affected. *Spastic type CP* refers to pathology localized in the cerebrum. Predictably, overactive stretch reflexes and loss of voluntary control are observed, especially in distal portions of the limbs. These symptoms are prototypical to conditions that affect the communication pathway between the cerebral cortex and the neurons in the anterior gray horns of the spinal cord.

While spastic CP is the most common type, *athetoid type CP* is the second most frequent. *Athetosis* is one of the common symptoms observed when the basal nuclei of the cerebrum are the focal points of damage. The hallmark symptom of involuntary movement is observed in the person with athetoid type CP, especially slow sinuous movement in the distal parts of the extremities. Unstable muscle tone may also be present.

The focal point of the third most frequent type of CP, *ataxic CP*, is the cerebellum. Common symptoms include uncoordinated movements, difficulty in learning how to walk, and difficulty maintaining balance. Pastpointing is also observed in this group (e.g., they may overstep while descending stairs). They may also have trouble acquiring and utilizing joint sense information to coordinate movements.

Seizure Disorders

Epilepsy is the most common cause of a series of symptoms characterized by the random and transitory discharge of neurons in the CNS. A *seizure,* however, is frequently caused by another disorder, substance abuse, or a metabolic imbalance. Seizures may be a symptom of almost any lesion to the CNS, especially the brain. Only when the seizures recur on their own and with no other apparent cause is the diagnosis epilepsy considered.

Epilepsy may be primary or secondary. Seizures experienced after head injury, for example, would be classified as *secondary epilepsy*. If the epilepsy has no identifiable etiology, then it is classified as *primary epilepsy*. Epileptic seizures are also categorized according to severity. The old classification system for seizures (e.g., grand mal, petite mal, aura) has given way to a system of classification that considers the progression of the seizure. The newer system divides seizures into two categories based on whether it occurs in one or both hemispheres. *Partial seizures* involve only one cerebral hemisphere; *generalized seizures* involve both hemispheres. The partial category is further delineated by referring to the severity of the symptoms—*simple* refers to a seizure with no loss of consciousness and *complex* refers to seizures that induce a loss of consciousness.

Either of the partial type seizures may progress to a generalized seizure. Motor symptoms are common with the generalized category seizure. A tonic-clonic seizure is the most frequent type of motor pattern in the generalized seizure category. Formerly called grand mal seizures, *tonic-clonic seizures* are usually preceded by a simple seizure, and then the more severe, involuntary contractions, which may be accompanied by voiding of bladder and bowel.

Therapeutic Recreation and Neurological Impairments

Head Injuries

Symptoms displayed by persons with head injuries may vary dramatically, depending on the extent and severity of the lesion as well as individual differences (Stumbo & Bloom, 1990). Conditions that may result from a head injury are difficult to predict. The variability of common problems makes planning and intervention even more challenging. Nevertheless, some problems following head injury are more frequent than others. Damage to the frontal and temporal lobes is more usual, especially with a closed head injury. Three areas of the cerebrum are preferentially found to sustain lesions: deep blood vessels supplying the basal surface of the cerebrum and axons that connect the two cerebral hemispheres, the frontal lobe, and the temporal lobe. Krane (1994) has translated each of these lesions into specific, behavioral and cognitive problems common among persons with head injuries:

- Injury to *deep blood vessels* compromises the blood supply to deep cerebral structures and some brainstem structures, which is correlated with difficulties in processing large amounts of information and sustaining attention
- Damage to the *inferior surface of the temporal lobe* leads to memory deficits and difficulties in learning
- Bruising of the *frontal lobe* can cause problems with social appropriateness and emotions, as well as abstract thinking

The variability of symptom presentation challenges the TR Specialist to anticipate problems and plan successful programs with the head-injured population. One useful, global assessment commonly part of the assessment subsequent to head injury is the Rancho Los Amigos Cognitive Functioning Scale. The Rancho scale is comprised of eight levels of function, ranging from comatose and unresponsive (Level I) to purposeful, appropriate, independent behavior (Level VIII). Predictably, mid-range levels are assigned to greater or lesser functional behavior (e.g., Level VI, confused but appropriate). The scale is referenced throughout the TR literature (e.g., Carter, Van Andel & Robb, 1995, pp. 250–251; Stumbo & Bloom, 1990, p. 71).

The findings of Fazio and Fralish (1988) provide a point of departure for planning TR programs for persons with head injuries. They surveyed 70 programs of late rehabilitation and transition for persons with head injury and found that the top five goals for this population were to develop basic social skills, to decrease social isolation and withdrawal, community reintegration, independent leisure involvement, and to enhance verbalization and self-expression. Many of the goals discovered in the Fazio and Fralish (1988) study are consistent with the interventions described under the therapy, leisure education, and recreation participation sections that follow.

Spinal Cord Injury

Spinal cord injury (SCI) presents a unique sequelae in comparison to clients with MS, CP, or head injury. Unlike persons with head injury and the later stages of MS, persons with SCI are mentally lucid and relatively stable psychologically. Unlike CP, SCI is an acquired condition. Unlike MS, SCI is not progressive.

The health of a person with SCI tends to be stable with the exception of the development of complications. Although SCI can happen to anyone, the typical profile of a person with SCI is that of a young male involved in a traffic accident who has many years remaining to live. Following SCI, the person is also likely to be unemployed or underemployed.

This profile confers certain advantages and disadvantages on the strategies for the delivery of TR services to persons with SCI. For instance, more likely than not the client will retain a wish to remain physically active postinjury. This attitude creates an environment favorable for the development of an aggressive program of fitness, physical activity, and sport among this group. However, the same conditions may result in considerable frustration if the client is no longer able to act on his wishes to continue an active lifestyle, or if the client cannot successfully negotiate the barriers to participating in an active leisure lifestyle.

The approach to TR with disability groups assumes that the interface between leisure and the client is through an intervention program. However, the work of Kleiber and colleagues (Kleiber, Brock, Lee, Dattilo & Caldwell, 1995) took a different point of departure, presenting an overlooked aspect of the relationship between leisure and disability—leisure is not only relevant to the rehabilitation (through participation in TR programs), but also relevant to the illness.

Kleiber et al. (1995) completed a qualitative interview study of 20 subjects with SCI. All of the subjects (75% male, mean age = 32.2 years) had participated in clinical TR programs while in rehabilitation. The study wished to determine the extent to which leisure figured into each subject's experiencing of SCI. Leisure activities were hypothesized to be part of the experience of the illness to the extent that leisure activities were among the defining characteristics of the self (e.g., fisherman, jogger).

The results of Kleiber et al. (1995) supported their hypothesis: Dialogue about leisure figured prominently in subjects experiencing of their lives after SCI. In particular, loss of ability, disruption of relationships, dependence on others, and relapse were the themes discovered.

When subjects talked about the *loss of ability and skills* following SCI, they often described it in terms of the loss of abilities in leisure activities. The perception of loss of ability affected the amount of enjoyment derived from the activity, and the affirmation of competence that was derived from the activity before injury. Even when the client could find a way to reestablish participation in a previously favored activity, the satisfaction derived from the activity was not as high as before the injury. Perceived constraints were blamed for the decrease in leisure satisfaction.

The quality of leisure activities suffered from the *disruption of the relationships* that had been established through leisure participation (e.g., teammates in a softball league were friends), and the quality of the experience predicated upon relationships and interpersonal dynamics (e.g., playing catch with your son). The disruption of relationships compounds the person's loss of immediacy (associated with the loss of ability) and the sense of belonging and community interaction that comes with complete mobility.

The third theme discovered by Kleiber and associates (1995) was that of *dependence on others*. Having to ask for assistance to participate in leisure activities was enough to discourage many from participation. Negotiation with others and acceptance of the necessity of adaptive equipment created a significant psychological hurdle. The dependence on others clearly created an environment conducive to perceptions of helplessness.

A second interview with subjects following discharge revealed *relapse* as a theme. After discharge from rehabilitation, subjects were confronted with the realities of the real world and the lack of accommodations that they had experienced while in rehabilitation. Relapse was most salient among leisure activities that were cultivated and rediscovered during rehabilitation. Reacquiring competence in a former, favored, leisure activity only to discover a less than accommodating situation in their actual living circumstances was especially discouraging for many of the subjects interviewed. The unfortunate and frequent reaction was to gravitate to more passive, in-home activities that required little if any adaptation and accommodation.

The authors concluded that losses and changes in leisure figured significantly in describing the experience of the injury. This may be the case because of the psychological properties associated with leisure experience: self-identity, perceptions of competence, enjoyment, and friendship. Drawing on symbolic interactionism (Samdahl, 1989) the authors argued that leisure activities are containers of psychological meaning. The impact of the loss of these ascribed meanings through the loss of leisure or the change in participation dynamics defines an impairment such as SCI.

Multiple Sclerosis

The conventional measure of impairment for persons with *multiple sclerosis* (MS) is the Expanded Disability Status Scale (EDSS) developed by Kurtzke (1983). The scale ranges from no or little disability to marked disability and mortality. A higher number indicates more impairment. Because the lower extremities are preferentially affected, a crude division of the EDSS may be made based on ambulatory capability. Patients with scores of less than five remain independent in ambulation; those scoring five or higher are largely defined by degree of impairment in ambulation.

Programming goals are subject to change based on the responsiveness predicted from the EDSS. Interventions using some modalities will be more successful with lower EDSS scores because of higher function. Furthermore, because of the unpredictability of MS and its progression, the therapeutic recreation (TR) professional may have to adjust estimates of the client's functional capabilities if exacerbations are pronounced (i.e., even though the client may be in active therapy, impairment may continue). This discouraging fact of life for the MS client makes programmatic responses to the disorder frustrating for the therapist. How is one to know if progress has been made if the net improvements are neutralized by an exacerbation of the illness?

No easy answers are apparent, other than advising the therapist to be well-aware of possible exacerbations and anticipate episodes from time to time. The net effect on TR programming is that the goals for the client will have to remain fluid, subject to change depending on whether the person is experiencing an attack or in remission. The amount of return during remission is as important as the frequency and intensity of exacerba-

tions. Treatment goals may be less ambitious if return during remission falls short of preonset function. Conversely, if return is nearly complete, but symptoms are slow to regress, constant monitoring will signal the TR Specialist when to adjust goals in a more aggressive manner.

Moreover, the TR Specialist must remain cognizant of the fact that most persons with MS do not die of MS; they expire from the same disorders as the rest of the population (e.g., heart disease, stroke). However, because of the functional impairment associated with MS, they are at risk of acquiring a host of chronic and acute conditions that may threaten health. Hence, interventions designed to prevent secondary disabilities and conditions (e.g., heart disease, depression) seem the appropriate companion to those designed to address the primary symptoms of the disorder.

Cerebral Palsy

Several general principles are useful to the TR Specialist beginning work with clients with CP in any of the service delivery settings. Persons with CP, especially children and those with more severe cases of CP, are characterized by a persistence of several primitive reflexes (e.g., startle reflex) that prove to be dysfunctional (Jansma & French, 1994; Sherrill, 1986). Primitive reflexes are normally integrated at an early age in the able-bodied individual and normal postural responses then develop. Persistence of primitive reflexes inhibits the emergence of normal reactions and interferes with normal motor activities.

Some interventions to address the persistence of primitive reflexes may be implemented during the therapy phase of service delivery and through community-based programs that cooperate with adapted physical education efforts during the developmental years. These steps may be applicable during any phase of service delivery because primitive reflexes may, necessitate continued management of adverse effects on normal motor activity (e.g., functional positioning in a wheelchair is one method for managing primitive reflexes and spasticity that may be implemented regardless of the TR service setting).

Persons with CP frequently present with multiple disabilities (Jansma & French, 1994; Sherrill, 1986). Common disabilities secondary to CP include communication difficulties, visual or auditory deficits, difficulties in learning, and mental retardation.

The general health of persons with CP is usually stable. In contrast to cases of MS or head injuries, the client with CP will have persistent but predictable levels of impairment over a sustained period of time. While persistent symptoms frustrate curative efforts, stability of general health and primary symptoms makes goals and interventions easier to develop and implement. This is in sharp contrast to MS, where exacerbations are difficult to predict and deterioration may occur even during active and otherwise effective treatment.

Therapy

The therapy aspect of intervention is divided according to disability groups. Persons with disabilities often present with similar problems, though each may differ in magnitude (e.g., spinal cord injury resulting in paraplegia versus quadriplegia).

Head Injuries

Rehabilitation for persons with head injuries often takes a considerable amount of time (Kwan & Sulzberger, 1994). The amount of time head trauma takes to reconcile itself is a matter of patience on the part of the client and the rehabilitation team. Research indicates that the amount of effort directed toward therapy must be in excess of customary norms for therapeutic change to occur. The expedited treatment received under the current managed care approach to healthcare and rehabilitation, however, does not portend well for persons with head injuries. The following review of interventions with persons who have sustained significant head injuries supports a longer, more patient rehabilitation initiative. Much of the work to be accomplished is feasible in community-based settings.

In 1989, Dordel found that 8–20 hours of exercise, physical activity, or sport per week were needed for 10 weeks to 7 months to produce significant improvement in clients. Marked improvement was found in standing and walking, posture and balance, endurance, motor control, and precise movement.

Likewise, Kunstler and Sokoloff (1993) learned that intensive TR using corrective exercises, adaptive sports (e.g., adapted swimming, walking, weight training), games and crafts, community reorientation, and leisure counseling translated into dramatic gains. A 20-year-old male with a head injury improved strength endurance, and balance and developed realistic goals and new interests resulting in functional improvements. He removed his leg brace and was able to walk up to one mile, developed new leisure interests (e.g., model

building, jogging), began community college, and started to work part-time. Consistent with Dordel's work, Kunstler and Sokoloff found that the therapeutic initiative had to be intensive (3–5 days per week at a rate of 3–5 hours per day for 6–36 months of treatment) to realize the gains.

The data from Dordel and Kunstler and Sokoloff must be considered suggestive, not definitive. First, both studies were case studies: Dordel had two subjects and Kunstler and Sokoloff reported only one of five subjects that had experienced a head injury. Second, if researchers find intensive rehabilitation to be successful with clients with head injuries, then the treatment threshold may become an obstacle to TR service delivery. Cost/benefit issues are the legacy of managed healthcare. Large sample findings may support the work of Dordel and Kunstler and Sokoloff, but will the healthcare community be willing to pay the price? The healthcare community must answer the question: How long is long enough? Third, even if compelling evidence is discovered, the burden of rehabilitation may fall to creative, community-based programs that can be run on an outpatient, fee basis (e.g., aquatics programs).

Unlike the work Dordel and Kunstler and Sokoloff, Stumbo and Bloom (1990) suggested potential cognitive gains that may be realized through calculated use of games and activities that place a premium on cognitive processing capabilities. Each game may be presented in a simplified manner until the client attains mastery over the information load in the environment. The games also provide for progression—adding more information demand to the environment as the client can tolerate.

Stumbo and Bloom suggested three treatment goals: improving problem-solving ability, improving memory skills, and increasing attention span. The use of positive reinforcement to manage behavior (Jansma & French, 1994) and the use of other environmental cues (e.g., hand signals, see Howard & Claiman, 1994) may help to call the client's attention to socially inappropriate behavior during the activities.

Relative to the goal of increasing attention span, the TR Specialist must be aware of the amount of stimuli in the recreation activity environment. Noise (irrelevant stimuli) in the environment must be reduced to a minimum when beginning an activity. The chances of enhancing social skills in a group are not feasible until the client can focus on the activity at hand and interact with only one other individual. When the client can attend to the activity and be socially appropriate with one other person, then another person may be added to the group (i.e., adding more stimuli to the activity environment).

For example, a music appreciation program may be conducted with a variable sized group, from two to six ideally. Asking questions at the end of each session can quantify the attending competence of the client. The number of correct answers, averaged over several sessions, may then serve as a marker for adding more stimuli to the environment (e.g., taking the person to a concert in the community or adding more members to the group).

Spinal Cord Injuries

In 1992 Youngkhill Lee developed a theoretical framework for understanding the role of TR (and leisure) relative to SCI. Using qualitative methods, Lee and associates attained a fundamental understanding of the role of TR in the lives of persons with SCI. Lee, Brock, Dattilo, and Kleiber (1992) suggested that TR had the potential for helping the person with SCI re-story his or her life. Lee, Dattilo, Kleiber, and Caldwell, (1996, p. 210) later referred to the use of re-storying when the "imagined future becomes doubtful." *Re-storying* involves adaptation and adjustment of a life story narrative that we all write for ourselves in our mind's eye. Re-storying is the client's effort to make sense out of the SCI, adjust the life story narrative to the impairment, and restore a sense of meaning and purpose to life.

Lee et al. (1992) also maintained that TRS could intervene with the clients by helping them understand the preinjury lifestyle and the significance of leisure in that lifestyle. As suggested previously in the Kleiber et al. (1995) study, leisure figured prominently in the meaning of the person's preinjury life—many significant aspects of personal identity and psychological profile were symbolized by the meanings imputed by persons to the leisure lifestyle. Leisure lifestyle, especially the active lifestyle led by most young people, has an important impact on post-injury adjustment, "...particularly important when that lifestyle centered on embodied activity [e.g., sport, exercise, physical activity]" (Lee et al., 1992, p. 205). One's sense of continuity and connection with the past and its historical context have been disrupted. Hence, Lee et al. (1992) concluded that re-storying may be what happened during various TR interventions when adjustment was judged to be successful. Especially when the client has relied on embodied activities, imaginative programs can help the person rewrite the life story, either through new activities or adaptations of old favorites.

Lee et al. also concluded that understanding of the person's preinjury lifestyle provided insight into the significance of leisure activities in the person's life story narrative. After injury some activities may no longer be part of the person's life story or the activities may be reestablished as part of the narrative in an adapted form, through partial participation, with the assistance of adaptive equipment, or by relying on someone else for assistance.

To test the validity of Lee's theory, Caldwell and Lee (1994/1995) investigated the role of TR in rehabilitation of persons with SCI. Twenty subjects (mean age = 30.2 years) with SCI (7 with paraplegia, 13 with quadriplegia) participated in qualitative interviews to describe their perceptions of the role of TR in rehabilitation. Several themes emerged from the data, indicating that TR:

- Provided hope and a sense of future possibilities (people recognized they could still participate in some preinjury activities)
- Provided information, education, and adaptive resources (identified of leisure resources made available through participation in TR)
- Facilitated skill development (acquired of skills through instruction and practice)
- Encouraged and motivated (interaction skills persuaded clients to try activities)
- Developed confidence (participated in leisure activities that resulted in perceptions of self-efficacy)
- Provided aspects of leisure experience (convinced clients that they had choices in their free time, that they could still enjoy life, and that all former activities were not lost)
- Assisted in coping and adjusting to disability (helped subjects cope with apprehensions associated with community outings and adjust to the realities imposed by the impairment)
- Facilitated community integration (prepared the individual for return to the community and coping with life changes)

Even though the subjects in this study judged TR effective, they had a few negative comments about their experience. Although TR was perceived as beneficial, the potentials for leisure experienced during rehabilitation were rarely realized after discharge. This contradiction of leisure experiences led to feelings of disappointment, anger, and frustration on the part of the subjects. Subjects complained that this phenomenon may make adjustment more difficult.

Caldwell and Lee (1994/1995) used Nelson's (1990) theory of reintegration to understand the role of TR in rehabilitation of patients with SCI in a more general manner. Although Caldwell and Lee did not find any role of TR reported by their subjects that matched Nelson's first phase (buffering) many of the roles elicited from subjects correlated with the remaining three phases of reintegration: transcending, toughening, and launching.

Transcending refers to assisting the person in overcoming intrinsic barriers and culturally imposed stereotypes. Caldwell and Lee argued that the TRS acted as an "ideology" pusher, being persistent with the person with SCI and encouraging participation in seemingly inaccessible activities.

Toughening follows transcending—the client experiments with activities (new and old, unassisted and adapted). Compensations and relying on the assistance of others slowly helps the person delimit his sphere of leisure operation, and defines the psychological margins of participation. The limits of participation are further elaborated during the toughening phase through adaptations, accommodations, and approximations to unassisted activities.

The final phase of *launching* was best illustrated through outings designed to promote autonomy and push the edges of independent leisure lifestyle. Through negotiation with the external world (e.g., using adaptations, asking for assistance) the clients tested the effectiveness of skills and strategies learned during rehabilitation.

Lee et al. (1996) used data from the same 20 subjects to investigate the continuity of previous leisure activities during early postinjury (i.e., during rehabilitation and shortly after discharge from rehabilitation). The authors began by capitalizing on Kagawa-Singer's (1993) innovative model, which is based on a two-dimensional concept of health: physical status and social function. Lee and colleagues (1996) maintained that even though the person with a SCI cannot reestablish his or her complete preinjury life, he or she can reestablish and even exceed his previous level of social function. Thus, the person with a SCI affirms health by "...the degree to which one is able to be satisfactorily engaged in social activities in spite of physical limitations" (Lee et al., 1996, p. 212). Further, the authors maintained leisure participation represented a health promoting activity because it induces perceptions of social competence and integrity of social ability. Not surprisingly, their findings were consistent with those of Caldwell and Lee (1994/1995). They identified three major themes: seeking continuity as an aspiration of adjustment, seeking continuity through approximations to preinjury activities, and accommodating for continuity.

The first theme identified in the interview data by Lee and associates (1996) was *seeking continuity*. This represented an attempt by subjects to reconnect to their preinjury leisure lifestyle. However, seeking continuity was the expression of a wish to return to preinjury activities—an emerging awareness—and not the actual accomplishment of the preinjury lifestyle. Nevertheless, seeking of continuity served to energize and motivate the subjects to try favorite past activities and later to explore new activities. The mere possibility of returning to some preinjury activities may be interpreted as an attempt to piece together a part of the life story and avoid complete re-storying. Seeking continuity is most consistent with Caldwell and Lee's (1994/1995) earlier interpretation of the same data—that TR was perceived as a source for hope and the sense of future possibilities.

The next theme reported by Lee et al. (1996) was *establishing a sense of continuity*. Subjects participated in activities interpreted as similar to but not identical to preinjury participation. The authors called this the approximation of preinjury activity. The approximation of previous participation style seemed to be adequate to establish continuity between past, present, and future. Approximating previous participation may be interpreted as a realization that some part of the person's previous life story narrative may still be valid, despite the impairment.

Reconciliation between preinjury participation and current realities was captured in the final interview theme identified by the authors (Lee et al., 1996). *Accommodating for continuity* was attained through repeated bouts of participation and negotiation with the environment to attain leisure aspirations. Modifications such as changing the activity, the behavior, or the context of participation reconciled the limitations of SCI with the motivation to return to the preinjury lifestyle.

Lee et al. (1996) asserted that if these data were broadly applicable to the greater population of persons with SCI, then early adaptation to SCI involves a period of adjustment. Furthermore, leisure appeared to figure prominently in early adjustment as the person aspires to past capabilities, reestablishes connection to past leisure activities, and finally accommodates to present limitations in order to adjust successfully.

Further data confirming Lee's theory of adjustment to SCI through leisure were provided in the text of a case study of a quadriplegic male reported by Blake (1991). The young man (age 24) was readmitted to a rehabilitation program for treatment of secondary complications (e.g., substance abuse, incontinence). He explored leisure options (seeking continuity), selected activities to try out (made efforts to reestablish continuity), and finally accommodated for continuity by adapting a previously favored activity—skiing using an Arroya sit ski.

Some studies (e.g., Lyons, 1987; Coyle & Kinney, 1990) contradict the findings of Lee and his team. Instead of continuity, these studies indicated that subjects with SCI report less participation in active pursuits, more isolated, homebound activities, and more passive recreation. This apparent contradiction may be explained by the fact that many surveys have examined the quantitative aspects of leisure (how much) in preference to the qualitative aspects (psychological meaning) of leisure. Because young people are most likely to participate in active leisure, and are more likely to sustain a SCI, a reduction in the frequency of activity comes as no surprise. But as Lee and his team suggested, leisure can still be part of the adjustment to the SCI if social ability through leisure can be established.

A more serious concern with Lee's theory of adjustment to SCI through leisure relates to the long-term adjustment to SCI and the role played by leisure; however, data do not appear to support this concern. For instance, Coyle, Lesnik-Emas, and Kinney (1994) found no significant difference in leisure satisfaction or life satisfaction among groups (n = 91) who differed in time since SCI injury. The average length of disability was 9-and-a-half years. Consistent with predictions from Lee's theory, leisure satisfaction was significantly positively correlated with life satisfaction. Moreover, this finding confirms that the quality of the leisure experience had not deteriorated since the time of injury. Likewise, Caldwell and Weissinger (1993) reported that number of years since discharge did *not* predict boredom in leisure among subjects with SCI.

Similarly, Crewe and Krause (1990) studied the long-term adjustment of persons with SCI (n = 154; mean time passed since injury = 21 years). Social activity, life satisfaction, and social life were found to be stable after 11 years. These data indicate that psychological profiles were acceptable, even though other studies have reason to believe that absolute frequency of participation in active leisure may well have declined in 11 years. Crewe and Krause concluded that the immediate period following injury may provoke the most adaptation and adjustment on the part of the individual. The data further suggest that if the person can negotiate the near-term adjustment to SCI, chances are good that psychological health can be maintained in the long run. Collectively, the findings pertaining to the long-term adjustment to SCI suggest that Lee's theoretical model may be quite robust.

Groff and Dattilo (1994) reported a study of adolescents who sustained SCI. The 9 subjects (ages 10–18) were interviewed and the transcripts were analyzed for emergent themes. The themes were similar to those identified by Lee et al. (1996): adjustment to SCI, friendships, and focusing on the present. Some of the aspects of Lee's theoretical model may be recognized in the reports of Groff and Dattilo's subjects, such as the importance of social function to overall health (emphasis on friendships) and the use of negotiation to adjust to impairment.

Although Lee's insight into SCI marks a significant development, other aspects of SCI must be considered to complete our understanding of the role of leisure and TR with SCI. Most salient are the complications and secondary conditions that plague persons with SCI. Urinary tract infections, incontinence, skin lesions, transient pain, and contractures number among the most frequent physical complications following SCI. The psychological fallout from these physical complications includes depression, social isolation, and boredom. Consideration of frequent secondary conditions and the role of TR service in addressing secondary problems follows.

Researchers in TR have focused on the psychological sequelae of physical complications. For instance, estimates of probable clinical depression associated with the development of secondary complications range from 21% (Coyle, Shank, Kinney & Hutchins, 1993) to about 33% (Berryman et al., 1991; Coyle et al., 1994). Further, because of the absence of employment opportunities and the leisure profile of persons with SCI (e.g., inactive, passive, isolated, home-bound leisure), many have excess time on their hands (Caldwell & Weissinger, 1994; Coyle et al., 1993). Boredom is a frequent complaint and a precursor for the development of other negative conditions, such a depression and the practice of risky health behaviors (e.g., smoking).

Coyle et al. (1993) studied 48 subjects with SCI who developed physical complications (e.g., urinary tract problems). Measures of personal, family, and social leisure were negatively correlated with depressive symptoms. Santiago, Coyle, and Kinney (1993) urged the use of leisure activities with cases of relapse and secondary complications among the SCI population and not simply during the (relatively) acute rehabilitation phase. Leisure participation may serve to insulate the subject from negative psychological concomitants of physical complications. However, the greater the impairment the less the expressed interest in personal, family, and social leisure; subjects with quadriplegia were significantly less interested than those with paraplegia (Coyle et al., 1993). This suggests that the TR Specialist may need to anticipate more efforts in the direction of motivation to energize participation of those most impaired by SCI.

Caldwell and Weissinger (1994) conducted a secondary analysis of data reported earlier by Caldwell, Adolph, and Gilbert (1989). They were able to predict 21% of the variance in leisure boredom scores in their subjects with SCI after discharge from rehabilitation. In order of strength of explanation, perceived competence in leisure, income, comparative leisure satisfaction, and leisure participation were negatively related to boredom in leisure. The implications are consistent with the findings of Coyle et al. (1993) that leisure participation and favorable perceptions of leisure experiences may neutralize negative emotionality, in this case boredom. This association is less of a surprise because excess time and passive leisure contribute to boredom in the first place.

Exercise may prove to be beneficial for persons with SCI relative to both psychological distress (e.g., depressive symptoms) and the prevention of secondary conditions associated with an enforced sedentary lifestyle. Coyle and Santiago (1995), for example, found that 12 weeks of aerobic exercise practiced by a small sample of persons with physical disabilities was associated with a significant decrease in depressive symptoms compared to control subjects with physical disabilities. These results are encouraging but need further verification because of several methodological problems in the study design. Subjects self-selected into exercise and control groups (i.e., participated only if interested), and the groups were quite heterogeneous with respect to disabilities represented (e.g., two with paraplegia in the exercise group, seven with paraplegia in the control group). Nevertheless, the results should motivate further study concerning the psychological benefits of exercise for persons with physical disabilities in general, and for persons with SCI specifically.

While findings have suggested that persons with SCI may benefit from regular exercise in a manner similar to that of able-bodied individuals, researchers have discovered some important differences. First of all, the prospects for improvement are greater in persons who have experienced less impairment (e.g., persons with paraplegia are more apt to benefit than persons with quadriplegia) (Davis, 1993; Figoni, 1993). Persons with paraplegia have a training advantage over those with higher spinal cord impairment because they retain more functional muscle mass that may be stimulated by exercise. This creates a greater demand on the heart to support muscular activity than in those with

quadriplegia who may only retain function of proximal muscle of the upper extremities (e.g., muscles of the shoulder girdle).

Besides the sheer amount of muscle mass that is unavailable for exercise because of paralysis, many of the problems associated with SCI relate to ANS dysfunction. The sympathetic division of the ANS stimulates cardiac response to aerobic exercise. Recall that the sympathetic division of the ANS is located at thoracic and lumbar levels. Spinal cord section at high thoracic and cervical levels denies the sympathetic division of the spinal cord input from higher centers in the brainstem responsible for adjustment to exercise (e.g., increased cardiac output). Therefore, the heart is unable to respond to additional demands placed on it to deliver blood to working muscles.

The sympathetic division is also responsible for stimulating sweating to cool the body during exercise. Compromise of sympathetic tone mitigates against a normal sweating response during aerobic exercise. This causes blood to accumulate (pool) superficially in the skin to compensate for the absence of sweating during exercise. Blood also tends to pool in the lower extremities because of paralysis of lower extremity muscles that normally squeeze on veins and force blood back toward the heart. (See Chapter 14, Cardiopulmonary System for discussion of the skeletal muscle pump.)

Furthermore, blood in arteries is normally redirected from organs to skeletal muscles during exercise by constriction of arteries leading to organs and dilation of blood vessels leading to skeletal muscles doing the work. This shunting mechanism is controlled the sympathetic division of the ANS, which is unavailable to persons with high thoracic or cervical lesions. The arteries leading to viable muscles still seem to dilate, but those to organs do not seem to compensate by constricting. Hence, the shunting of arterial blood with its rich oxygen supply is incomplete. The slowed return of blood to the heart and the impaired shunting mechanism serve to limit response to aerobic exercise in two ways. First, the failure of the arterial system to completely compensate by redirecting blood to working muscles causes exercise induced hypotension (i.e., excessively low blood pressure). Second, this causes earlier than normal fatigue, nausea, and dizziness.

Despite the challenges of exercise for persons with SCI, researchers (Davis, 1993; Figoni, 1993) remain positive about the benefits of exercise, especially in preventing or retarding development of secondary problems (e.g., heart disease, progressive atrophy, further loss of mobility). Within limits even the person with high thoracic and cervical injury can benefit, but

TRS should recognize:

- Response to aerobic exercise is limited
- Improvements in aerobic health are likely attributable to adaptation of muscles rather than significant training of the heart as in able-bodied persons
- Improvements in strength of functional muscles should approach that of normal individuals of the same age and gender

The benefit of improved strength through exercise and adaptation of functional muscles to aerobic exercise likely will translate into improved functional ability and capability to retain some competence in activities of daily living (Davis, 1993; Figoni, 1993). Programs focusing on muscle strength are simpler and safer to implement and tax the person's ability less than conventional aerobic exercise.

Innovative techniques have been used to involve more muscle mass and to improve venous return to the heart. For instance, Figoni and Glaser (1993) combined electrically stimulated leg contractions using a stationary bicycle with an arm ergometer. The subject was a 27-year-old male with a cervical lesion. Researchers were able to evoke a higher cardiac response than in the past. This was later verified by the same researchers (Figoni & Glaser, 1995a). By involving 14 subjects with quadriplegia in various exercise protocols, they demonstrated higher cardiac output with the combined arm/leg protocol than with an arm only or electrically stimulated leg only exercise training protocols.

Figoni and Glaser (1995c) also reported that the combined arm/leg training program of 15 weeks (at three times per week) produced significant improvement in aerobic variables, but not in central cardiovascular parameters (e.g., heart rate during training). The authors concluded that the training effects observed were likely a result of peripheral factors (e.g., muscle adaptation to exercise).

Although the technology necessary to support and safely implement aerobic training among persons with SCI is not widely available for field use, the results are promising. Further, the same studies have uncovered some simple and helpful strategies that may be used to improve exercise among persons with SCI. A slightly reclined posture has been shown to influence venous return to the heart (Figoni & Glaser, 1993). This suggests that tilting seats back slightly in exercise devices (e.g., using inclined stationary bicycles) or having the person exercise in a supine position (e.g., bench press instead of upright press in weightlifting) would improve performance. In addition, wearing

elastic stockings and an abdominal binder during exercise (Figoni & Glaser, 1993) puts external pressure on the venous system, assisting venous return to the heart. Finally, immersion in a fluid environment would put favorable ambient pressure on the lower extremities and abdominopelvic structures to augment venous return to the heart (Figoni & Glaser, 1993).

Multiple Sclerosis

Traditional recommendations for persons with MS to avoid exercise and physical activity are being reexamined. Some evidence suggests that mild to moderate forms of exercise do not aggravate symptoms, but may result in noticeable improvements in fitness that may translate into improved functional ability. Exercise, physical activity, and sport participation may retard deconditioning that is part of the disease progression and may help maintain optimal physical function to ward off the development of secondary conditions (Ponichtera-Mulcare, 1993).

As with any exercise program, a health screening and consultation with a physician are necessary prior to the introduction of an exercise program for persons with MS. The added incentive for the health screening for persons with MS relates to the fact that in some cases the individual may manifest contra-indications for exercise. For instance, Ponichtera-Mulcare (1993) reviewed the literature and reported that some persons with MS have adverse cardiac and blood pressure responses to exercise. This is likely a result of the involvement of some of the ANS centers in the brainstem and ANS pathways to the spinal cord.

These cases should not discourage attempts to introduce mild to moderate exercise into the treatment regime of persons with MS—only to serve as a reminder to approach such situations with appropriate caution (e.g., having a physician present during initial workouts to monitor the client's response to exercise). Knowing the risk profile of persons with MS who are more likely to experience adverse responses to exercise will help the professional anticipate difficulties and flag high-risk situations. Risk factors for adverse responses to exercise include cardiac and blood pressure instability at rest, level of impairment (those with higher EDSS scores are more at risk), and length of disease.

Ponichtera-Mulcare (1993) found compelling evidence in the literature in support of exercise for clients with MS, if functional symptoms are minimal (i.e., low EDSS score). She concluded that persons with minimal MS symptoms can exercise in a manner similar to healthy age-matched subjects. Scant evidence supports the improvement in skeletal muscle function in persons with MS, but data support improvement of aerobic fitness variables following training by MS subjects. Certainly, individuals with minimal functional impairment are capable of participation in exercise, calisthenics, and swimming.

Subsequent to Ponichtera-Mulcare's (1993) review, Ponichtera-Mulcare, Mathews, Glaser, and Gupta (1995) compared the performance of 10 subjects with MS (minimal impairment; EDSS mean=1.7) to 10 age-matched controls without MS. Subjects were compared on exercise responses using legs only, arms only, and legs and arms in combination. Predictably, subjects without MS performed better than the 10 subjects with MS. But the authors learned that the exercise using legs and arms in combination was apt to result in the most benefit for persons with MS. Using the leg/arm technique, subjects with MS attained their highest heart rate peak at 91% of predicted maximum. (Non-MS subjects attained an average heart rate peak of 96% of predicted maximum.)

Petajan, and associates (1996) later implemented the leg/arm technique with more success. Fifty-four subjects with MS were randomly assigned to treatment and control conditions. The treatment group trained for 15 weeks for three 40-minute sessions per week. The exercise group improved on bowel and bladder control and measures of aerobic fitness (e.g., maximum oxygen consumption), and other measures of functional fitness (e.g., upper and lower extremity strength, skin folds, blood cholesterol profile). Subjects in the exercise group also perceived less anger, depression, fatigue, and improved social interaction, emotional behavior, home management, and recreation participation following the intervention.

Since most persons with MS are not likely to be hospitalized throughout most of the course of the disease process, contact with TR is most likely in a community-based setting. The exercise principles derived from the Ponichtera-Mulcare et al. study (1995) and Petajan et al. (1996) offer guidance for the implementation of a mild to moderate exercise program for persons with MS in a TR setting. The leg/arm technique offers the advantage of greater cardiopulmonary responsiveness and metabolic demand. The basic principles include the following:

- MS affects the lower extremities more, hence, incorporation of combination leg/arm techniques provides a precise adaptation to symptom presentation. Involving the upper extremities will advance the effectiveness of the exercise.

- Using the leg/arm technique will spread the workload over more muscle mass and decrease the onset of fatigue and stress. Involving all functioning extremities in unison will also increase the potential workload.

- The leg/arm method is consistent with many functional activities and tasks of daily living that require coordinated movement of both upper and lower limbs.

Given the advantages of the leg/arm combination technique, *aquatic activities* represent one practical, field-based analog to the sophisticated modifications necessary to use all four limbs in unison. Not surprisingly, aquatic-based exercise studies on MS have been reported, though the number of subjects has been small. (Review of pertinent studies of aquatic therapy with persons diagnosed with MS can be found under "Specific Programs and Protocols in Therapy.")

Little research has examined the relationship between activities and the emotional concomitants secondary to MS. One report by Heininger (1994) provides tentative encouragement for the use of exercise in this regard. Heininger surveyed 58 subjects with MS and learned that perceived level of fitness was correlated with self-esteem. Future studies should ascertain the level of function of participants with MS (EDSS scores) to better inform the practitioner of the breadth of application of the results. In the absence of functional assessment and given the risks for cardiac and blood pressure abnormalities, the reader must assume that the subjects were experiencing only minimal involvement (i.e., little functional impairment).

Cerebral Palsy

Persons with CP are infrequently seen in rehabilitative settings after childhood for several reasons. First, the disorder is not usually progressive in nature. Second, rehabilitation efforts are usually maximized during the developmental period through direct service in traditional therapy, or more often through developmental programs associated with public schools. Third, problems secondary to CP may affect the health status of the person with CP following the developmental period (e.g., skin lesions, contractures). In the latter cases, the TR Specialist may find the adult with CP in an acute therapy setting.

Despite the deinstitutionalization of persons with disabilities in general, cases of severe CP in company with other significant impairments (e.g., severe mental retardation) may require long-term custodial care.

Young children with CP may also be seen in clinical, rehabilitative settings.

Goals for persons with CP in a clinical therapy setting may find application in leisure education efforts through outpatient and community TR programs. Primary goals are designed to correct the symptoms that present in different forms of CP: delayed ambulation, abnormal reflexes, and hypertonic or hypotonic muscles (Jansma & French, 1994; Sherrill, 1986).

Besides proper positioning, transfer, and carrying techniques, the TR Specialist may employ proactive interventions. Play activities emphasizing basic movements and movement exploration and object control activities (toy play) may prove to be useful interventions (Sherrill, 1986) for preambulation skills (e.g., crawling, balance). Motor gyms and adapted obstacle courses are sometimes used at younger ages.

Normal postural reactions may be trained through motor activities in different positions. Beginning with lying in prone and supine positions, activities on a mat may train static and dynamic pathways and responses. Playground activities and apparatus may be used as the child demonstrates competence with motor control and balance. Safety should remain a primary concern, and surfaces surrounding and supporting playground equipment should meet appropriate safety regulations. Adequate supervision should also make falls and accidents unlikely. Crawford (1989) has reported on some work with children with CP in playgrounds (see "Leisure Education").

Proper positioning is important for the TR Specialist to understand, even though it is not a major clinical function of TR. When a client with CP completes the TR program, he or she should be returned to nursing, physical therapy, or occupational therapy in the correct position. This means that close observation of the client should be made before removal from the wheelchair to assure return to the chair in the proper position. General principles for positioning (Jansma and French, 1994, p. 237) include: provide support of key body parts (e.g., neck, shoulders, hips, vertebral column), work in front of the client instead of off to the side to inhibit asymmetrical reflexes, take extra time for relaxation training, refrain from forcing range of movement, and offer slow, gradual physical assistance.

Later in the developmental period, clinical programs should turn to the improvement of strength, range of motion, and fitness as goals for interventions (Sherrill, 1986). The rationale for moving on to the fitness related goals is that progress in terms of addressing primary symptoms may have plateaued, and that intervention should now turn toward consolidating gains and maxi-

mizing motor abilities that are present through strength and endurance training.

Program goals likely to continue throughout life pertain to management of spasticity, ataxia, or athetosis. Sherrill (1986) offers guidance to the therapist relative to these common symptom patterns. She suggests frequent range of motion and stretching. Because flexors, adductors and medial rotators ("antigravity muscles") are most affected by spasticity and contractures, augmenting extensors in recreational activities is the preferred course of action. Emphasizing reciprocal movements through aquatic activities and dance are especially effective with cases of marked spasticity.

For persons exhibiting symptoms of athetosis, relaxation is very important to minimize troublesome involuntary movements. Both ataxic and athetoid symptoms increase the risk of falls later in life. Hence, balance training may be useful, although safety precautions are a must (e.g., soft surfaces to fall on, doing activities in recumbent or kneeling positions). In contrast to those with spastic symptoms, those with athetosis should work (motorically) in a symmetrical manner, holding positions, starting and stopping frequently to minimize interruptions from involuntary movements.

Secondary benefits from regular recreation participation (especially recreational exercise) include increased productivity at work, prevention of secondary disorders, and control of risk factors for the development of chronic conditions (e.g., osteoporosis).

Because many persons with CP who are employed work at manual, physically demanding tasks, fitness is essential. Some authorities (Jansma & French, 1994) recommend that they may need to be more fit just to accomplish everyday movements (e.g., working in a constant condition of hypertonic muscles).

Persons with CP run comparable risk of developing some chronic conditions (e.g., heart disease) and additional risk for other chronic conditions (e.g., osteoporosis and postural abnormalities). Hence, regular exercise and physical activity is needed to avoid or delay the onset of secondary disorders as well.

The good news for adults with CP residing in the community is that regular exercise is feasible and effective. Pitetti, Fernandez, and Lanciault (1991) studied the effects of an 8-week aerobic exercise program on several physiologic markers of fitness. Participants exercised twice weekly for 30 minutes per session at a rate of 40–70% maximum effort. The seven adult subjects (average age=30.5 years) demonstrated significant gains in physiologic work capacity by the end of the training program. The training program was safe and implemented without incident. Unfortunately, only one subject continued to exercise after completion of the training.

Nevertheless, the results demonstrate the promise of a recreationally based exercise program. Following customary health screening and clearance, similar programs should be feasible within a clinical or community TR setting. Outcome variables may have to be adjusted from physiologic measures to functional outcome measures. (See examples in Chapter 11, Muscular System, under the protocol for frailty.)

Furthermore, exercise programs for persons with CP and accompanying disabilities hold the promise of being equally effective, at least in the case of CP with mental retardation. Winnick and Short (1991) compared the fitness of subjects with CP to those with CP and mental retardation and found no significant differences between the two groups. Almost the same amount of fitness was explained with three derived factors: skinfold, grip strength, and speed/endurance.

Specific Programs and Protocols in Therapy

Head Injuries

Three protocols specific to head injuries were found in the literature: two developed at Rancho Los Amigos Hospital (one pediatric and one adult) and one developed at the Santa Clara Medical Center (Land, Marmer, Mayfield, Gerski & Murphy, 1989). The protocols are based on a rehabilitation approach and are organized into three phases that require progressively more function from the patient.

The pediatric protocol aims to promote old and new recreational skills, develop appropriate behavior for leisure participation, create positive socialization experiences, and enhance functional independence. *Phase One* orients the child and provides a sampling of the activities offered through the TR program. All activities in Phase One are within the agency and the client may function at a maximally assisted level or may not be able to participate at all. *Phase Two* requires higher cognitive functioning than Phase One, with maximally assisted to minimally assisted levels of cognitive function necessary for participation. In addition to encouraging participation in all activities within the agency, the client is now eligible for structured community-based programs. Cognitive function for *Phase Three* is at a supervised/independent level.

Goals include community reintegration and application of the leisure functioning skills acquired in Phase One and Phase Two.

Likewise, the Rancho protocol for adults with head injuries is progressive and involves three levels, but reports exclusion criteria. To be eligible, the client must exhibit some functional communication, and be assessed at functional Level VI on the Rancho Los Amigos scale (confused but appropriate). Similar to the progression with pediatric cases, the adult version of the protocol requires only minimal function for Phase One, which provides information about activities and encourages involvement.

Assuming the client responds favorably to the Phase One initiatives and improves in cognitive function, then Phase Two may be introduced. Phase Two programs increase information processing loads placed on the client by adding stimuli to the client's environment. Appropriate behavior is expected, group/social activities are added, and patients must attend to environmental information enough to show an interest.

Phase Three requires higher cognitive function capabilities, including application of skills learned through earlier participation, self-initiation, decision making, problem solving, and better memory. The goal of Phase Three is independent leisure functioning. From activity selection and planning to implementation, all activity-related responsibilities are assumed by the client in a best case scenario. Obviously, not all cases will attain complete independent leisure functioning as an endpoint, but this remains the goal.

The protocol developed by Santa Clara Valley Medical Center (Land et al., 1989) capitalizes on some aspects of the Rancho Los Amigos approach. Specifically, the Santa Clara initiative employs the Rancho Los Amigos scale to assign patients to specific interventions. The advantage of the Santa Clara approach is that it provides for involvement for all levels of cognitive function subsequent to head injury. For example, Level III patients are only able to give a localized response to specific stimuli, and even this is inconsistent. Nevertheless, the TR Specialist may discover the "hot" stimuli for a given patient at Level III and evoke prefunctional skills that the treatment team may build upon (e.g., consistently moving an extremity in the direction of a family picture or colorful balloon). Reality orientation may be included for Level III patients along with one step commands. Simple games (e.g., matching games) that may be demonstrated by the therapist may also prove to elicit meaningful behavioral responses.

The Rancho Los Amigos and Santa Clara protocols each provide for progression, although progression may not always be realized. The approaches are both based upon the assumption that intervention must begin with the functional capabilities the client currently possesses and gradually increase the information load and cognitive processing demands placed on the client's nervous system. Increments in processing demands are accomplished by adding to the complexity of the environmental array (e.g., larger groups with more people to pay attention to, more complex games with several steps and rules, and reintegration into the community where problem-solving skills are needed to adapt to a less predictable environment).

Spinal Cord Injuries

The Rancho Los Amigos pediatric protocol for head injuries applies to SCI in children as well. A protocol for children and adults with SCI was developed at Santa Clara Medical Center (Land et al., 1989). The SCI protocol was designed as a three-phase program requiring progressively more responsibility from the patient. Likewise, the TR goals at each phase are progressively more ambitious:

- Phase One—orienting the patient with activities provided at bedside
- Phase Two—orienting the patient with advanced expectations for participation in all aspects of the TR program
- Phase Three—community orientation with the expectation that the patient will assume most responsibilities

The TR protocol maximizes the attainment of the patient's leisure lifestyle. Assessment precedes actual involvement in the program, with data acquired directly from the patient and from the family and friends if necessary. Phase One establishes initial contact with the patient through passive, bedside activities while the patient is in intensive care. The TRS monitors the patient for readiness for off-unit programs. Phase Two begins when the patient is medically stable and able to tolerate a wheelchair. The protocol during Phase Two requires full involvement of the patient in all activities. Activities generally focus on socialization, physical function, and endurance. Phase Three represents the culmination of progress through the protocol, and it proves to be the most thought-provoking aspect of the Santa Clara SCI protocol. The patient takes more responsibility for his leisure through a series of community outings. Opportunities for additional responsibility include making decisions, including the family in

activities, and participating in the planning of activities. Transition into the community culminates in referral to community-based programs.

Aquatic Therapy

Aquatic-based programs are widely applicable and apt to benefit most physical disabilities. The characteristics of water favor its use among persons with mobility impairments. Buoyancy adds support to immobilized limbs and body parts so that range of motion (passive or active) may be accomplished with less pain. The flotation and support afforded the trunk makes balance in the water easier for persons with cerebellar lesions (e.g., ataxic CP) as well.

Water's resistance increases muscular strength and endurance for many persons with neurological impairments (Broach & Dattilo, 1996). Resistance may also afford an optimal amount of stress on the skeleton for those at risk for developing osteoporosis secondary to conditions (e.g., SCI) that leave them unable to ambulate and carry on weight bearing activity. The theoretical and empirical evidence for the effectiveness of water with such persons is not as clear as for the effectiveness of aquatic therapy with other symptoms and impairments.

For some disabilities, aquatic activities may present an advantage or disadvantage relative to temperature. For persons with MS who tend to be heat sensitive, cooler temperatures afforded by water activities may delay the onset of fatigue. Alternatively, for persons with arthritis, warmer water temperature helps with joint mobility and pain. However, in cases of severe hypertension and profound cardiac impairment, aquatic activities may be unsuitable if water temperatures are too warm (Hurley & Turner, 1991). Likewise, active skin lesions are more susceptible to infection from water borne bacteria, making persons with decubiti poor candidates for an aquatic program until after healing is complete. The opinion on persons with incontinence is mixed. Some (Garvey, 1991) maintain that participation is feasible with correct timing, while others (Hurley & Turner, 1991) contend that incontinence makes the person ineligible for water-based activities.

The current managed healthcare movement urges consideration of aquatics programs. Broach and Dattilo (1996) maintained that because hospital stays are shorter, chronic conditions are more prevalent and take longer to rehabilitate, and some evidence exists that health insurers are willing to reimburse services

(Beaudouin & Keller, 1994), water-based exercise and activity programs are well-suited to TR service. Professionals in TR are positioned to take the initiative to deliver ongoing, community-based intervention of low risk and probable benefit for a sustained period of time to a broad array of disability groups. The community-based TR practitioner is especially well-positioned because the majority of aquatic resources are under the direction of community recreation programs. The effectiveness of aquatic-based therapies must be regarded as suggestive, however, because the available research on water-based activities and disorders of the nervous system deals mostly with small samples and a limited number of impairments.

Woods (1992) studied the effects of individualized aquatic-based exercise on two clients with MS. The program consisted of passive stretching, active assisted range of motion, resistance exercise, modified swimming strokes, and ambulation while in the water. The fluid environment of the pool offered many advantages: buoyancy and support, resistance, cooler temperature, and protection from falls (Broach, Groff, Yaffe, Dattilo & Gast, 1995; Peterson & Bell, 1995).

The first subject, a 46-year-old female client, was introduced into the program nine years postonset (Woods, 1992). Treatment goals included improving trunk stability, maintaining function in her one minimally affected (upper) limb, and facilitating daily living skills. The subject participated in the program for three-and-a-half years. During that time, one hospitalization occurred and resulted in several months of cessation of the program. Over the course of treatment, symptoms did not worsen appreciably.

The second subject was a 43-year-old male. He began the program with some ability to ambulate but impaired balance, impaired vision, and general muscle weakness. The treatment goal for this case was to reduce spasticity. Five months of aquatic-based exercise three times per week resulted in significant improvements in walking (while in the water) and distance swam using a modified stroke and flotation device. Unfortunately he experienced a major exacerbation of symptoms and the program had to be temporarily suspended. Significant increases in spasticity and development of contractures required a change in treatment goals. The cases presented by Woods (1992) illustrate the promise and frustration that come with MS.

Broach et al. (1995) reported the results of an aquatic-based exercise program for three subjects with MS. The treatment described by Broach and her colleagues was more standardized than in the Woods

(1992) study, but the themes were similar. Subjects participated in a 45-minute program of water-based exercise twice a week for 20 weeks. Significant improvements in endurance and gross motor ability were noted. The improvements in functional fitness corresponded to improvement in functional tasks that involved gross muscle activity (e.g., riding a bike, climbing stairs, vacuuming). The absence of improvement in fine motor tasks and function may have been a result of the nature of the training program (focusing in gross muscle activity in preference to fine motor activity) and/or the nature of the disease (preferentially affecting distal muscles in the extremities).

In an earlier study, Gehlsen, Grisby, and Winert (1984) assessed the effects of a 10-week water aerobics class (swimming and water-based calisthenics) on the upper and lower extremity strength of 10, ambulatory subjects with MS. Subjects exercised at 60% to 75% maximum heart rate (typical for cardiovascular training in able-bodied adults). Significant and consistent improvement across several levels of resistance was evident for upper extremities. However, the results were mixed for the lower extremities, with improvement reported at some intensities of resistance, but not others.

Broach, Groff, and Dattilo (1997) reported an aquatic therapy intervention with four young adult subjects with paraplegia. The researchers introduced aquatic therapy using a multiple baseline design, wherein subjects begin the program at slightly different times to serve as temporary controls. The intervention focused on swimming instruction and practice using an adaptive swimming method. Three of the subjects completed the 15-week program at a rate of 3 times per week for 1 hour per session. However, one subject participated in the program for only 10 weeks because of scheduling conflicts with school. Subjects completed a 12-minute aerobic swimming test before practice swimming portion of each session. Endurance increased noticeably, but vital capacity did not change. Relative percent of body fat decreased as well.

Beaudouin and Keller (1994) interviewed subjects with disabilities following an aquatics program. The responses indicated perceived benefits of the program, especially related to fitness and socialization. Although subject disabilities are not reported in detail, some individuals with SCI and head injury did participate in the aquatic intervention. They reported that evaluation of the program showed the strength, endurance, and flexibility improved along with psychological measures (e.g., depressive symptoms). However, the report does not make it possible to associate specific changes with specific types of impairments.

The general picture of aquatic interventions for persons with neurological impairments is positive and promising. Research indicates that interventions may systematically produce an array of physical changes associated with primary problems (e. g., spasticity) and secondary problems (e.g., depression) of persons with disorders of nervous tissue. This is consistent with the favorable results of aquatic therapy for persons with skeletal and joint disorders reported previously.

Leisure Education

Head Injuries

Stumbo and Bloom (1990) showed continuity in programming by demonstrating goals commonly associated with therapy—such as problem solving, better memory, and improved attention span—through a program of leisure education. Problem solving may be addressed through the use of leisure scenarios, narratives about real challenges the person may face relative to leisure participation in the community. Leisure experience diaries were suggested as a means to improving memory. Use of discussion groups requires the individual to selectively attend to communication from others in the group. Furthermore, the group setting also affords the person an opportunity to practice social skills (e.g., eye contact, active listening).

Several studies converge on the topic of community reintegration for persons with head injuries. Baker-Roth, McLaughlin, Weitzenkamp, and Womeldorff (1995) reported the case of a 30-year-old female who sustained a head injury. The case highlights the active, facilitative role played by the TR Specialist in the client's transition back in to the community over the course of 3 years. The client regressed into some previously contraindicated behaviors (e.g., depression and marital problems led to a resumption of substance abuse) during this time, while making slow but steady progress toward independence. Self-esteem and confidence improved as participation in active recreational pursuits supported the functional gains that resulted in ambulation. The subject adjusted to stress more readily, often using leisure activity as a coping device. Some of the activities introduced by the TR Specialist failed, as the client was not physically or emotionally prepared to handle the activity demands (e.g., tennis). However, progress continued and the client assumed responsibility for most of her leisure choices and the details prerequisite to participation. She still sought occasional support from the TRS at the time the case study was published.

The actions of the TRS opened windows of access to community resources necessary to satisfying leisure participation. Techniques used by the TRS included providing information about safe community programs, identifying financial resources (e.g., activity scholarships), facilitating transportation alternatives, and educating service providers about underserved groups.

The findings of Baker-Roth et al. (1995) are consistent with a number of other papers. The endpoint of the intervention attained by the client in Baker-Roth et al. was an almost independent, self-determined leisure lifestyle. However, a state of being empowered is useless unless the client has the capabilities to act on that freedom. Further, Howard and Claiman (1994) remind practitioners that "...being empowered does not necessarily mean going it alone" (p. 20). The crucial feature of a transition/facilitator role is to be cognizant of when to let the client take control. As a general rule, the TR specialist should err on the side of empowering the client, even though it may sometimes result in failure, as it sometimes did in the case study described previously.

Likewise, Kwan and Sulzberger (1994) maintained that acting as a bridge to community resources was an appropriate role for the TRS when working with persons with head injuries. They listed many of the same techniques articulated by Baker-Roth and associates, such as providing information about resources and joint programming initiatives between clinical and community-based agencies.

Follow-up through transition programs and use of liaison personnel (as in the Baker-Roth et al. case study) is consistent with another recurring theme in the head injury literature: complete rehabilitation in the case of persons with head injuries takes longer than the norm (e.g., Krane, 1994). The lengthy recovery may be a function of the time needed for brain tissue to repair itself, the time needed for undamaged areas of the brain to take over the responsibilities of the damaged areas, the time premorbid conditions take to reemerge after discharge, the time necessary for adequate repetition for mastery of component tasks (Kwan & Sulzberger, 1994), or a combination of all of these factors. Whatever the reason, the literature is quite clear about the need for protracted rehabilitation efforts. Specific to TR intervention, the transition effort that spanned three years in the Baker-Roth et al. case study illustrates the long-term commitment needed for the effectiveness of interventions to emerge. Multiple methods and resources are also necessary to successful TR intervention because some of the activity experiments are bound to fail.

Other leisure education strategies have been less successful. Zoerink and Lauener (1991) reported on an experiment designed to determine whether values clarification was more effective than group discussion in inducing favorable changes in leisure attitudes, leisure satisfaction, and perceived freedom in leisure. Twelve subjects with head injuries were randomly assigned to values clarification and group discussion treatments. Researchers found no differences between the groups for leisure satisfaction, leisure attitudes, or perceived freedom in leisure. The authors attributed the nonsignificant findings to idiosyncratic differences between subjects and the reduction of statistical power associated with a small sample. The authors concluded that applied behavior analysis (single subject methods) might be more productive with this population because of the dramatic individual differences typical of this group.

Spinal Cord Injuries

Despite the fact that most persons with SCI are discharged back into the community following acute rehabilitation, little research has been completed to support the effectiveness of TR in facilitating the transition. The idea that TR should play a leading role in the reintegration of patients with SCI back into the community seems conceptually sound, however.

Zoerink (1997) reported the results of a survey of 43 orthopedically impaired adults residing in rural communities and found that leisure satisfaction was significantly and positively related to perceived health, but negatively correlated with depressive symptoms. Although the specific disabilities of the subjects were not reported, all had acquired impairments. Similar findings were reported earlier (Kinney & Coyle, 1992) in a sample of persons with a mix of disabilities (21% SCI). Leisure satisfaction was the most significant predictor of life satisfaction.

Several reports, however, have revealed that persons with SCI are less active than their able-bodied peers, and more inclined to passive, solitary, and homebound recreation. This state of recreation participation (or nonparticipation) exists even though more than two-thirds of subjects in one study reported that they had an excess of time on their hands (Coyle et al., 1993). Further, some research lends insight into the reasons for the lower than acceptable quality of recreation among persons with SCI. Obviously, the injury alone presents a continuing challenge to the leisure repertoire of the person with SCI long after discharge.

This is confirmed in papers by Coyle et al. (1993), Coyle and Kinney (1990), and Caldwell, Adolph, and Gilbert (1989). Lack of ability and lack of skill are reliably reported among the leading barriers to recreation participation. However, lack of ability because of the practical limitations imposed by SCI is not the same as the limit imposed by lack of skill.

Lack of skill relates not as much to the impairment as to the lack of opportunity, resources, instruction and adaptation prerequisite to participation. Clearly, lack of ability attributable to the real limitations imposed by the impairment is addressed by short-term and long-term rehabilitation efforts. But lack of skill is an educational matter, not wholly attributable to physical limitation. Coyle et al. (1993) found that lack of skill was the second most frequently reported barrier to participation among the subjects with health problems secondary to SCI. Caldwell et al. (1989) also confirmed that lack of skill was a significant barrier for their 155 subjects with SCI in a survey subsequent to discharge back into the community.

After studying boredom among subjects with SCI, Caldwell and Weissinger (1994) stated:

> Emphasizing opportunities for free choice (self-determination) in TR programs without initial attention to elevating levels of perceived competence may be ineffective in assisting persons to develop fully satisfying leisure. (p. 23)

A similar theme was identified by Caldwell and Lee (1994/1995) following analysis of qualitative interview data from 20 subjects with SCI: The conundrum of building an aspiration to a leisure lifestyle while in rehabilitation that may not be achieved after discharge into the community.

Caldwell et al. (1989) conducted follow-up phone interviews with 155 persons with SCI after discharge. They discovered that those subjects who had participated in leisure counseling (leisure counseling included assessment, skill development, community orientation, counseling, and resource information) felt better prepared to deal with free time. But those same subjects who participated in leisure counseling also said that they felt more bored, less satisfied, and reported more internal barriers to leisure participation. Caldwell et al. (1989) explained these rather contradictory findings in a manner similar to Caldwell and Lee (1994/1995) five years later. They argued that leisure counseling raised expectations of the subjects that the community could not satisfy, skills may not have been developed to an optimal extent, and the communities may not have been as receptive as anticipated.

The studies of Coyle et al. (1993), Caldwell et al. (1989), and Caldwell and Weissinger (1994) do not provide an inspiring picture of recreation for persons with SCI in the community. They demonstrate that lack of skill consistently appears on lists of significant barriers provided by persons with SCI. These data further indicate that more attention should be directed toward the acquisition of skills and competence in specific activities as well as the street smarts and advocacy talents necessary to access recreation opportunities in the community.

Hedrick (1985, 1986) reported one of the few research efforts designed to learn more about the effectiveness of leisure education with persons with SCI. Fifteen children (average age 13.2 years) with physical disabilities (specific disabilities not reported) participated in a tennis instruction and participation program in the community. Subjects were randomly assigned to one of three groups: homogeneous learning and performance (neither experience was integrated), homogeneous learning and heterogeneous performance (only the performance phase was integrated with nondisabled peers), and heterogeneous learning and performance (both experiences were integrated). Subjects were assessed on tennis skills and perceived competence.

Subjects in the heterogeneous learning and performance group did not experience significant gains in skill, whereas the other two groups did. Subjects in the homogeneous learning/heterogeneous performance group faired better in perceived competence, especially physical competence. Hedrick (1985) concluded that persons with physical disabilities might learn more and feel better about their competence if they acquired skills in a segregated environment before being integrated into a regular sport participation setting. He further explained that subjects may have been more anxious in the heterogeneous learning condition because they had not yet acquired the skill. Hedrick speculated that once comparable skill was acquired in a segregated setting, the differences between the participants in an integrated setting would not be as salient, thus easing the integration effort and increasing the prospects of tolerance and acceptance by nondisabled peers.

Further analysis of these data confirmed earlier suspicions. Nondisabled peers were asked their perceptions of the competence of the subjects with physical disabilities. The pattern of perceptions was identical to the perceptions of the subjects of themselves—subjects in the homogeneous learning/heterogeneous performance and the homogeneous learning/homogeneous performance groups received higher appraisals of tennis efficacy from their able-bodied peers than subjects in the heterogeneous learning/heterogeneous performance condition. Again, Hedrick concluded that integrating adolescents with physical disabilities with able-bodied peers who are markedly more skilled served to inhibit the formation of favorable perceptions and the acquisition of tennis skills.

Hence, the person with a physical disability needs leisure education to acquire knowledge and skills necessary for satisfying participation in leisure activities. The need for leisure education includes both the short-term (e.g., while in acute care and rehabilitation) and the long-term (e.g., after discharge into the community). Furthermore, if Hedrick's findings are more broadly applicable, then skills and competencies should be developed in a segregated setting. Once suitable competence is developed, the person can be integrated with a reasonable expectation of acceptance as an equal. Hedrick's findings further imply that the adolescent with a physical impairment that limits mobility must possess the capability to reciprocate in terms of activity-specific behaviors and competencies if he/she expects integration to be genuine and not just empty compliance with regulations. To *reciprocate* means to execute requisite leisure skills at an acceptable level of competence for a given activity.

The need for further research in leisure education for persons with SCI is unmistakable. Successful adaptation and adjustment of the client to the community depend on more in-depth knowledge of the dynamics of successful transition back into the community and the role leisure plays in that transition. If TR is not successful in teaching and enhancing leisure skills and competencies, then the client is preordained to underachieve and articulate resentment of TR for promoting expectations of a satisfying leisure lifestyle after discharge (Caldwell et al., 1989)

Cerebral Palsy

Because CP is considered a developmental disorder, students with CP are eligible for considerable service through the public schools. While the child is eligible for educational services from ages 3–21, community-based TR may support the efforts made within the schools. This may occur in several ways. The community program may serve as a provider of the resources needed for some programs (e.g., aquatic exercise). Many public schools do not have the resources to offer all of the recreational, exercise, and physical activity programs that may benefit the student. In this case, simple networking and consultation may benefit the student.

Most public schools count reintegration and transition into the community among the goals for the student with CP. Independent or semi-independent community dwelling is facilitated if the student has contact with community resources before graduation. Leisure education may be part of transition education near graduation. Mahon and Bullock (1992) have successfully implemented leisure education with other disability groups, and Luken (1993) has described a program of leisure education to aid the transition of persons with psychiatric impairments back into the community. These models may be applicable for persons with CP.

Once the students with CP have graduated from the public schools, they often become productive members of the community. Leisure education may continue, including programs of instruction (e.g., swimming lessons), adaptations needed for participation, or initiatives designed to ease integration into regular program participation.

Instruction through leisure education programs for persons with more severe involvement may encompass some of the same goals listed under the "Therapy" section of this chapter. Instruction in exercise, sport, and aquatic participation may support the goals of decreasing risks for developing secondary impairments, controlling spasticity, or increasing strength and endurance. For instance, Crawford (1989) implemented leisure skills instruction and reinforcement to induce use of playground equipment among a small group of children with severe handicaps. Among the subjects were two children with both ataxic CP and mental retardation. The 7-year-old improved use of one piece of playground equipment, but not with a second. The 10-year-old subject showed interest in two pieces of apparatus, but did not learn how to use either. Those subjects who learned how to use a new piece of apparatus were also those who improved their social skills.

Recreation Participation

Head Injuries

Potter, Smith, and Finegan (1994) interviewed 22 persons (mean age 31) with head injuries following discharge and collected data pertaining to their leisure activities before and after injury. They found that social activities fell by 62%. Those able to maintain a higher level of social involvement had full-time jobs. The authors reasoned that full-time employment supported more involvement in social leisure because of the contacts originating on the job, and because of the income which could be used to secure access to more social activities. Also those employed full-time were likely less impaired functionally, although the Potter et al. study did not report level of functional impairment for their subjects.

The results of Harwood and Smale (1990) were consistent with the findings of Potter et al. (1994). Data about preinjury and postinjury recreation participation were gathered from teenage subjects (mean age 17) who had experienced head injuries. Like Potter and associates, Harwood and Smale found a dramatic drop in the amount and quality of leisure participation. A 50% decline in active recreation participation was accompanied by a 44% increase in passive activities. Likewise, support from various sources seemed to make a difference. In this case, family involvement was positively correlated with the most active participation patterns.

Together, the work of Potter et al. and Harwood and Smale further the argument for a variety of support networks as the person with a head injury makes the transition into the community. "The results indicated that continued support following discharge is necessary for the adolescent to reestablish his or her independent leisure lifestyle" (Harwood & Smale, 1990, p. 5). Moreover, data on recreation participation patterns following cessation of active treatment and leisure education serve to demonstrate the therapeutic role that may fall within the responsibilities assumed by the community TR professional.

Spinal Cord Injuries

Coyle and Kinney (1990) produced the most comprehensive survey of recreation participation among persons with SCI. They interviewed 790 persons with a variety of physical disabilities (most frequently reported: 23% SCI, 16% CP, 11% MS, 11% visually impaired). Less than one third (31%) worked either full-time or part-time, and most reported having an excess amount of time on their hands. Consistent with earlier reports, passive, homebound, solitary activities accounted for much of the leisure repertoire profile of the sample. Reading (23%), television (19%), socializing (15%), individual, noncompetitive sports (11%), and music/art appreciation (8%) were the most frequently reported activities. Surprisingly, 41% said they participated in an integrated activity, but 46% could not identify at least three accessible facilities. Satisfaction with leisure was further mediated by some contextual variables. Those with an acquired disability were less satisfied with leisure than subjects with congenital disabilities, and subjects with more severe impairments were less satisfied with their leisure.

Coyle and Kinney (1990) maintained that the sedentary profile of leisure reported by their subjects with physical disabilities did not distinguish them significantly from the profile of leisure customarily reported by a cross-section of the U. S. population. Nevertheless, given the scientific evidence that supports the health benefits of a more active leisure lifestyle, advocacy and creative programming seem to be in order with respect to upgrading to quality of the typical leisure profile of a person with a physical disability. On the other hand, these data bring into question the earlier conclusion that the long-term adjustment of persons with SCI was fairly good—do the results indicate satisfaction for the long term, or resignation?

Cerebral Palsy

Considerable research has accumulated about elite athletes with CP. The results may lend insight into the nature of attitudes, motives, and psychological benefits that all persons with CP may derive from sport and exercise participation. Persons with CP that participate in competitive sports at the highest level present an almost identical psychological profile as athletes who are not disabled.

Two important psychological variables that determine quality of life for persons with disabilities are self-actualization and self-concept. Sherrill and Rainbolt (1988) found similar self-actualization profiles between athletes with CP and able-bodied athletes. Likewise, Sherrill, Hinson, Gench, Kennedy, and Low (1990) learned that the self-concepts of 158 young athletes (52 were CP) were within normal ranges for total score and subscale scores on a standard self-concept inventory.

Cooper, Sherrill, and Marshall (1986) compared two groups of 165 total athletes with CP on attitudes toward physical activity. One group was comprised of ambulatory subjects; the other group consisted of athletes with CP who were nonambulatory. No differences were discovered between two groups of athletes with CP on various dimensions of attitude toward physical activity.

While these results serve to support the potential for some persons with CP to transcend their disabilities and share common ground with their peers without disabilities, not all of the news is good. Inevitably, all athletes need to either cease participation in their sport or compete at a lower level of performance. When ending a sport career, the athlete with CP may be in for a considerable letdown.

Martin, Adams-Mushett, and Smith (1995) studied the 57 adolescent swimmers with disabilities (24 with CP) and found that they had a strong self-identity, moderate to strong social identity, and strong competitiveness and goal orientation. The data also showed that the subjects had a strong desire to attain their competitive goals. In sum, Martin et al. concluded that they had a strong athletic identity and that their sport was very important to them. However, Martin et al. argued that the reliance on sport alone for self-identity may make them more susceptible to psychological problems when unable to participate. Hence, encouraging a diversity of leisure interests may help to minimize the letdown associated with cessation of any one activity.

Some data also suggest another way athletes with CP differ from their nondisabled peers. Dummer, Ewing, Habeck, and Overton (1987) examined the causal attributions that 147 athletes with CP used to explain their performances. To their surprise the customary internal, stable attributions for successful performance were not consistent among participants. Athletes made use of both stable and unstable attributions. Winners were more likely than losers to use both internal and external attributions for success, contrary to the literature. Those athletes who reported that they were satisfied with their performance (regardless of win or loss) were also more apt to say that they felt good about their performance (e.g., tried hard, enjoy competition, able to meet the challenge). Satisfaction with performance (win or lose) was the best predictor of persistence in a sport in this sample.

Like the balance of the population, however, most persons with CP do not participate at an elite level— recreational participation is the norm. Blinde and McClung (1997) studied the effects of a variety of physically active, recreational pursuits of 23 subjects (of the 23, 6 had CP, 4 were head injured, 5 were paraplegic, 3 were quadriplegic). Qualitative interviews were used to gather data about the physical self after participation in activities they selected for 5–10 weeks. Some subjects, however, extended their participation for a longer period of time. Several themes emerged from the interview data. Subjects experienced their bodies in new ways, enhanced their perceptions of their own physical attributes, redefined their physical capabilities, increased their confidence to pursue new activities, enhanced perceptions of social-self, expanded social contacts, and initiated social activities in other contexts.

Blinde and McClung (1997) concluded that the physical demands of the activities offered even at a recreational level were sufficient to provoke important and positive changes in psychological states. They attributed success of the program to five key factors. First, the activities gave the subjects a sense of control they did not normally perceive in everyday life. Second, most of the activities were new ones for the subjects. Third, companions were provided for instruction and support of each subject's efforts. Fourth, social development was fostered through participation in integrated settings as much as possible. Finally, necessary transportation was provided to circumvent one of the most frequently cited obstacles to participation in the literature—transportation problems.

Sports for Persons with Neurological Impairments

One way in which a more active leisure lifestyle manifests itself among persons with physical disabilities is through a sporting career. Physical and psychological benefits are apt to accrue as a result of participation in active, sports pursuits.

Certainly, the type of health benefit depends on the nature of the sport and practice associated with preparation for competition. For example, weightlifting competition would improve muscular strength, whereas long-distance competitions for persons in wheelchairs would be more likely to contribute to muscular endurance and cardiovascular fitness. The physical and psychological benefits of sport participation among persons with physical disabilities are represented by the leading motive for participation (fitness) reported in one study (Brasilie, Kleiber & Harnisch, 1991).

The psychological benefits of sport participation for persons with physical disabilities are similar to those of able-bodied peers who participate in sport. Porretta and Moore (1996/1997) reviewed the literature relevant to the psychology of sport participation by persons with physical disabilities. Their report was organized according to disability group (e.g., neuromuscular, CP). They concluded that "...with few exceptions to date, the results of sport psychology research with persons possessing disabilities are similar to results obtained in studies with nondisabled athletes" (p. 89). The psychological picture of athletes with physical disabilities was consistently one that mirrored that of able-bodied athletes with respect to self-actualization, self-esteem, self-concept, attitude toward physical activity, and mood.

Patrick (1986) compared novice wheelchair athletes (n = 10), veteran wheelchair athletes (n = 12), and nonathletes in wheelchairs (n = 12) before and after a competition. Novice wheelchair athletes showed significant improvement in both self-concept and acceptance of disability compared to veteran wheelchair athletes and nonathletes. Though very tentative because of design and power limitations, Patrick's findings point optimistically toward early psychological benefit from sport participation for persons with disabilities.

Motives for participation were studied by Brasilie et al. (1991) when he asked 158 athletes with disabilities and 116 athletes without disabilities a series of questions about their motives for participation. The reasons for sport participation were compared for persons with and without disabilities and correlated highly ($r = 0.83$). In the same study, responses were subjected to factor analysis to identify motivational sets that would contribute to a more parsimonious understanding of sport motivation. Five factors—fitness incentives, ego incentives, task incentives, social integration incentives, and social affective incentives—were identified. The factors were most associated with an intrinsic, task-motivated orientation toward sport. Importance of the sport to the participant was the best predictor of the motivational factors.

Reporting on the cessation of sport participation, Martin (1996) sketched a framework for understanding and investigating the topic. He maintained that *transition theory* provides a sound method for understanding the potential positive and negative factors surrounding transition out of a sporting career by person with disabilities. Three types of transitions are possible when moving out of a sporting career. An anticipated versus unexpected transition mediates the ease of change, with unanticipated cessation (e.g., a career-ending injury) leading to the most difficulty in adjustment. A change may be anticipated but not occur and be the source of adjustment problems, as in the case of a person not making a team. Chronic hassle transition is caused by recurrent injuries that take a toll and frustrate the athlete.

Martin used findings for able-bodied athletes to infer possible scenarios for athletes with disabilities transitioning out of a sport. Unanticipated transitions present the greatest adjustment challenge for able-bodied athletes. Furthermore, persons with a stronger sport identity have more difficulty ceasing active sport involvement. Martin maintained that athletes with disabilities may be more at risk for adjustment problems attributable to strong sport identity. He reasoned that because persons with disabilities experience pronounced underemployment and unemployment and are thereby deprived of a work-related identity, they are more likely to invest a major portion of their identity in sport.

Martin also outlined several strategies for easing the adjustment to the cessation of a sporting career that may be implemented by TR Specialists:

- Encourage diversification of interests
- Generalize mental skills developed in sports
- Teach coping skills through leisure education
- Help the retired athlete find other roles within the sport (e.g., coaching)
- Volunteer in support of the sport

Practical Applications

Autonomic Hyperreflexia (Autonomic Dysreflexia)

This condition is common in persons with SCI at mid-thoracic levels and higher. Usually, input from the brainstem (medulla oblongata) vasomotor center regulates sympathetic stimulation (T1–L2 segments of the spinal cord) of the vascular system. Normally sympathetic stimulation causes constriction through contraction of the involuntary muscle in the walls of blood vessels. The net effect raises the blood pressure of the individual. In the person without a spinal cord lesion this response serves a useful purpose because the hypertension can be regulated and is only a temporary response to an emergency or threat. However, in the person with SCI, parts of the sympathetic division in the thoracic and lumbar segments of the spinal cord are isolated from the input from the vasomotor center. The result is a condition known as autonomic hyperreflexia— a rapid and uncontrolled elevation in blood pressure.

The condition should be treated as an emergency and addressed immediately. Symptoms follow a clear pattern. Besides elevated blood pressure and a slowed heart rate, external evidence of autonomic hyperreflexia includes the following symptoms above the level of the lesion: flushed skin, profuse sweating, headache, and anxiety. Piloerection (gooseflesh) is also commonly observed below the level of the lesion.

Following contact with the appropriate medical staff, the practitioner should bring the person into a full, upright position (or at least elevate the head) and remove all binding (e.g., leg hose, abdominal binders). If possible, the bladder should be emptied.

Temperature Regulation and Postural Hypotension

Problems with temperature regulation and postural hypotension (excessively low blood pressure) are also common problems for persons with SCI. The TRS should be vigilant for dizziness, excessive sweating, and pale appearance—all signs of possible postural hypotension. Postural hypotension may be avoided by slow changes in posture. The TRS should monitor the wearing apparel of persons with SCI carefully to assure adequate cooling in warm conditions, and sufficient clothing to prevent chilling in cooler temperatures.

Incontinence

Inability to control voiding is a common problem for persons with neurological impairments, especially those that involve the spinal cord (e.g., SCI, spina bifida). Normal bladder function relies on inhibition of the involuntary muscle of the bladder wall (the detrusor muscle) to allow for filling. The reflex voiding center is located in sacral segments of the spinal cord. Sacral segments of the spinal cord also innervate the external sphincter to allow for voluntary control of voiding. Normal voiding consists of low pressure filling and storage and complete emptying of the bladder.

Neurogenic spastic bladder is the more common type of incontinence. In persons with SCI above sacral segments, control of voiding is disrupted because the brainstem control center is no longer connected with the reflex-voiding center. The result is involuntary contraction of the bladder via the voiding reflex, which remains functional. Voiding often occurs well before complete filling. This is combined with incomplete emptying, which puts the person at greater risk for infections of the urinary system and damage to the kidneys and bladder.

Neurogenic flaccid bladder is caused by a low SCI in the sacral segments or spina bifida. Unlike spastic bladder, the person with flaccid bladder experiences complete filling of the bladder and even overfilling because the voiding reflex is disrupted with sacral levels of damage to the spinal cord and supporting structures.

Although not a central concern of the TRS, bladder management may be necessary during recreational activities, especially on extended, off-site trips. This may be as simple as providing a private place for self-catheterization. Clean and careful procedures should be used at all times in emptying collection devices to avoid infection of the urinary system. The practitioner should acquire knowledge of each client's bladder program and idiosyncrasies prior to intervention, especially in preparation for extended trips.

Bowel elimination is regulated by structures comparable to those for urination. However, bowel programs are subject to some advantages. Elimination of the bowel is less frequent and can be timed more consistently than bladder voiding in the normal adult. Dietary management can support regulation of the bowel (e.g., extra fiber, high fluid intake). Artificial stimulants may also supplement elimination. Again, the TR Specialist should take bowel programs into consideration when planning activities.

Seizures

Safety is the major concern during a seizure episode, especially when the practitioner is in the field with a client. Keeping the person clear of furniture and other environmental obstructions is essential. If the individual does not end the episode spontaneously after a short time, medical support should be contacted immediately. In any case, a seizure episode should be reported to the medical staff for documentation and evaluation of drug management protocols. Drug compliance is often essential to successful management of seizures. The TR Specialist should be cognizant of existing drug management during planning and be prepared to assure compliance if the client must take the drug during recreational activity, especially on trips off-site. Noncompliance with drug management is the most frequent cause of recurrence of a seizure.

Head Injuries

Interventions with persons with head injuries should be expected to run longer than other groups of persons with disabilities before observing effectiveness of treatment. Krane (1994) has discussed the following strategies for working with persons with head injuries:

- Persons with head injuries usually respond better to consistent and quiet feedback rather than unsystematic reinforcement
- If the choice is one of understimulation or risking overstimulation, err on the side of too little stimulation (the person may have difficulty attending to more stimuli and sources of information in the environment)
- Memory compensation strategies may be necessary (use reminders, detailed calendars, name badges and other simple strategies to reduce the demands on memory and decrease the risk of overstimulation)
- Develop socially appropriate strategies for dealing with stress through recreation and physical exertion

Cerebral Palsy

Positioning and transportation strategies are essential to successful implementation of recreation programs for persons with CP. Proper lifting and transfer techniques are essential to the safety of both the therapist and the client. Thorough planning and preparation can eliminate or minimize the need for actual physical lifting of the client. For instance, good candidates for programs off-site should have minimal transfer skills (e.g., from wheelchair to bus seat), be accompanied by appropriate support staff trained in transfers and transportation, or be able to articulate clear directions for transfer and manual transportation in the event of an emergency (e.g., evacuation of a recreation site because of a fire). The TR Specialist can ease the working relationship with the client by integrating postural exercise into the regular activities or setting aside a time to work on specific tasks.

Chapter Summary

This chapter examined the nervous system and addressed the following key concepts:

- Nervous tissue is the most complex in the body. For this reason, it does repair itself very well.

- The nervous system is responsible for thought and movement control as well as for maintenance of the body's internal environment.

- A wide variety of disorders may affect the nervous system. The extent and severity of the impairment is depends on the area damaged.

- Recreational-level exercise programs are feasible and effective with most persons with a variety of neurological impairments.

- Research suggests that leisure activities may be crucial to successful transition from pre-injury to postinjury lifestyle.

- Programs for persons with brain injuries have better results when an "intensive" approach is used and outcomes focus on deficits in memory, attention, processing, and emotional instability.

References

Baker-Roth, S., McLaughlin, E., Weitzenkamp, D., and Womeldorff, L. (1995). The impact of a therapeutic recreation community liaison of successful re-integration of individuals with traumatic brain injury. *Therapeutic Recreation Journal, 29*, 316–323.

Beaudouin, N. M. and Keller, M. J. (1994). Aquatics solutions: A continuum of services for individuals with physical disabilities in the community. *Therapeutic Recreation Journal, 28*, 193–202.

Berryman, D., James, A., and Trader, B. (1991). The benefits of therapeutic recreation in physical medicine. In C. P. Coyle, W. B. Kinney, B. Riley, and J. W. Shank (Eds.), *The benefits of therapeutic recreation: A consensus view* (pp. 235–288). Ravensdale, WA: Idyll Arbor.

Blake, J. G. (1991). Therapeutic recreation assessment and intervention with a patient with quadriplegia. *Therapeutic Recreation Journal, 25*, 71–75.

Blinde, E. M. and McClung, L. R. (1997). Enhancing the physical and social self through recreational activity: Accounts of individuals with physical disabilities. *Adapted Physical Activity Quarterly, 14*, 327–344.

Brasilie, F. M., Kleiber, D. A., and Harnisch, D. (1991). Analysis of participation incentives among athletes with and without disabilities. *Therapeutic Recreation Journal, 25*, 18–33.

Broach, E. and Dattilo, J. (1996). Aquatic therapy: A viable therapeutic recreation intervention, *Therapeutic Recreation Journal, 30*, 213–229.

Broach, E., Groff, D., and Dattilo, J. (1997). Effects of an aquatic therapy program on adults with spinal cord injuries. *Therapeutic Recreation Journal, 31*, 159–172.

Broach, E., Groff, D., Yaffe, R., Dattilo, J., and Gast, D. (1995). Effects of aquatics therapy on physical behavior of adults with multiple sclerosis. *Symposium on Leisure Research Abstracts*, 26.

Caldwell, L. L., Adolph, S., and Gilbert, A. (1989). Caution! Leisure counselors at work: Long term effects of leisure counseling. *Therapeutic Recreation Journal, 23*, 41–49.

Caldwell, L. L. and Lee, Y. (1994/1995). Perceptions of therapeutic recreation among people with spinal cord injury. *ATRA Annual, 5*, 13–26.

Caldwell, L. L. and Weissinger, E. (1993). Factors influencing free time boredom in a sample of persons with spinal cord injuries. *Therapeutic Recreation Journal, 28*, 18–24.

Carter, M. J., Van Andel, G. E., and Robb, G. M. (1995*). Therapeutic Recreation: A practical approach* (2nd ed.). Prospect Heights, IL: Waveland.

Cooper, M. A., Sherrill, C., and Marshall, D. (1986). Attitudes toward physical activity of elite cerebral palsied athletes. *Adapted Physical Activity Quarterly, 3*, 14–21.

Coyle, C. P. and Kinney, W. B. (1990). Leisure characteristics of adults with physical disabilities. *Therapeutic Recreation Journal, 24*, 64–73.

Coyle, C. P., Lesnik-Emas, S., and Kinney, W. B. (1994). Predicting life satisfaction among adults with spinal cord injuries. *Rehabilitation Psychology, 39*, 95–112.

Coyle, C. P. and Santiago, M. C. (1995). Aerobic training and depressive symptomatology in adults with physical disabilities. *Archives of Physical Medicine and Rehabilitation, 76*, 647–652.

Coyle, C. P., Shank, J. W., Kinney, W., and Hutchins, D. A. (1993). Psychosocial functioning and changes in leisure lifestyle among individuals with chronic secondary health problems related to spinal cord injury. *Therapeutic Recreation Journal, 27*, 239–252.

Crawford, M. E. (1989). The development of age appropriate outdoor playground behaviors in severely disabled children. In F. N. Humphrey and J. H. Humphrey (Eds.), *Recreation: Current selected research* (pp. 91–108). New York, NY: AMS Press.

Crewe, N. M. and Krause, J. S. (1990). An eleven-year follow-up of adjustment to spinal cord injury. *Rehabilitation Psychology, 35*, 205–210.

Davis, G. M. (1993). Exercise capacity of individuals with paraplegia. *Medicine & Science in Sports & Exercise, 25*, 423–432.

Dordel, H. J. (1989). Intensive mobility training as a means of late rehabilitation after brain injury. *Adapted Physical Quarterly, 6*, 176–187.

Dummer, G. M., Ewing, M. E., Habeck, R. V., and Overton, S. R. (1987). Attributions of athletes with cerebral palsy. *Adapted Physical Activity Quarterly, 4*, 276–292.

Fazio, S. M. and Fralish, K. B. (1988). A survey of leisure and recreation programs offered by agencies serving traumatic head injured adults. *Therapeutic Recreation Journal, 22*, 46–54.

Figoni, S. F. (1993). Exercise responses and quadriplegia. *Medicine & Science in Sports & Exercise, 25*, 433–441.

Figoni, S. F. and Glaser, R. M. (1993). Arm and leg exercise stress testing in a person with quadriparesis. *Clinical Kinesiology, 46*, 25–36.

Figoni, S. F. and Glaser, R. M. (1995a). Development of a hybrid exercise system for spinal cord injured individuals. Abstracts of research papers presented at the annual ACTA Clinical Scientific Conference 1994.

Figoni, S. F. and Glaser, R. M. (1995b). Peak physiologic responses of trained quadriplegics during arm, leg, and hybrid exercise in upright and reclined postures. Abstracts of research papers presented at the annual ACTA Clinical Scientific Conference 1994.

Figoni, S. F. and Glaser, R. M. (1995c). Training effects of upright hybrid exercise on peak physiologic responses in quadriplegics. Abstracts of research papers presented at the annual ACTA Clinical Scientific Conference 1994.

Garvey, L. A. (1991). Spinal cord injury and aquatics. *Clinical Management, 11*, 21–24.

Gehlsen, G., Grisby, S., and Winert, D. (1984). Effects of an aquatic fitness program on the muscular strength and endurance of patients with multiple sclerosis. *Physical Therapy, 64*, 653–657.

Groff, D. and Dattilo, J. (1994). Adolescents with spinal cord injuries: attitudes toward leisure and recreation. *Symposium on Leisure Research Abstracts,* 19.

Harwood, M. and Smale, B. J. (1990). Recreation, rehabilitation, and the leisure independence of head injured adolescents. *Symposium on Leisure Research Abstracts,* 57.

Hedrick, B. N. (1985). The effect of wheelchair tennis perception and mainstreaming upon the perceptions of competence of physically disabled adolescents. *Therapeutic Recreation Journal, 19*, 34-46.

Hedrick, B. N. (1986). Wheelchair sport as a mechanism for altering the perceptions of the nondisabled regarding their disabled peers' competence. *Therapeutic Recreation Journal, 20*, 72–84.

Heininger, E. J. (1994). The relationships among perceived physical fitness, physical activity patterns and self-esteem for individuals with multiple sclerosis. *Symposium on Leisure Research Abstracts,* 20.

Howard, C. and Claiman, B. (1994). Leisure lifestyle planning: One path to empowerment for individuals who have sustained an acquired brain injury. *Journal of Leisurability, 21*, 23–25.

Hurley, E. and Turner, C. (1991). Neurology and aquatic therapy. *Clinical Management, 11*, 26–30.

Jansma, P. and French, R. (1994). *Special Physical Education: Physical activity, sports, and recreation.* Englewood Cliffs, NJ: Prentice-Hall.

Kagawa-Singer, M. (1993). Refining health: Living with cancer. *Social Sciences and Medicine, 37*, 295–304.

Kennedy, D. W. (1985). Using leisure activities blank with spinal cord-injured persons: A field study. *Adapted Physical Activity Quarterly, 2*, 182–188.

Kinney, W. B. and Coyle, C. P. (1992). Predicting life satisfaction among adults with physical disabilities. *Archives of Physical Medicine & Rehabilitation, 73*, 863–869.

Kleiber, D. A., Brock, S., Lee, Y., Dattilo, J., and Caldwell, L. (1995). The relevance of leisure in an illness experience: Realities of spinal cord injury. *Journal of Leisure Research, 27*, 283–299.

Krane, A. (1994). Traumatic Brain Injury: What follows the "Miraculous Survival." *Journal of Leisurability, 21*, 3–9.

Kunstler R. and Sokoloff, S. (1993). Clinical effectiveness of intensive therapeutic recreation: A multiple case study of private practice intervention. In M. P. Lahey, R. Kunstler, A. H. Grossman, F. Daly, S. Waldman, and F. Schwartz (Eds.), *Recreation. leisure, and chronic illness: Therapeutic recreation as intervention in healthcare* (pp. 23–30). New York, NY: Haworth.

Kurtzke, J. F. (1983). Rating neurological impairment in multiple sclerosis: An expanded disability status scale (EDSS). *Neurology, 33*, 1444–1452.

Kwan, W. and Sulzberger, A. (1994). Issues and realities in brain injury, leisure and the rehabilitation process: Input from key stakeholders. *Journal of Leisurability, 21* (2), 26–33.

Land, C., Marmer, A., Mayfield, S., Gerski, M. K., and Murphy, C. (1989). *Protocols in therapeutic recreation.* Alexandria, VA: NRPA.

Lee, Y., Brock, S., Dattilo, J., and Kleiber, D. (1992). Leisure and adjustment to spinal cord injury: Conceptual and methodological suggestions. *Therapeutic Recreation Journal, 27*, 200–209.

Lee, Y., Dattilo, J., Kleiber, D. A., and Caldwell, L. (1996). Exploring the meaning of continuity of recreation activity in the early stages of adjustment for people with spinal cord injury. *Leisure Sciences, 18*, 209–225.

Long, K., Meredith, S., and Bell, G. W. (1997) Autonomic dysreflexia and boosting in wheelchair athletes. *Adapted Physical Activity Quarterly, 14*, 203–209.

Luken, K. (1993). Reintegration through recreation. *Parks and Recreation*, 28, 52–57.

Lyons, R. F. (1987). Leisure adjustment to chronic illness and disability. *Journal of Leisurability*, 14, 4–10.

Martin, J. S. (1996). Transitions out of competitive sport for athletes with disabilities. *Therapeutic Recreation Journal*, 30, 128–136.

Martin, J. J., Adams-Mushett, C., and Smith, K. L. (1995). Athletic identity and sport orientation of adolescent swimmers with disabilities. *Adapted Physical Activity Quarterly*, 12, 113–123.

McAvoy, R. H., Schatz, E. C., Stutz, M. E., Schluin, S. J., and Luis, G. (1989). Integrated wilderness adventure: Effects on personal and lifestyle traits of persons with and without disabilities. *Therapeutic Recreation Journal*, 23, 50–64.

Mahon, M. J. and Bullock, C. C. (1992). Teaching adolescents with mild mental retardation to make decisions in leisure through the use of self-control techniques. *Therapeutic Recreation Journal*, 26, 9–26.

Murray, M. (1994). My father's head injury: How we coped. *Journal of Leisurability*, 21, 10–16.

Nelson, A. L. (1990). Patients' perspectives of a spinal cord injury unit. *SCI Nursing*, 7, 44–63.

Patrick, G. D. (1986). The effects of wheelchair competition on self-concept and acceptance of disability in novice athletes. *Therapeutic Recreation Journal*, 20(4), 61–71.

Petajan, J. H., Gappmaier, E., White, A. T., Spencer, M. K., Mino, L., and Hicks, R. W. (1996). Impact of aerobic training on fitness and quality of life in multiple sclerosis. *Annals of Neurology*, 39, 432–441.

Peterson, J. L. and Bell, G. W. (1995). Aquatic exercise for individuals with multiple sclerosis. *Clinical Kinesiology*, 48, 69–71.

Pitetti, K. H., Fernandez, J. E., and Lanciault, M. C. (1991). Feasibility of an exercise program for adults with cerebral palsy: A pilot study. *Adapted Physical Activity Quarterly*, 8, 333–341.

Ponichtera-Mulcare, J. A. (1993). Exercise and multiple sclerosis. *Medicine and Science in Sports and Exercise*, 25, 451–465.

Ponichtera-Mulcare, J. A., Mathews, T., Glaser, R. M., and Gupta, S. C. (1995). Maximal aerobic exercise of individuals with multiple sclerosis using three modes of ergometry. *Clinical Kinesiology*, 48, 4–13.

Porretta, D. L. and Moore, W. (1996/1997). A review of sport psychology research for individuals with disabilities: Implications for future inquiry. *Clinical Kinesiology*, 50, 83–93.

Porth, C. M. (1990). *Patho-physiology: Concepts of altered states* (3rd ed.). Philadelphia, PA: Lippincott.

Potter, J. S., Smith, R. W., and Finegan, J. F. (1994). Leisure participation among individuals with traumatic brain injury following discharge from a transitional facility. *Journal of Leisurability*, 21, 34–42.

Samdahl, D. M. (1989). A symbolic interactionist model of leisure: Theory and empirical support. *Leisure Sciences*, 10, 27–39.

Santiago, M. C., Coyle, C. P., and Kinney, W. B. (1993). Aerobic exercise effect on individuals with physical disabilities. *Archives of Physical Medicine & Rehabilitation*, 74, 1192–1198.

Sherrill, C. (1986). *Adapted physical education and recreation: A multidisciplinary approach*. Dubuque, IA: Brown.

Sherrill, C., Hinson, M., Gench, B., Kennedy, S. O., and Low, L. (1990). Self-concepts of disabled youth athletes. *Perceptual and Motor Skills*, 70, 1093–1098.

Sherrill, C. and Rainbolt, W. (1988). Self-actualization profiles of male able-bodied and elite cerebral palsied athletes. *Adapted Physical Activity Quarterly*, 5, 108–119.

Stumbo, N. J. and Bloom, C. W. (1990). The implications of traumatic brain injury for therapeutic recreation services in rehabilitation settings. *Therapeutic Recreation Journal*, 24, 64–79.

Weiss, C. R. and Jamieson, N. B. (1988). Hidden disabilities: A new enterprise for therapeutic recreation. *Therapeutic Recreation Journal*, 22, 9–17.

Winnick, J. P. and Short, F. X. (1991). A comparison of the physical fitness of nonretarded and mildly mentally retarded adolescents with cerebral palsy. *Adapted Physical Activity Quarterly*, 8, 43–56.

Woods, D. A. (1992). Aquatic exercise programs for patients with multiple sclerosis. *Clinical Kinesiology*, 45, 14–20.

Zoerink, D. A. (1997). Exploring the relationship between leisure and health of adults with orthopedic disabilities living in rural areas. *Symposium on Leisure Research Abstracts*, 11.

Zoerink, D. A. and Lauener, K. (1991). Effects of a leisure education program on adults with traumatic brain injury. *Therapeutic Recreation Journal*, 25, 19–28.

CHAPTER 13
SENSORY SYSTEMS

Sensory systems rely on specialized receptors that respond to specific stimuli and then send that sensation to the brain for interpretation. Sensory systems represent a broad array of specialized receptors that detect stimuli in the external and internal environments. Sensory receptors inform us about light (vision), vibration (hearing), touch, temperature, and pain (skin). We can also detect other stimuli, such as proprioception (e.g., joint position, muscle tension, muscle stretch). This chapter focuses on visual and auditory impairments and also briefly discusses the skin.

Sensory systems have several characteristics in common. *Receptors* are specialized to respond to one or only a few stimuli. Therefore, the sensory receptor for light (retina) will not respond to auditory stimuli. The receptor is associated with a *nerve fiber*. The nerve fiber transmits the sensory information to the brain (cerebrum) for detection and interpretation. The *cerebral cortex* has designated areas set aside for the identification and interpretation of sensory information from various systems. Visual information is interpreted by the occipital lobe of the cerebral cortex, auditory information by the temporal lobe, and pain information (from the skin) by the parietal lobe.

Anatomy of the Sensory System

Visual System

Each eye is located in the bony orbit on the anterior portion of the skull. Six *extraocular muscles* arise from the orbit and insert into the outer layer of the eye. These skeletal muscles allow for voluntary direction of the gaze. Three cranial nerves—oculomotor, trochlear, and abducens—share innervation of the extraocular muscles.

The *conjunctiva*—a thin, transparent, protective membrane—lines the exposed portion of the eyeball and the inner surface of the eyelid. The conjunctiva is the structure affected by the condition conjunctivitis (commonly known as pink eye).

Three layers called *tunics* comprise the eyeball (see **Figure 13.1**). An outer *fibrous tunic* has two parts—the cornea and the sclera. The *cornea*—the exposed anterior part—curves anteriorly (convex) and serves to

refract (bend) light as it enters the eye. The unexposed, posterior portion—the *sclera*—comprises an ample complement of fibers that present a tough, protective, external surface.

The second tunic of the eyeball, the *vascular tunic*, contains the choroid, ciliary body, and iris. The *choroid* comprises a generous array of vascular tissue lining the inner part of the sclera. It is highly pigmented and thus gives a brownish color to the unexposed part of the eyeball. On its anterior extent, the vascular tunic thickens into a *ciliary body*. Ciliary (involuntary) muscles within the ciliary body attach to the lens by way of tendons. The degree of contraction of the ciliary muscles determines the shape of the lens, and the shape of the lens affects how much the light rays refract when they enter the eye. The third part of the vascular tunic, the *iris*, is continuous with the choroid and represents the colored portion of the eyeball. It has an opening in the center called the *pupil*. The pupil constricts or dilates according to the lighting in the external environment and the response of smooth muscles that control the size of the opening.

The third, inner tunic, the *retina*, does not line the entire internal extent of the eyeball, but covers just the choroid portion of the vascular tunic. The retina contains the sensory receptors for light, the rod cells and cone cells.

As seen in Figure 13.1, the eyeball also contains two cavities filled with fluid—one anterior and one posterior. The fluid of the anterior cavity, the *aqueous humor*, is watery and produced on a constant basis. The fluid of the posterior cavity, the *vitreous humor*, is more gel-like and not produced on a constant basis. The vitreous humor holds the retina firmly against the choroid of the vascular tunic. Together, the aqueous humor and vitreous humor determine the intraocular pressure of the eye.

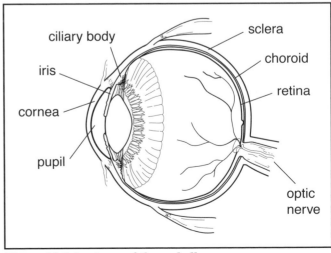

Figure 13.1 Anatomy of the eyeball

The neural pathway for light information includes the optic nerve, a portion of the thalamus, with connection to the occipital lobe. Some fibers terminate in the midbrain to help coordinate the response of the body to light information.

Auditory System

Hearing and equilibrium (balance) receptors are situated close to one another—auditory information and balance information are both carried by the eighth cranial nerve (vestibulo–cochlear nerve). Not surprisingly, balance problems are often associated with hearing impairments. The hearing mechanism comprises three parts—the outer ear, the middle ear, and the inner ear (see **Figure 13.2**).

The *external auditory canal* and the *tympanic membrane* (eardrum) comprise the *outer ear*. Sounds produce vibrations in the air that travel down the external auditory canal. The vibrations cause the tympanic membrane to move back and forth.

The tympanic membrane is attached to three small bones referred to as *auditory ossicles* (malleus, incus, stapes). The ossicles are situated in the second part of the auditory mechanism, the middle ear. A canal leading from the back of the throat (pharynx) to the middle ear, the *Eustachian tube*, allows for the equalization of air pressure within the middle ear.

The third of the three middle ear ossicles, *stapes*, attaches to a structure known as the oval window. The *oval window* marks the beginning of the inner ear. Both hearing and balance receptors are situated in the inner ear. Likewise, the eighth cranial nerve transmits impulses for both audition and equilibrium from the inner ear to appropriate structures in the brain.

The sensory receptors for balance and hearing work in a similar manner, although each responds to a different stimulus. The utricle, saccule, and the three semicircular canals represent the sensory receptors for static and dynamic balance. The cochlea of the inner ear possesses hair cells that transform vibrations into nerve impulses. Depending on which part of the cochlea is stimulated, different sounds will be heard. Sounds travel at a rate referred to as *frequency*, measured in *hertz* (Hz). Sounds also have the characteristic of loudness, measured in *decibels* (dB).

The eighth cranial nerve transmits impulses for hearing to the temporal lobe for detection and perception and to the midbrain for somatic responses and adjustments to sounds. The neural pathway for hearing, therefore, includes the eighth cranial nerve, a relay in the thalamus, with fibers then projecting to the auditory cortex of the temporal lobe.

Within the utricle and saccule are *hair cells* that respond to forces of gravity and movement instead of vibration. The hair cells are associated with nerve fibers that comprise the eighth cranial nerve. Displacement of the hair cells stimulates the nerve and transmits an impulse. Vestibular (balance) information then travels to the medulla oblongata of the brainstem for automated responses and adjustments to disturbances of balance. Balance information is also sent to the cerebellum for processing and integration with other joint sense information.

Skin System

The functions of the skin system include *protection*—it serves as a physical barrier because of the immune activity that takes place in its deeper layers and it protects deeper structures from excessive exposure to ultraviolet radiation (sunlight)—and *regulation of fluid levels and temperature*. The function of interest for the purposes of the present chapter, however, is the skin as a *sensory receptor*.

The skin is organized into three layers. The most superficial layer is known as the *epidermis*. It is comprised of four to five layers of cells that serve as the first barrier to germs and other undesirable substances and stimuli. The second layer of the skin, the *dermis*, comprises many different sensory receptors, including receptors for pain, touch, temperature, and pressure. Unlike the epidermis, the dermis contains a rich blood supply. In addition, the dermis is often the focal point of an initial immune response to a virus or other germs (e.g., the redness, swelling, and irritation that accompany a cut

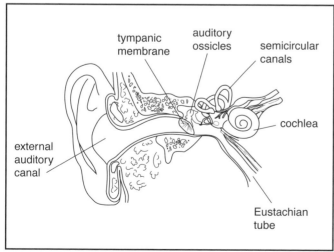

Figure 13.2 Outer, middle, and inner ear

on the finger). The third and deepest layer of the skin is known as the *subcutaneous* or *hypodermis*, which contains abundant adipose tissue, blood vessels, and nerve supply.

Normal Development

The eye develops from both the embryonic ectoderm (part of the embryonic brain) and mesoderm around the fourth week of gestation. At this time an invagination (known as the optic vesicle) forms. Its proximal portion narrows to become the optic stalk. A depression in the surface ectoderm overlying the optic vesicle deepens and eventually becomes the lens vesicle. At the same time the optic vesicle differentiates into a two-layered optic cup. These two layers eventually become the retina. Blood vessels establish themselves in a groove along the optic cup. These vessels eventually become the vessels that supply the retina. The stalk that attaches the optic cup to the embryonic brain evolves into the second cranial nerve—the optic nerve. Surrounding mesoderm cells differentiate into the remaining two layers of the eyeball—the choroid and the sclera.

The ear begins to develop in fetal life about the same time as the eye (around the fourth week). The ear involves all three germ layers—ectoderm (surface and neural), mesoderm, and endoderm. The inner ear develops from surface ectoderm, from symmetrical structures on each side of the embryonic brain (otic placodes). Each placode sinks deep into the mesoderm and changes into otocysts. The otocysts differentiate into both the cochlea and inner ear balance mechanisms—utricle, saccule, and three semicircular canals. The eighth cranial nerve derives from surrounding tissue of the embryonic brain, serving both balance and hearing as the vestibulo-cochlear nerve. The middle ear ossicles are derived from the mesoderm and first appear as mesenchymal condensations near the developing otocyst. About the same time development of the Eustachian tube begins. The external auditory canal is formed from surface ectoderm in the vicinity. By the eighth week the outer, middle, and inner ear structures are identifiable and correctly positioned.

The skin develops from embryonic ectoderm and mesoderm cells. The ectoderm differentiates into the multiple cell layers of the epidermis. Accessory structures develop from the surface ectoderm as well, including the hair, glands, and fingernails. Undifferentiated cells of the mesoderm, mesenchymal cells, form the dermis. As mesodermal cells differentiate into connective tissue cells, fibers (e.g., collagen, elastin) are produced, lending strength and resilience to the skin.

All of these events are completed by the eleventh week of fetal life.

Primary Disorders of the Sensory Systems

Visual System

Vision is commonly evaluated by assessing how well the individual can distinguish forms on an eye chart expressed as a ratio of what the individual can see to what normally sighted persons can see. Hence, 20/20 vision means the person can see at 20 feet what a normally sighted person can see at 20 feet. Other degrees of visual impairment are expressed in like manner: travel vision (5/200-10/200), motion perception (3/200-5/200), light perception (less than 3/200) (Carter, Van Andel & Robb, 1995). The legally blind person can see at 20 feet what the normally sighted person can see at 200 feet, or 20/200 vision. Complete inability to see light is exceptional; legal blindness and the other associated visual impairments have more to do with loss of functional vision.

Visual impairment may relate to problems with the lens and its capacity to focus an image on the retina. When the image focuses in front of the retina, the condition known as *myopia* (nearsightedness) results. When the image focuses behind the retina, *hyperopia* (farsightedness) results. The lens may also have irregularities on its surface that disrupt its capability to focus an image on the retina—an *astigmatism*. *Presbyopia* is usually associated with aging as a result of a loss of elasticity of the lens—the lens is no longer able to refract light rays enough to hit the retina. This is usually noticed first when viewing close objects because the light from close objects must be bent more to hit the retina. The use of prescription glasses, which assist the person's own lens, can typically correct these conditions.

Another usually correctable disorder is a *strabismus*. When the extraocular muscles do not focus both eyes on the same point, various visual problems can result. *Diplopia* (double vision) is a common problem for the person with a strabismus. Depending on the severity and cause of the strabismus, various surgical procedures are available to correct the condition.

Like presbyopia, several other visual impairments are associated with the aging process. A *cataract*, for instance, is a clouding of the lens or cornea of the eyeball. Cataracts are the leading cause of blindness, with the onset of the deterioration of vision typically occurring as the person ages. Few cataracts are congenital, most are found in older adults. Surgical correction has proven successful.

Glaucoma is another visual impairment associated with the aging process—second to cataracts as a leading cause of blindness. Glaucoma involves an excessive build-up of pressure in the aqueous humor of the anterior chamber of the eyeball. More fluid is produced than recycled and pressure gradually increases. The added pressure may damage blood vessels that supply the retina or it may affect the optic nerve. Glaucoma may occur as early as age 40 and may cause blindness.

Macular degeneration is not common until around age 70. The *macula* is the part of the retina where vision is the sharpest (sometimes referred to as central vision). A reduced blood supply to the macular area of the retina results in a gradual loss of central vision.

Retinopathies cause a deterioration in the nerves supplying the retina (the optic nerves). *Diabetic retinopathy* is found in persons who develop late onset diabetes mellitus or non-insulin-dependent diabetes mellitus (NIDDM). With NIDDM, the patient experiences changes in the blood vessels that supply the retina, eventually causing minute hemorrhages that lead to a deterioration of the retina. The other leading cause of a retinopathy is a poorly regulated oxygen environment for a premature infant who must receive oxygen support until his or her respiratory system matures. A traumatic blow to the head or directly to the eye may also affect the retina, causing it to detach from underlying layers. A *detached retina* is less frequently caused by a tumor or vascular afflictions. *Retinitis pigmentosa* is a genetic disorder that also affects the retina. The first and classic sign of the disorder is difficulty seeing at night. Accordingly, the person with retinitis pigmentosa experience deterioration of rod cells initially, followed by cones cells later.

Secondary problems associated with sensory impairments may be more limiting functionally than the actual loss. For instance, Skaggs and Hopper (1996) reviewed the literature pertaining to school-age children with visual impairments and found that they presented with consistently lower levels of physical fitness (e.g., cardiovascular, muscular endurance, balance, motor performance). The authors reasoned that the lack of opportunity, lack of qualified instructors, and limited programs in the public schools may provide part of the answer. They cited research that indicated that segregated environments provided more opportunity for regular exercise and physical activity. The authors also indicated overprotection by parents and teachers as an environmental factor that may limit development of psychomotor skills and abilities among children with visual limitations.

Auditory System

Batshaw (1997) estimates that one third of hearing impairments are genetic, and about one third acquired. While an estimated 70 genetically determined syndromes cause congenital hearing impairments, the final one third of cases are idiopathic—of unknown cause.

Like visual impairments, hearing impairments can be gauged according to the degree of functional loss on a standardized assessment. Hearing losses are measured according to the loudness (in decibels) required to be heard by the patient. As shown in **Table 13.1**, functional descriptions accompany each type of hearing impairment (adapted from Carter et al., 1995, pp. 306–307; see also Bullock & Mahon, 1997, pp. 223–224). As a benchmark, normal conversation is usually between 45–55 dB (Batshaw, 1997).

Auditory impairments may be conductive or sensory/neural. *Conductive impairments* involve the external and/or middle ear. *Sensory/neural losses* involve the inner ear, the eighth cranial nerve, the pathway from the inner ear to the auditory cortex, or the auditory cortex of the temporal lobe.

Common causes of acquired hearing impairments include infections, meningitis, premature birth, anoxia/hypoxia, auditory trauma, and hyperbilirubinemia. An explanation of some of the more common syndromes and causes follows.

Otitis media, a middle ear infection, is caused by germs that travel up the Eustachian tube from the pharynx to the middle ear. Repeated cases of otitis media may cause the middle ear ossicles to be less responsive to sounds, or it may lead to the formation of scar tissue, which lessens sensitivity to sounds. *Cholesteatoma* may

Impairment	Decibels	Example
Slight	27–40 dB	Cannot understand faint speech
Mild	41–55 dB	Understands conversation 3–5 feet away
Moderate	56–70 dB	Understands loud conversation
Severe	71–90 dB	May not hear voices 1 foot away, but may understand speech with amplification
Profound	91+ dB	Only aware of vibrations

Table 13.1 Examples of hearing impairments

also result from repeated perforation of the tympanic membrane, causing tissue from the external ear to invade the middle ear and immobilize the auditory ossicles. Habitual middle ear infections can lead to more serious conditions, such as otosclerosis. *Otosclerosis*, which is associated with the middle ear, involves the bony labyrinth of the inner ear and immobilization of the auditory ossicles. Repeated experiences with otitis media, cholesteatoma and otosclerosis may cause a conductive hearing loss.

Mastoiditis also begins with a middle ear infection, but in this case the infection spreads to the air cells in the mastoid process situated in the temporal bone. Unfortunately, the mastoid air cells are situated in close proximity to the cochlea of the inner ear. As a result of mastoiditis, the inner ear may be damaged and lead to a sensory/neural hearing loss. Another inner ear problem, *Meniere's Disease*, is associated with the aging process, but its exact cause remains unknown. The patient typically presents with both hearing loss and balance difficulties (vertigo). The hearing loss tends to be progressive and often is accompanied by a ringing in the affected ear (tinnitus).

People adapt to hearing impairments in many ways depending upon the extent of hearing loss, the environmental support system, and the preferred method of communication. For some individuals (persons with slight, mild, or moderate hearing impairments) a hearing aid may be of assistance. Most hearing aids have three parts—a microphone, an amplifier, and a receiver. The TRS should make certain the person has the device properly affixed to the ear, either externally or within the external auditory canal. Usually, a simple reminder will suffice. For others, an alternative communication system may be necessary, such as using manual communication, speech reading (oralism), or some combination of both (total communication).

The TRS should be sensitive to the deaf culture—the values and attitudes of persons with hearing impairments who have been socialized into manual communication as their preferred communication modality. Manual communication is not simply a communication system, but a social construction that represents a history for persons with hearing impairments—a time when they constructed their own culture because of the lack of access to mainstream society. Often, inclusion efforts show a preference for oralism or total communication. Supporters of the deaf culture and its manual communication method argue that mainstream society did not value the inclusion of people with hearing impairments enough to make accommodations until recently. They further maintain that they should not be forced to adapt their communication method simply because the law (American's with Disabilities Act) now requires accessibility and accommodation of public services. The staunchest supporters of deaf culture maintain that the rest of society should have to adapt and learn manual communication, instead of the other way around. Other alternative communication devices must be made available at public accommodations according to ADA, such as telecommunication devices for deaf persons (TDD) and other communication alternatives (e.g., interpreters, decoders). Clearly, preferred communication method and the deaf cultural values need to be considered when the TRS programs for persons with auditory impairments.

Similar to children with visual limitations, children with hearing impairments experience constraints with respect to accessing opportunities for regular physical activity, sport, and exercise. In the absence of a physiologic reason, children with auditory impairments have performed below average on some fitness tests (Goodman & Hopper, 1992). However, Goodman and Hopper concluded that "HI [hearing impaired] children and youth are more similar than dissimilar to H [hearing] children and youth in psychomotor abilities, with the exception of balance" (1992, p. 232). Further, they maintained that balance problems were not unexpected because of the anatomical and developmental associations between vestibular and auditory systems. The explanation for areas of deficit performance related to fewer opportunities, language delay, low self-concept, and resistance to inclusion from the deaf community (Goodman & Hopper, 1992).

Skin System

In fulfilling its protective function, the skin is often injured. One such injury is a *burn*. Children and young adults are the most frequent victims of burns (Carter et al., 1995). Thermal injuries are assessed according to the amount of surface area involved and the severity, determined by the layer(s) of skin affected. *First-degree burns* affect the outer epidermis of the skin. They are painful and produce considerable redness and swelling. *Second-degree burns* affect both the epidermis and dermis. If widespread, this type of injury may cause shock resulting from rapid fluid loss. Blistering and infections may also accompany the second-degree burn. The most severe thermal injury, the *third-degree burn*, affects all three layers of the skin—epidermis, dermis, and hypodermis. It may even involve other soft tissue structures, such as muscle. Symptoms include a charred appearance without pain (all nerve fibers and pain receptors have been destroyed).

The magnitude of injury may be assessed by applying the "rule of nines" (Carter et al., 1995). The upper extremities and head count for 9% of the body surface each. The anterior part of the trunk and the posterior part of the trunk each count as 18% of the body surface. The lower extremities each count for 18% of the body surface.

Therapeutic Recreation and Disorders of the Sensory Systems

Only on rare occasions will the TRS encounter a patient in a clinical setting admitted exclusively for treatment of a visual or auditory impairment. More often, persons with multiple disabilities will exhibit difficulties with sensory processing. Examples include older adults with various functional impairments such as diabetes and diabetic retinopathy, or an older adult who has sustained a hip fracture and may also present with balance and hearing difficulties.

Equally as exceptional is the TRS who works with persons with visual or auditory impairments in a segregated environment, such as a special school for the blind or deaf. A much more likely scenario would involve the person with a sensory impairment visiting a community recreation center to enroll in a class or activity available to all members of the community. Hence, this section focuses on therapeutic recreation (TR) interventions associated with inclusive recreation for persons with visual and auditory impairments, and programs that prepare the person with a sensory impairment for an inclusive experience. Therapy focuses on identification and treatment of secondary problems frequently associated with sensory impairments. TRS involvement with thermal injuries is presented, as well as research-based interventions relative to some specific secondary problems.

Secondary Problems with Visual Impairments

Common secondary problems among persons with visual impairments include low fitness, obesity, cognitive developmental delay, and poor sensory awareness (Carter et al., 1995). Low fitness and obesity were alluded to above as problems for children with

visual impairments, often relating to accessibility of programs and opportunities. Cognitive deficits are associated with limitations in communication channels for learning. Sensory awareness problems (i.e., difficulty detecting stimuli) may be attributable to poor awareness of body parts and the function of each (Carter et al., 1995).

Carter et al. (1995) and Batshaw (1997) agree that blindisms are a major obstacle to the inclusion of persons with visual impairments in regular recreation programs and leisure education within the community. Blindisms represent a series of unusual behaviors thought to be attributable to attempts on the part of the individual to stimulate himself. Blindisms include eye rubbing, waving the fingers in front of the eyes, rocking, assuming rigid positions, and other self-stimulating behaviors. Carter et al. (1995) also maintain that persons with visual impairments miss important social cues and contextual gestures that help with understanding during verbal communication. Persons with visual impairments may not appear to be socially appropriate as a result. Batshaw (1997) reports that children with visual impairments appear to play with less imagination. Play activities are more stereotyped and routine than that of sighted peers.

Diabetes mellitus, especially the adult, later onset form (NIDDM) is associated with the development of retinopathy. Evidence supports regular exercise in conjunction with dietary and medical management to decrease the likelihood of complications from NIDDM. Certainly this suggests a clear role for the TRS in guiding the patient with NIDDM in a program of moderate intensity, recreational level exercise.

Interventions with Visual Impairments

Dattilo (1988) successfully assessed the music preferences of three elementary school children with severe mental retardation. Two of the children also had significant visual impairments. Children were allowed to express their music preferences by depressing switches that allowed them to choose between paired samples of music. Data pertaining to the choices they made among the music pairs demonstrated that they were available to show clear and systematic preferences for music.

Data consistently show low fitness and obesity as problems among persons with visual impairments. Recent studies have demonstrated that persons with visual impairments are as capable of attaining similar benefits from exercise as their sighted peers. Blessing, McCrimmon, Stovall, and Wiliford (1993) exposed children with visual disabilities (ages 8–18) to a 16-week aerobic exercise program and found a significant improvement in cardiovascular and body composition fitness among the participants. In a second study that employed 7 weeks of aerobic training, Ponchillia, Powell, Felski, and Nicklawski (1992) discovered that subjects with congenital blindness improved cardiovascular fitness, body composition, and abdominal strength following the program.

Because competent performance sport and physical activity is self-reinforcing, techniques designed to enhance competent performance may be useful to TR practitioners. Hanrahan, Grove, and Lockwood (1990) exposed visually impaired athletes to several sport psychology techniques (e.g., mental skills training) designed to enhance their performance. Qualitative data were gathered about the subjects' preferences for specific techniques. Relaxation techniques were universally beneficial for all of the athletes in the study. Idiosyncratic preferences for other techniques showed that each of the mental training methods was liked by some but not all of the athletes. Some preferred the body awareness exercises, while others preferred creating their own musical tapes or goal setting.

Exercise has also proven useful as part of a complete lifestyle management program designed to minimize the probability of complication from diabetes. Weitzman (1993) described an exercise program that may be implemented for persons with diabetes, including warm-up and cool-down phases as well as strength, aerobics, and flexibility components. Weitzman was careful to caution readers that exercise for this type of client should be accompanied by glucose monitoring before and after exercise. To this precaution we add that exercise should be implemented within the greater context of a total lifestyle management program, which may include other components besides exercise, such as dietary management, stress management, cholesterol monitoring, and weight reduction.

Secondary Problems with Auditory Impairments

Secondary problems common to persons with auditory impairments vary somewhat from those found in association with visual impairments. We have already noted that children with auditory difficulties perform similar to their peers with hearing on most physical fitness and performance measures, with the exception of balance. Hence, secondary problems for persons with auditory impairments are more social in nature.

With regard to balance, Goodman and Hopper's (1992) review cited studies that consistently showed balance deficits in association with hearing impairments among children. Extending this conclusion to include older adults predicts Meniere's Disease with its accompanying symptoms of vertigo and balance difficulty.

Carter and her associates (Carter et al., 1995) chronicled secondary problems among persons with auditory impairments. They maintained that deafisms may be present in persons with hearing impairments just as blindisms are evident in persons with visual impairments, although deafisms do not seem to be as frequent. Like blindisms, deafisms are unusual and inappropriate behaviors that make it difficult for the person to blend into social situations in an inconspicuous manner. Deafisms include a shuffling gait, restlessness, and balance problems. However, there is not complete agreement on whether balance problems should be considered a deafism.

Expressive language and inability to read the social context make communication difficulties the leading secondary problem for persons with auditory impairments. Batshaw (1997) maintained that the person with a hearing impairment misses important social interactions. And Carter et al. (1995) remind the reader that prelingual (before language and speech) hearing losses have an even more pronounced effect on social appropriateness and expressive language. Social inappropriateness may take many forms, including interrupting conversations, difficulty expressing emotions in an appropriate manner, and misreading the social context (Carter et al., 1995).

Add to these social problems the difficulties parents have in establishing behavioral expectations for their children with hearing impairments (Batshaw, 1997) and one can begin to appreciate how a person with an auditory impairment comes to exhibit socially inappropriate habits, even in the absence of cognitive and emotional disability.

Interventions with Auditory Impairments

Goodman and Hopper (1992) suggest several recreation-level exercises and activity programs to help train persons with auditory impairments on static and dynamic balance. *Dynamic balance* may be improved using movement exploration (most appropriate with younger children), dance, tumbling, gymnastics, martial arts, and tai chi. *Static balance* may be improved through simple practice—standing on one foot (eyes open) or balancing on both feet (eyes shut). Static balance may even begin with the patient on his or her knees to minimize risk.

Interventions for assisting with social problems of persons with hearing impairments are not abundant. Some of the more promising research qualifies as leisure education and/or recreation participation and will be covered in those section.

One outdoor experience with campers with hearing impairments did prove to be beneficial. Luckner (1989) took 10 persons with deafness on a 10-day wilderness adventure experience. Physical conditioning in preparation for the trip was followed by long-distance cross-country skiing. Luckner reported significant gains in self-concept among the participants, which persisted at a 2-month follow-up.

Schick and Gale (1995) exposed preschool children with hearing impairments to different story-telling methods (two different types of manual communication and a combination of the two). The students interacted more with peers when they were read the stories using American Sign Language than either of the other two modes of communication. The researchers believed that this research may have implications for language development and learning because some writers speculate that language delay is to blame for learning delays once hearing impaired children enter school.

Interventions with Burn Patients

Carter et al. (1995) suggest that the role of the TRS in working with burn patients relates to three goals: disfigurement, limited mobility, and pain. An example of an intervention in pain management follows.

Kelley, Jarvie, Middlebrook, McNeer, and Drabman (1984) investigated the effectiveness of play choice and positive reinforcement on the perceived pain of two children during rehabilitation from significant thermal injuries. The children, ages 4 and 6, were allowed to choose cartoons to view during a painful procedure and were rewarded with stars placed on a chart if they were able to cry less. The children exhibited fewer pain-related behaviors, thus making the process go faster. Physical therapist and mother's ratings of pain, anxiety, and cooperativeness of each child were all favorably affected by the intervention. The authors concluded that the treatment may have worked because of the diversionary characteristics of the recreational activity—the viewing of the cartoons competed with the painful stimuli for the child's attention, decreasing the saliency of the painful stimuli. Although tentative the results are

promising relative to the contribution that the TRS may make in the management of pain using TR activities.

Leisure Education

The TRS is much more likely to work with persons with sensory impairments in community recreation environments than in clinical settings. Leisure education and recreation participation interface well with community TR goals and inclusion efforts.

Visual Impairments

Batshaw (1997) suggests educational priorities for children with visual impairments that may guide leisure education efforts by the TRS. He recommends that educational efforts focus on five areas when working with children with visual difficulties:

- Set-up stimulating environments
- Develop motor skills
- Provide structure to play
- Stimulate residual vision
- Use behavior modification to reduce blindisms

He urges educators to set up *stimulating environments*, using varied textures, audible goals, source balls, and sound producing toys. Batshaw's second educational priority for children with visual impairments is to *develop motor skills*. While the young person remains in the public school system, a coordinated effort between the public schools and the TRS in the community may work best to address motor and fitness deficits through a program of physical activities, sports, and development of regular exercise habits. Play and social skills training may need extra attention. To the extent that children with visual impairments exhibit developmental delay, TRS practitioners may be wise to follow Loovis' (1985) recommendation to provide structure to play so that the children may learn (e.g., through role modeling) the correct manner in which to play with preferred toys. Research reported by Loovis (1985) in an earlier chapter noted that many of the children show marked preferences for certain toys but seemed to play with them in unconventional ways. Batshaw's (1997) remaining two educational priorities for children with visual impairments are ongoing and relevant to adults with visual impairments as well. Any residual vision should be stimulated. This goal may be realized through the careful planning and implementation of activities to place some demand on residual sight (e.g., using large print). Batshaw also urges the use of behavior modification to reduce blindisms and assist with the development of socially appropriate skills. Some techniques used with persons who have sustained a head injury may apply here (e.g., have a signal to alert the person of inappropriate behavior).

Auditory Impairments

Batshaw (1997) also suggests educational priorities for children with auditory impairments that the TRS may integrate into leisure education:

- Establish clear expectations
- Emphasize clear communication
- Provide social skills training
- Increase leisure outlets
- Enhance self-determination

Because children (and less frequently adults) with hearing impairments use motoric displays to express emotions and frustrations, Batshaw emphasizes that educators and parents should establish *clear and appropriate behavioral expectations*. Carter et al. (1995) and Bullock and Mahon (1997) join Batshaw in their endorsement of the importance of *communication* as an educational priority for this group. While Batshaw maintains that hearing losses result in the loss of important social interactions, Carter et al. and Bullock and Mahon recommended teaching important communication skills, such as enunciating words clearly, maintaining eye contact, and repeating parts of the conversation as needed (this includes writing the message in some instances). *Social skills training* (Carter et al., 1995) should also be part of a complete leisure education effort for persons with hearing impairments. Learning objectives may stress the appropriate expression of emotions, reading social contexts, and not interrupting conversations. The final recommendation pertains directly to leisure activities. Persons with hearing impairments need to *increase their leisure outlets* (Carter et al., 1995), and accordingly *enhance their perceptions of self-determination*. Acquisition of leisure skills to afford competent participation in social, creative, and expressive activities also serves to underscore the preceding learning priorities as well. For instance, the acquisition of more leisure skills will enhance the person's prospects to engage in social interactions so that she may practice reading the social context.

The educational literature also revealed one study designed to determine the factors that affect the inclusion of children with hearing impairments in a regular classroom. To the extent that the leisure environment resembles a learning environment, some or all of the following strategies may apply. Afzali-Nomani (1996) surveyed classroom teachers and special educators and asked them to identify conditions associated with favorable outcomes relative to academic performance, social adjustment, and self-esteem of students with hearing impairments. The researcher found that genuine interactions between students with and without hearing impairments were vital. Allowing the student to use manual communication and peer students and teachers learning how to sign also enhanced the experience for the student with a hearing impairment.

Afzali-Nomani (1996) also found that when placement was based on need (rather than monetary factors) and that when a range of placement options was included, the student was more likely to thrive in the educational setting. This finding is consistent with a principle emphasized in earlier chapters: skill acquisition is sometimes best achieved in a segregated learning environment, with integration following acquisition and practice to attain a level of competence. Smaller classes worked better than larger ones. Authentic teacher support and parental support were vital to the success of the educational effort.

The research findings with respect to balance have been consistent—showing a predictable problem with equilibrium among many persons with hearing impairments. The intent is not necessarily to remedy the balance deficit. Rather, the TRS may teach skills to *prevent or retard the onset of balance problems*. More generally, because of the prevalence of balance difficulties among persons with hearing impairments, the activity planning should include consideration of the balance requirements of all activities implemented for persons with auditory problems.

Practical Applications

Guidelines for Persons with Visual Impairments (Adapted from Bullock & Mahon, 1997)

Ask before helping. Not all persons with visual impairments want your help all the time. The TRS also shows respect for the person's right to self-determination by asking if help is needed.

Do not shout. The person with a visual impairment does not necessarily have trouble hearing.

Identify yourself. We would not presume to anonymously interject ourselves into a situation with a person without introducing ourselves; we should treat the situation with a person who has a visual impairment in an identical manner. The TRS may also use the introduction and identification as a staff member to lend credibility to the assistance and to set the person's mind at ease.

Respect guide dogs. Although we may want to establish trust with the person we are assisting by befriending their guide dog, the dog is there for a purpose. Different persons handle this situation in different ways, and the TRS needs to respect whether the person considers the animal a pet to be shared, an adaptive device necessary to negotiating the environment, or some combination of the two. Respect the animal as you would the person's property.

Provide orientation. Use the clock method to describe the position of key environmental objects, doors, and windows. For instance, the teacher is at 12 o'clock, the windows are at 3 o'clock, the door is at 11 o'clock, and the rest of the class is behind you between 3 and 9 o'clock.

Use physical guidance with consent. The TRS should be familiar with the sighted-guide method. After obtaining consent, the guide presents her arm (usually the right) for the subject to grasp. The guide walks about one half step ahead of the person at a comfortable pace (don't drag, pull, or push) and may describe key environmental features during movement (e.g., curbs, steps, and other key environmental features). When approaching a door, make certain to place the subject on the hinged side of the door and open the door into the subject's free hand. Guidance to a seat involves placing the subject's hand on the back of the seat, and may include some description if the seat is unusual (e.g., a desk in a classroom). (For more details on the sighted-guide method, see Bullock & Mahon, 1997, pp. 216–217).

Guidelines for Persons with Auditory Impairments (Adapted from Bullock & Mahon, 1997)

Ask before helping. This rule applies for all persons with sensory impairments; many consider their impairment an inconvenience rather than a disability. Accordingly, they often want to manage themselves rather than accept assistance. This right to self-determination needs to be respected.

Speak clearly. Many persons with hearing impairments use total communication. Signing and clear articulation of words (not necessarily speaking louder) provide multiple channels of communication that the person may use to complete the message.

Be expressive to augment the message. Try communicating without gesturing to begin with, adding gestures on a trial basis if needed. Gesturing can appear condescending and patronizing if not used in a judicious and timely manner. Modeling behaviors and skills may prove to be a useful accompaniment to clearly articulated verbal instructions.

Reduce noise. This is especially necessary when presenting new information or explaining safety precautions. The TRS wants the participant to concentrate on the message. Some verification may be necessary to ascertain whether the instructions were understood and comprehended. The TRS may wish to ask the participants to demonstrate the correct behavior or skill to assess understanding. Alternatively, the TRS may request simple feedback, such as a verbal summary of what was presented, to ascertain the person's understanding of the message.

Position yourself for effective communication. If the participant does not have any residual hearing, then facing the person before trying to communicate is essential. Adequate lighting is also a consideration, but make certain not to stand in a position with excessive back lighting.

Speak to the person. Remember that the person with the hearing limitation is part of the group and deserves the same attention you would give to any group member. Do not talk to a companion about the person with the hearing impairment, as if the person was not even present or cannot understand.

Repeat as needed. Become accustomed to trying over if the message is not understood on the first attempt. Be persistent and be patient; if the communication is worthwhile, then so is the effort needed to send an accurate message. See how the person with the hearing limitation feels about writing the message if parts of the conversation are not easily understood. You may even wish to make short notes for the person if you accompany them to a lecture where conversation among the audience members is not appropriate.

Adapt as necessary. Try the activity or program without adaptation first unless the initial attempt presents serious risk to the participants. When used, adaptations should be kept as simple as possible—using flags to signal the beginning and ending of a game or competition, flickering the lights in a classroom to gain attention, dismiss the class, or indicate a transition in the activity.

Chapter Summary

This chapter examined the sensory systems and addressed the following key concepts:

- Sensory systems include receptors specialized to register a sensory modality, nerves to convey the impulse back to the central nervous system, and areas in the brain to interpret the sensations.

- Visual impairments do not usually mean the person cannot see. Rather, most visual impairments interfere with functional vision; vision necessary to independent functioning and quality of life.

- Auditory impairments are divided into conductive and sensori-neural problems. Conductive deficits are more amenable to correction, although there has been remarkable progress with correction of sensori-neural impairments in the recent past.

- Thermal injuries vary according to the number of layers of the skin affected and the extent of the trauma. Acute threat is related to shock, chronic danger is related to infection.

- Children and adolescents with auditory and visual impairments are often below par in motor ability and fitness, most likely because of latent barriers to inclusion in mainstream opportunities during the developmental years.

- Some evidence suggests that recreational activities can be useful in assisting children in coping with pain during procedures associated with thermal injuries.

References

Afzali-Nomani, E. (1996). Educational conditions related to successful full inclusion programs involving deaf/hard of hearing children. *American Annals of the Deaf*, *140*, 396–401.

Batshaw, M. L. (1997). *Children with disabilities* (4th ed.). Baltimore, MD: Paul H. Brookes.

Blessing, D. L., McCrimmon, D., Stovall, J., and Wiliford, H. N. (1993). The effects of regular exercise programs for visually impaired and sighted schoolchildren. *Journal of Visual Impairment*, *87*, 50–52.

Bullock, C. C. and Mahon, M. J. (1997). *Introduction to recreation services for people with disabilities*. Champaign, IL: Sagamore Publishing.

Carter, M. J., Van Andel, G. E., and Robb, G. M. (1995). *Therapeutic Recreation: A practical approach* (2nd ed.). Prospect Heights, IL: Waveland.

Dattilo, J. (1988). Assessing music preferences of persons with severe disabilities. *Therapeutic Recreation Journal*, *22*, 12–23.

Goodman, J. and Hopper, C. (1992). Hearing impaired children and youth: A review of psychomotor behavior. *Adapted Physical Activity Quarterly*, *9*, 214–236.

Hanrahan, S. J., Grove, J. R., and Lockwood, R. J. (1990). Psychological skills training for the blind athlete: A pilot program. *Adapted Physical Activity Quarterly*, *7*, 143–155.

Kelley, M. L., Jarvie, G. J., Middlebrook, J. L., McNeer, M. F., and Drabman, R. S. (1984). Decreasing burned children's pain behavior: Impacting the trauma of hydrotherapy. *Journal of Applied Behavior Analysis*, *17*, 147–158.

Loovis, E. M. (1985). Evaluation of toy preference and associated movement behaviors of preschool orthopedically handicapped children. *Adapted Physical Quarterly*, *2*, 117–126.

Luckner, J. L. (1989). Effects of participation in an outdoor adventure education course on self-concept of hearing-impaired individuals. *American Annals of the Deaf*, *134*, 45–49.

Ponchillia, S. V., Powell, L. L., Felski, K. A., and Nicklawski, M. T. (1992). The effectiveness of aerobic exercise instruction for totally blind women. *Journal of Visual Impairments*, *86*, 174–177.

Schick, B. and Gale, E. (1995). Preschool deaf and hard of hearing students' interactions during ASL and English storytelling. *American Annals of the Deaf*, *140*, 363–368.

Skaggs, S. and Hopper, C. (1996). Individuals with visual impairments: A review of psychomotor behavior. *Adapted Physical Activity Quarterly*, *13*, 16–26.

Weitzman, D. M. (1993). Promoting healthful exercise for visually impaired persons with diabetes. *Journal of Visual Impairment and Blindness*, *87*, 361–364.

Wilhite, B. C. (1995). Leisure involvement and social acceptance in youth with and without disabilities. *Symposium on Leisure Research Abstracts*, 29.

CHAPTER 14
CARDIOPULMONARY SYSTEM

The cardiopulmonary system actually represents two systems: the *cardiovascular system* (heart and blood vessels) and the *pulmonary (respiratory) system* (lungs and bronchi). The cardiovascular system and the respiratory system share one very essential task in common: gas exchange. The cardiovascular system transports gases attached to red blood cells (erythrocytes) while the respiratory system exchanges carbon dioxide for oxygen in the capillary beds that surround the air sacs (alveoli) in the lungs. Both systems are also "tube" systems designed to transport fluids and gases throughout the body. The cardiovascular system is made up not only of tubes (blood vessels) but also fluid (blood) and a pump (the heart). Likewise, the respiratory system is comprised of tubes (bronchioles) and organs (lungs).

Cardiovascular System

Functions

Besides figuring prominently in gas exchange, the cardiovascular system performs several other functions. It transports nutrients to tissues for a variety of metabolic functions, exchanging them for waste products voided through respiratory, urinary, and digestive systems. Some of the constituents of blood serve a protective function. *White blood cells* defend the body by destroying various microorganisms and debris. Some white blood cells function in the immune mechanism. *Platelets* help with clotting to prevent excess loss of blood. The cardiovascular system also transports *hormones*, substances secreted by endocrine glands that precipitate changes in the function of target tissues and glands (see Chapter 15, Visceral Systems).

Anatomy

Blood

Formed elements (red blood cells, white blood cells, platelets) and fluid comprise the blood. Together, formed elements make up about 45% of the total blood volume. This figure, customarily referred to as the *hematocrit*, serves as a routine indicator of normal health.

The process of blood cell formation, *hemopoiesis*, and is especially crucial in maintaining a proper hematocrit. Red blood cells only live for about 3 months and must be continuously replaced by hemopoiesis. Red blood cells, therefore, must be continuously formed in the bone marrow of some bones; they are broken down and destroyed when worn out by the liver and the spleen. White blood cells form in bone marrow and in the lymph nodes of the lymphatic system. Platelets also form in bone marrow, though they are parts of larger cells known as *thrombocytes*.

Plasma, the fluid portion of blood, is mostly water (about 90%) with a few plasma proteins. Plasma volume is sensitive to the balance of fluids throughout the body (e.g., plasma volume may increase if there is an excess of fluid in the intercellular matrix of surrounding tissues).

Heart

The *heart*—the pump of the cardiovascular system—supplies the force behind the blood to propel it to its various destinations. It is located in the center of the thoracic cavity, called the *mediastinum*. Like most of the visceral organs of the ventral body cavity, the heart has its own protective membrane, the *pericardial sac*. Situated in the pericardial sac, posterior to the sternum, and anterior to the vertebral column, the heart is afforded considerable protection from external trauma.

In cross-section, the heart takes on a pattern similar to that of the tube systems from which it was derived (see "Normal Development"). It consists of a characteristic outer layer of connective tissue (*epicardium*), a middle layer of involuntary (cardiac) muscle (*myocardium*), and an inner layer of epithelial tissue (*endocardium*). The thickness of the myocardium varies depending on the chamber; those chambers that must send blood to the lungs or into systemic circulation have the thickest layer of cardiac muscle.

The heart is a four-chambered pump (see **Figure 14.1**). The upper chambers, the *atria* pump blood to the lower chambers. Because the blood is delivered from the atria to chambers inferior in position, gravity assists the process. Accordingly, the myocardium is not as thick because it does not have to work as hard to deliver blood to its destination.

In contrast, the myocardium of the *ventricles* (lower chambers) is noticeably thicker and more prominent in cross-section. The ventricles have to work much harder to deliver blood to its destination. The right ventricle has to pump blood to the lungs on either side of the heart. The myocardium of the left ventricle is thicker yet because it has to pump blood into the systemic circuit—delivering it to all of the tissues of the body. Hence, the left ventricle has to exert enough force on the blood it pumps to drive it upward against gravity to the brain, and inferiorly to the tips of the toes. Furthermore, the extensive vascular network that the left ventricle must pump blood through presents a significant amount of resistance because of the friction produced when the blood, a relatively viscous fluid, passes along the surface area made up of the inside of the vessels.

The right side of the heart is generally regarded as the pulmonary circuit because it pumps blood to the lungs. More specifically, it pumps the deoxygenated blood it receives to the lungs where carbon dioxide can be exchanged for oxygen and returned to the left heart. In contrast, blood returning to the left atrium from the lungs is now fully oxygenated. The left heart (specifically the left ventricle) drives the oxygen-rich blood out to tissues where oxygen may be exchanged with carbon dioxide and the whole process repeats itself. Oxygen-poor blood, high in carbon dioxide, is returned to the

right atrium where it is then pumped to the lungs by the right ventricle, and so on.

Figure 14.1 also illustrates several important vessels that enter or exit various chambers of the heart. *Veins* bring blood to the heart, and *arteries* take blood away from the heart. Three major vessels return deoxygenated blood to the right atrium: the *superior vena cava* (draining the head and upper extremities), the *inferior vena cava* (draining the lower extremities and most of the ventral body cavity), and the *coronary sinus* (draining the heart itself). The pulmonary trunk (an artery) exits the right ventricle and takes blood from the heart to the lungs. The oxygen-rich blood from the lungs returns to the left atrium by several pulmonary veins from each of the lungs. Finally, the aorta begins the delivery of oxygen-rich blood from the left ventricle to all structures in the body, including the heart muscle itself.

The name given to the process by which blood vessels deliver oxygen-rich blood to the myocardium of the heart and return deoxygenated blood to the right atrium is *coronary circulation*. Coronary arteries and veins (e.g., the coronary sinus mentioned earlier) run across the surface of the heart, usually between the chambers of the heart. The coronary arteries especially are affected by heart disease and are the most common focal point of an occlusion or vascular lesion that precipitates a heart attack (myocardial infarction).

The muscle of the heart (cardiac muscle) looks very much like skeletal muscle in its gross appearance, with striations and other similarities. Cardiac muscle has several other properties, however, that distinguish it from skeletal muscle—the most important being the property of *autorhythmicity* (i.e., the origin of the heartbeat is intrinsic). The heart regulates its own basic rate of contraction. It beats in the absence of external stimulation from nerves because it contains a specialized structure (the sinoatrial node) that sets the basic heart rate. The Autonomic Nervous System (ANS) can increase the heart rate and cardiac output (in response to an emergency or as necessitated by exercise) or decrease the heart rate and output (to conserve energy), but the basic heart rate is determined by structures intrinsic to the heart.

A typical cardiac cycle at rest follows a predictable sequence of events. The two upper chambers contract in unison, driving blood into the lower chambers. This atrial contraction takes about 0.1 seconds. Powerful ventricular contraction follows and takes somewhat longer, about 0.3 seconds. A quiescent period of about 0.4 seconds ends one complete cardiac cycle. If the demand for cardiac output is increased then the quies-

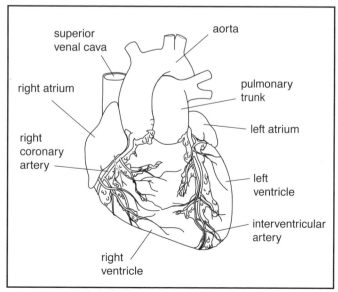

Figure 14.1 Structure of the heart

cent period is decreased and the heart rate increases. The heart may also increase its force of contraction to adjust to an increased demand for blood from tissues, pumping more blood with each beat (e.g., during exercise).

Figure 14.2 illustrates a record of the cardiac cycle. The inflections on the horizontal line indicate different events in a single heartbeat. For instance, the QRS complex represents ventricular contraction. This record is called an electrocardiogram (ECG or EKG).

Inside the heart exist four valves (not shown) that help regulate the flow of blood through the heart in a systematic fashion. When the ventricles contract the valves between the atria and ventricles close to prevent regurgitation of blood back into the atria from the ventricles. These are the atrioventricular valves (AV valves; also called the tricuspid valve on the right and the bicuspid valve on the left). During the quiescent period the blood that has been pumped into the pulmonary trunk and the aorta from right and left ventricle respectively obeys gravity and starts to return back into the ventricles. The semilunar valves between the pulmonary trunk and right ventricle and the aorta and the left ventricle close to prevent regurgitation of blood back into the ventricles from the two vessels. Many times, cardiovascular disease affects the integrity of the valves and causes dysfunction of the heart without directly precipitating a heart attack.

Blood Vessels

Blood vessels that carry blood to the heart are called *veins* and those that carry blood away from the heart are known as *arteries*. Veins and arteries are similar in that the same three layers of tissue—an outer layer of connective tissue (*tunica externa*), a middle layer of smooth muscle (*tunica media*), and an inner layer of epithelium (*tunica intima*)—comprise each of them.

The thickness and tissue composition of each layer serve to distinguish veins and arteries.

In contrast to veins, arteries are generally thicker-walled, mostly because of a greater compliment of smooth muscle within the tunica media. The primary reason for the difference in thickness is pressure—blood ejected into the arterial system from the ventricles of the heart is under more pressure than the blood returning to the heart in the venous system. The vessels adapt to the pressure demands accordingly. This is also why blood pressure is determined largely by the amount of resistance in the arteries, not the veins.

Blood tends to collect in the venous system and make slow progress back to the heart, in contrast to the rapid delivery of blood to tissues in the arterial system. Almost 60% of the total blood volume is contained within the venous system at any one time. This presents several problems for effective circulation—primarily how to accommodate the extra blood volume and how to return blood to the heart against gravity when there is very little pressure/force left behind the blood to drive it back to the heart.

The answer to the first problem is rather simple: There are more veins than arteries. Arteries are only found deep to other structures, whereas veins are found both superficially and deep. Hence, space to accommodate the added blood volume is available in the venous system. Another mechanism for accommodating the extra fluid volume in the venous side is an alternative circulation system known as the lymphatic system.

The second problem of returning blood against gravity is more challenging, and the venous system has two mechanisms for meeting this challenge. First, many veins pass through skeletal muscles. When the skeletal muscle contracts (even slightly) the vein collapses because of its thin walls, thus "milking" the blood toward the heart. This mechanism is commonly referred to as the *skeletal muscle pump*. Second, many veins are outfitted with one-way valves that allow blood to flow only toward the heart. Together, the skeletal muscle pump and the one-way valves return venous blood gradually back to the heart.

The basic pattern of arterial distribution in the body can be seen in **Figure 14.3** (p. 270). Arterial distribution can be divided into several logical categories based on the area supplied. *Coronary circulation* was mentioned earlier as the system that supplies blood to the heart. *Pulmonary circulation* accounts for the exchange of blood between the heart and the lungs that results in the oxygenation of blood on return to the heart. *Cerebral circulation* refers to the blood vessels that supply blood to the brain (mostly the internal carotid arteries).

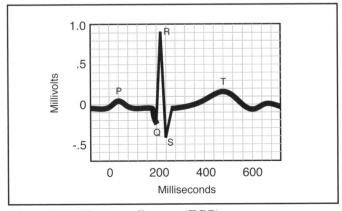

Figure 14.2 Electrocardiogram (ECG)

Branches of the same vessels that supply the brain also supply superficial structures of the head and neck.

Branches of the aorta supply the remaining areas of the body. The subclavian and its branches supply the upper extremities (brachial, radial, ulnar arteries) and supplement cerebral circulation (vertebral artery). The aorta arches posteriorly and to the left, then descends deep within the ventral body cavity, giving off branches that supply structures in the thoracic cavity (intercostal arteries) and the abdomino–pelvic cavity (renal, hepatic, celiac trunk, superior mesenteric, and inferior mesenteric arteries). The descending aorta (abdominal aorta) then splits at about the level of the fourth lumbar vertebra to form the two common iliac arteries to supply arterial blood to the pelvis and the lower extremities through its major branches (femoral, tibial, fibular arteries).

For the most part deep veins parallel the arteries (e.g., femoral arteries and femoral veins). There are more veins than arteries, however, and the extra veins are primarily those that may be seen with the naked eye just under the skin. Collectively, known as superficial veins, they account for the extra veins needed to accommodate the extensive blood volume that pools in the venous system. Figure 14.3 gives a good idea of the distribution pattern of deep veins, but not the distribution of superficial veins.

The venous system has another characteristic that distinguishes it from the arterial system: hepatic portal circulation. *Hepatic portal circulation* refers to direction of venous blood from the digestive system into the liver and then from the liver into the inferior vena cava for return to the right atrium of the heart. The hepatic portal mechanism allows blood that carries the products absorbed from the digestive system to pass through the liver first. This process allows the liver to filter out some harmful substances (e.g., alcohol, foreign bacteria) and to store carbohydrates in the form of glycogen for later use.

As indicated previously, blood pressure is primarily determined by the resistance on the inside of vessel walls in the arterial system. The pressure is far greater in the arterial system because it receives the full force of blood ejected from the powerful ventricles (primarily the left ventricle) and arteries contain a generous amount of smooth muscle that allows for vasoconstriction (narrowing of the lumen of the vessel) or vasodilation (widening of the lumen of the vessel). The pressure exerted by ventricular activity and the resistance provided by the arteries are the major determinants of blood pressure.

Blood pressure is measured by a *sphygmomanometer* and expressed as millimeters of mercury (mm Hg). Normal blood pressure is expressed as *systolic pressure* (pressure in the arteries when the ventricles contract) over *diastolic pressure* (pressure in the arteries when the ventricles relax). Within reason, one would expect systolic pressure to be greater than diastolic. Normal blood pressure is 120/80 mm Hg. High blood pressure (hypertension) is a risk factor for cardiovascular disease because it puts extra strain on the heart by making it work too hard, and it compromises complete blood supply (perfusion) to peripheral structures and organs.

Lymphatic System

The *lymphatic system* intimately relates to the cardiovascular system in two ways. First, the lymphatic system produces some white blood cells that aid in the defense of the body and promote immunity. Second, the lymphatic system may be thought of as a supplementary circulation system, especially for the excess amounts of fluid volume that tend to back up in the venous system and surrounding tissue.

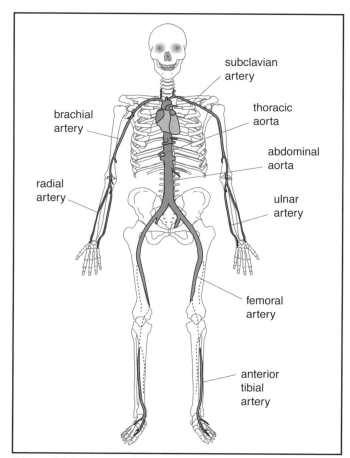

Figure 14.3 Pattern of arterial distribution

Excess fluid that drains into the lymphatic system (*lymph*) is similar in makeup to the plasma portion of blood. Most lymph drains from interstitial space (between the tissue cells) and returns to the venous system near the heart (into the subclavian veins). In this way the lymphatic system helps regulate the fluid volume that moves from the venous system into interstitial space. When the lymphatic and venous systems are overwhelmed, or when the heart begins to fail, fluid may collect in interstitial space and produce swelling in some areas of the body (*edema*).

The fluid lymph, lymphatic vessels, and lymphatic organs (mostly lymph nodes) compose the lymphatic system. The *lymph nodes* filter the lymph and produce white blood cells called *lymphocytes*. When a foreign microbe or virus overcomes the lymphatic system, some of the lymph nodes themselves may become infected and swell. This is what the physician checks for when palpating areas (e.g., the neck) that contain clusters of lymph nodes to determine whether you have a systemic infection or something more serious. Some forms of cancer are prone to migrate into the lymphatic system. Because of the distribution of the lymphatic system, the cancer cells may spread and affect sites secondary to the development of the original lesion, a process known as *metastases*.

Lymphatic vessels are similar to veins—thin-walled with one-way valves whose function is identical to the one-way valves of the venous system. Likewise, skeletal muscle contraction massages the lymph along its course while the one-way valves keep it moving in one direction—ultimately to be returned to the venous system near the heart.

Pulmonary System

Functions

Like the cardiovascular system, the primary function of the *pulmonary system* is gas exchange, although the focal point differs. The respiratory system is most concerned with the exchange between the external environment and the specialized structures in the lungs (alveoli) that exchange oxygen for carbon dioxide with the capillaries. The respiratory system has built-in protective reflexes—responses designed to protect the individual (e.g., coughing and sneezing). It also produces speech—as air passes through the larynx, respiratory structures alter the flow to produce the sounds, pitches, and tones of language.

Anatomy

The respiratory system is composed of a series of tubes ending in organs that contain the basic, functional unit of respiration: the *alveolus* or air sac. The respiratory system represents a series of structures designed to move air from the external environment into the lungs where the oxygen content may be delivered to red blood cells (*erythrocytes*) in exchange for carbon dioxide. The course of inspired air begins with the nasal cavity, then travels through the throat (pharynx), voice box (larynx), windpipe (trachea), bronchi, bronchioles, and alveoli.

Upper Respiratory Structures

Most of the upper respiratory structures (e.g., nasal cavity, larynx, trachea) are composed largely of cartilage. The upper respiratory structures conduct inspired air into the tubes leading to the lungs and inside of the lungs (the bronchi and the bronchioles). Upper respiratory structures do not have much capability to dramatically alter the flow of air into and out of the lungs.

Bronchioles

The most influential parts of the respiratory anatomy with respect to the regulation of airflow into and out of the lungs are the smaller tubes inside the lungs—the *bronchioles*. Unlike many of the structures of the upper respiratory tract, the bronchioles have a layer of smooth muscle that allows for modifications of the size of the lumen leading to the alveoli. The diameter of the bronchioles may be altered by stimulation of nerves from the ANS. Stimulation from the sympathetic division of the ANS will cause dilation of the bronchioles, whereas stimulation from the parasympathetic division will result in constriction.

Lungs

The *lungs* are reasonably symmetrical and quite elastic when the person is in good health. They are located on either side of the heart in the thoracic cavity, situated in lateral spaces named after the protective membranes that cover them: the *pleural cavities*.

Alveoli

The *alveoli*, the basic functional units of gas exchange, follow the principle of diffusion—the tendency for molecules to move from areas of high concentration to areas of low concentration. As erythrocytes pass near the alveoli the oxygen in the inspired air has a tendency to diffuse across the thin cell membranes of the alveoli and into the capillaries where the oxygen attaches to erythrocytes. In the opposite direction moves carbon dioxide, which is in high concentration in the capillary beds and low concentration within the alveoli. Diffusion again moves the molecules from areas of high concentration to areas low concentration—in this case within the alveoli.

Ventilation

Ventilation (breathing) refers to the movement of air into and out of the lungs—a prerequisite to gas exchange, but not the same as gas exchange. Air will move down a pressure gradient from areas of high pressure to areas of low pressure. Ventilation is a function of making the pressure inside the lungs less than the surrounding atmospheric pressure to allow for the movement of air into the lungs. Conversely, the exhalation of air is a result of increasing the pressure inside the lungs to slightly greater than the surrounding atmospheric pressure.

Inspiration is an active process; it requires muscle contraction. The muscles of respiration alter the pressure relationship between the ambient environment and the inside of the thoracic cavity. Intercostal muscles elevate the ribs, drawing them slightly forward to increase the anterior to posterior dimension of the thoracic cavity. The diaphragm pulls downward to increase the superior to inferior dimension of the thoracic cavity. Collectively these muscles reduce the pressure inside the thoracic cavity by increasing the dimensions of that space. Air then flows down the pressure gradient created, from the surrounding environment into the lungs.

In contrast, *expiration* usually does not require muscle contraction. Rather, expiration is normally a result of the rebound of the lungs because of their elastic quality. Elasticity means the ability to be distorted and then return to an original shape. This is exactly how the lungs increase pressure inside the thoracic cavity to greater than atmospheric and create a pressure gradient in the opposite direction—favorable for the movement of air out of the lungs. Labored expiration, as in exercise, is a function of the addition of contraction of some intercostal muscles and some of the muscles of the abdominal wall causing a more rapid elevation of pressure inside the thoracic cavity.

The ANS influences the respiratory system and thus influences ventilation. The *medula oblongata* sets the basic rate of respiration at about 15 per minute at rest for a healthy adult.

Normal Development

Like the balance of the cardiovascular system, the heart forms from the embryonic mesoderm. About week three of embryonic life, heart tubes form and move toward one another. They eventually fuse into a single heart tube, which is later partitioned into the chambers of the heart and the great vessels (e.g., aorta) associated with the heart. Circulation and pumping of the heart begin between the third and fourth week of embryonic life.

Fetal circulation largely depends on the relationship established between the mother and the growing infant. Shortly after implantation, a temporary organ (the placenta) forms. The *placenta*—partly maternal and partly fetal—serves as a focal point for gas and nutrient exchange. Gases are exchanged via diffusion of oxygen into fetal blood vessels and diffusion of carbon dioxide from fetus to maternal vessels within the placenta. Likewise, nutrients diffuse toward the infant and waste products toward the maternal vessels within the placenta. Literally, the mother breathes and eats for the infant.

Several organs, notably the lungs and liver, are bypassed by fetal arteries because they are not mature enough to function on their own until birth. Some congenital defects are associated with the persistence of these bypasses that are normal in fetal life, but dysfunctional after birth. Normally, pressure changes that take place with the infant's first breath cause the bypasses to close and establish normal circulation and respiration patterns.

The lungs and lower portions of the respiratory system evolve from the embryonic endoderm (inner layer of embryo) as an outpouching on the anterior surface of the future pharynx. The primary bronchi and trachea develop first, followed closely by progressively smaller bronchiole tubes. The alveoli start to develop only after the most distal portions of the bronchiole tube network forms. The alveoli and supporting lung tissue will not be completely formed until about the 26th week of gestation.

Primary Disorders of the Cardiopulmonary System

Cardiovascular System

Risk Factors

Risk factors for cardiovascular disease can be grouped into two general categories: those that can be changed (modifiable) and those that cannot (static). *Modifiable risk factors,* primarily lifestyle habits that can be addressed through education and monitoring (e.g., exercise and nutrition), include:

1. Hypertension (high blood pressure)
2. Obesity
3. Smoking
4. Sedentary lifestyle
5. Diabetes mellitus
6. Stress
7. Elevated blood lipids

Static risk factors include:

1. Gender (males have greater risk)
2. Age (older adults have greater risk)
3. Heredity (those with family history of CV have greater risk)

Risk factors for CV tend to overlap. For example, risk factors for coronary heart disease tend to be almost identical to risk factors for stroke. Also, many factors correlate highly (e.g., obesity and inactivity).

Chronic exposure to risk factors frequently results in the development of *atherosclerosis*, a type of *arteriosclerosis* (hardening of the arteries) Atherosclerosis typically presents as the accumulation of lipid and fibrous material on the inside of an artery. Over time, the size of the lesion increases and may cause impaired circulation in one of two ways. Atherosclerotic material may simply accumulate until it obstructs the vessel (a *thrombus*), or it may break loose and travel in the arterial system until it reaches a smaller vessel it cannot pass through and obstructs it (an *embolism*). In either event, the consequences may be dire if the obstruction prevents blood from reaching the heart, the brain, or other vital organs. Atherosclerosis is the leading cause of heart attacks and strokes.

The focal point of the obstruction determines the diagnosis, even though the precipitating etiology is the same. If the obstruction occurs in one of the coronary arteries, then the individual suffers a heart attack. If the obstruction occurs in the brain, then the person suffers a stroke. If the obstruction occurs in the other vessels, then the patient presents with peripheral vascular disease (e.g., occlusion of the femoral artery resulting from atherosclerosis causes compromised circulation to the lower extremity).

Hypertension

Hypertension (high blood pressure) may be considered a disease all by itself, or a risk factor that contributes to other disorders such as heart disease, stroke, and kidney disease. High blood pressure is determined quantitatively by a habitual reading of 140/90 mm Hg or higher. Risk factors for hypertension include obesity, smoking, stress, and family history.

Chronic hypertension causes the heart to work harder than normal. The cumulative wear and tear on the heart and blood vessels contributes to several cardiovascular pathologies. The heart must work harder to pump blood through a constricted arterial network, and the arteries suffer mechanical strain from the long-term exposure to excess pressure. Hypertension may also be implicated in more rapid formation of atherosclerotic lesions on the inside of the arterial network.

Coronary Heart Disease

The leading causes of *coronary heart disease* (CHD) include both static and modifiable risk factors that contribute to atherosclerosis. CHD ranges in severity from angina pectoris to myocardial infarction (MI).

Angina pectoris (or simply *angina*) means that the patient experiences pain over the sternum, left shoulder, arm, and jaw, although a general pressure over the entire chest wall may be present, too. Atherosclerosis in the coronary arteries usually causes angina and *ischemia* (impaired blood flow). The myocardium of the heart cannot function properly without enough oxygen and pain results, especially when the person undertakes more that the usual amount of physical exertion.

Angina may or may not be a warning sign of a heart attack, but the pathologic process is the same—occlusion of one or more coronary arteries from atherosclerosis deprives the myocardium of the oxygen necessary to do its work (i.e., pump blood via contraction). The difference between angina and a MI is a matter of degree—the extent of occlusion and the amount of heart muscle affected. Usually a thrombosis develops and occludes a portion of the heart muscle, depriving it of vital oxygen for a period of time sufficient to cause tissue death of that portion of the myocardium. If enough of the myocardium is deprived of oxygen, then death results.

Congestive Heart Failure

Many disorders can compromise the ability of the heart to pump adequate amounts of blood (heart failure). Etiologies include valve lesions, atherosclerosis, and myocarditis. *Congestive heart failure* involves one or more of these pathologies, resulting in a decrease in cardiac output and an accumulation of fluid in the body tissues (edema).

When the right heart fails (especially the right ventricle) blood backs up in the venous system. Osmotic pressure drives the fluid portion of blood into the body tissues, most pronounced in the lower extremities and the abdomen. As the condition persists, liver function may be disrupted because of the backup of blood volume into the portal system. *Cyanosis* (blue discoloration because of incomplete oxygenation of tissues) is often present in the later stages of the disease process, and the person fatigues easily.

With left heart failure, blood backs up into the lungs. *Pulmonary edema* develops, with pressure causing a seepage of fluid into the alveoli, impairing respiration. Cyanosis and *dyspnea* (shortness of breath) are symptoms. As with right heart failure, weakness and rapid onset of fatigue are present as the disorder exacerbates because of the inability of the left ventricle to deliver enough oxygenated blood to body tissues.

Patients with cardiac failure, such as those with congestive heart disease, are often categorized according to the amount of functional activity permitted. Rehabilitation and ongoing community programs use this classification system (see **Table 14.1**) to determine the extent of activity the person may safely participate in.

Cerebrovascular Accident (Stroke)

Strokes are attributable to the same pathological processes observed in the vascular system—thrombus, embolus, or hemorrhage of a blood vessel depriving (nervous) tissue of oxygen-rich blood. The etiology of a stroke follows a pattern similar to that of heart disease and peripheral vascular disease, with atherosclerosis (and its associated risk factors) most often the precipitating cause. Less frequently, emboli or hemorrhage of a cerebral vessel cause a stroke.

Alcohol abuse may also contribute to a vascular lesion in the cerebral arteries. Chronic abuse of alcohol

contributes to strokes because it is associated with hypertension, reduces blood flow to the brain, and may lead to the formation of an embolism in the heart that subsequently travels into cerebral circulation to occlude an artery.

An *aneurysm* (weakness in the wall) of a cerebral artery may also lead to a stroke. The affected artery protrudes laterally and is subject to sudden hemorrhage, resulting in a stroke. The vessel also promotes an abnormal circulation pattern because the channel disrupts laminar (smooth) flow, creating turbulence and encouraging clot formation. The aneurysm may also disrupt function if it presses on viable nervous tissue, leading to neurological symptoms. The etiology of an aneurysm is also atherosclerosis.

The motor impairments frequently associated with a stroke include contralateral hemiplegia or hemipariesis, accompanied by the signs of an upper motor neuron lesion (i.e., voluntary paralysis on the affected side, spasticity on the affected side, and a positive Babinski reflex). The extent of impairment correlates with the extent of injury to cerebral tissues.

Because each cerebrum exerts control over the opposite (contralateral) side of the body, the symptoms are contralateral to the side of the lesion. A stroke

Classification	Functional Ability Limitations
Class I	No limitation of physical activity Ordinary physical activity does not cause undue fatigue, palpitation, dyspnea, or anginal pain
Class II	Slight limitation of physical activity Comfortable at rest Oridinary physical activity results in fatigue, palpitation, dyspnea, or anginal pain
Class III	Marked limitation of physical activity Comfortable at rest Less than ordinary activity causes fatigue, palpitation, dyspnea, or anginal pain
Class IV	Inability to carry on any physical activity without discomfort Symptoms of heart failure or anginal syndrome may be present even at rest Discomfort increases with any physical activity

Table 14.1 Functional classifications of patients with cardiovascular disorders (American Heart Association http://www.americanheart.org)

affecting the left cerebrum or its tracts will cause right hemiplegia, and vice versa. In addition, *aphasia* (difficulty understanding or using language) may be present. If the trauma is associated with the dominant hemisphere (usually the left), cerebral areas controlling language may be involved.

Aphasia can involve any numbers of subskills utilized in language. *Expressive aphasia* occurs when the motor speech area on the dominant hemisphere (frontal lobe) is damaged. With expressive aphasia, the client can usually understand the spoken or printed word, but has difficulty articulating or writing accurately. Language in the client with expressive aphasia may be minimal, restricted to only very familiar phrases, and even these may not make any sense. The expression of nonexistent words (*jargon*) is not uncommon among those with expressive aphasia. Words may be correct but used inappropriately in this group as well. *Receptive aphasia* occurs when language and comprehension areas on the temporal lobe of the dominant hemisphere are infarcted. Mixed versions of aphasia are possible results of a stroke to the dominant hemisphere too. Clients with *mixed aphasia* exhibit symptoms of both expressive and receptive aphasia.

Strokes to the nondominant hemisphere often result in impairment of spatial orientation of the client. The patient may have problems orienting herself in space, locating her limbs in space, identifying the location of stimuli on the surface of her body, or perceiving depth. Stimuli received on the affected side may be overlooked or completely ignored.

Other Cardiac Disorders

Atherosclerosis alone or in combination with an MI, congenital abnormalities, and certain drugs (e.g., cocaine) may cause *disorders of cardiac rhythm*. As indicated previously, the basic heart rate is intrinsic to the heart, determined by specialized structures inside the heart. If these structures are deprived of blood, then the intrinsic conduction system of the heart is disrupted and the heart does not pump blood effectively.

Microbes, most commonly a virus, may infect the myocardium and cause inflammation of the heart muscle (*myocarditis*). Sudden death may result from cardiac failure if the disease is undetected or left to run its course. Inflammation may result secondary to rheumatic fever as well.

Rheumatic fever develops more often in children between the ages of 5 and 15 and is caused by a strep infection. The cardiac complications that may result are

preventable if the infection is treated promptly. For this reason cardiac damage that results from rheumatic fever is more common in impoverished areas. Along with the disruption of heart rhythm, the inner layer of the heart (the endocardium) and the valves of the heart may be affected by rheumatic fever.

The valves of the heart may narrow (*stenosis*) or not shut completely. The valves of the left heart—the bicuspid valve and the aortic semilunar valve—are most commonly affected. For instance, stenosis of the aortic semilunar valve causes the heart to work harder to push blood through the narrowed opening. Systolic blood pressure falls because of the inability of the left ventricle to maintain pressure behind the blood ejected through of the narrowed opening of the aortic semilunar valve. On the other hand, with regurgitation of blood back through an *incompetent aortic semilunar valve*, systolic pressure rises and diastolic pressure falls because of the leakage of blood back into the left ventricle. One symptom of an incompetent aortic semilunar valve is angina that results when the perfusion of blood into the coronary arteries is inadequate because of the leakage of blood from the aorta back into the left ventricle (instead of into the coronary arteries).

Congenital heart disorders can have genetic (e.g., chromosomal anomalies) or environmental (e.g., infections such as rubella) causes. The more common cardiac abnormality present at birth is a septal defect between the ventricles. The infant experiences distress because of the mixing of oxygenated blood from the left heart and the deoxygenated blood of the right heart. Pulmonary pressure may also increase. Incomplete peripheral circulation often results from congenital defects and causes cyanosis.

Pulmonary System

Asthma

Seen primarily in children and adolescents, *asthma* is usually precipitated by an allergy to some substance. The patient presents with an exaggerated response of the bronchi to the stimulus, with significant edema and mucus production. The bronchi become partially obstructed, leading to difficulty breathing (dyspnea) and breathing characterized by a wheezing sound. Ventilation becomes more difficult because the bronchi may go into spasm in response to the allergen. The TR Specialist usually will not see an individual with only asthma. However, the TR Specialist should be aware of any patients with multiple disabilities who also have asthma.

Emphysema

Emphysema is a more serious, nonreversible respiratory disorder associated with chronic cigarette smoking. Smoking causes the lungs to lose their elastic property, which is vital to the expiration of air. (Recall that normal expiration is primarily attributable to the elastic rebound of lung tissue.) The alveoli also expand and become progressively nonfunctional, often causing the barrel chested appearance attributed to patients with advanced emphysema. Dyspnea is significant in persons with advanced emphysema, as ventilation becomes labored.

Cystic Fibrosis

Most often fatal, *cystic fibrosis* is an inherited disorder of the exocrine system. Specifically, glands responsible for secreting mucus and sweat produce abnormal secretions that significantly impair respiratory function. The mucus produced is thicker than normal and accumulates on the inside of the bronchial tubes. This causes difficulties with ventilation. In some cases, complete obstruction of breathing can result. The sweat produced by a person with cystic fibrosis has a higher than normal salt content. Most persons with cystic fibrosis present with involvement of the pancreas, which fails to produce enough digestive enzymes to sustain proper nutrient absorption.

Lung Cancer

Like emphysema, most cases of *lung cancer* are attributable to cigarette smoking. Lung cancer is especially lethal (only a small fraction of patients survive even five years) because the patient is often asymptomatic until complaint of a persistent cough or bronchitis. Lung cancer is also apt to spread to other sites and affect other vital organs. (*Metastasis* is the term used to refer to the spread of cancer from one site to another. The most frequent sites of metastasis are the liver, brain, and skeleton.)

Cancer cells lead to impairment by competing with healthy tissues for limited resources and blood supply. The masses or tumors associated with cancer may also compress healthy tissues and cause dysfunction. For instance, tumors in the lungs compress healthy lung tissue and limit ventilation, leading to dyspnea. The pancreas may also be affected by lung cancer, resulting in weight loss and wasting in some skeletal muscle groups.

Treatment of lung cancer is usually aggressive and noxious, with many of the symptoms and loss of functional ability attributable to the treatments. Chemotherapy, surgery, and radiation therapy exert considerable stress on the body, making the person chronically fatigued and susceptible to opportunistic infections.

Sudden Infant Death Syndrome

Sudden Infant Death Syndrome (SIDS) is thought to be caused by respiratory dysfunction as well. The victim is an asymptomatic infant found dead after a nap or following sleep overnight. Various theories have attempted to explain the SIDS phenomenon, the most common have to do with abnormal respiratory control. As with atherosclerosis, researchers have identified a list of risk factors for the development of SIDS, which include premature birth, male gender, poor prenatal care, and a mother with a substance abuse problem.

Therapeutic Recreation and Cardiopulmonary Impairments

Cardiovascular System

Research pertinent to the effectiveness of therapeutic recreation (TR) interventions with patients with cardiopulmonary disorders is scarce, and few rehabilitation programs for this impairment include TR as a service component (McGuire, Young & Goodwin, 1996). Nevertheless, with the aging of society, the prevalence of cardiopulmonary disorders will likely continue to rise in the foreseeable future. Because most persons suffering an initial MI will survive (Gushiken, Treftz, Porter & Snowberg, 1986; McGuire et al., 1996), a considerable number of prospective clients await services designed to maximize functional recovery and minimize the likelihood for a second MI. The potential openings for TR intervention, therefore, lie in the area of risk reduction. *Risk reduction* activities correlate well with techniques already widely practiced in TR, including leisure education and lifestyle change. Risk factors TR may impact most include exercise, diet, and stress management (Carter et al., 1995; McGuire et al., 1996).

Exercise

Using *exercise* as a therapeutic modality for persons following a MI or for persons at risk for other cardiovascular diseases may cause further impairment if not applied properly. Proper screening and consultation with the primary care physician are prerequisite to beginning a mild to moderate intensity exercise program with recovering cardiac clients, or with those presenting with high risk factor profile (e.g., diabetes, smoker, sedentary, hypertensive). It is unlikely that the TRS would be involved in exercise prescriptions during the acute phase of recovery from a cardiac event; however, the patient may be exposed to mild to moderate intensity physical activity within the context of the regular TR program (e.g., walking, gardening, horseshoes). The treatment team and the client should be made aware of the nature of physical demands placed upon the client by the customary TR program so that contraindicated activities may be avoided. For instance, even mild activity may be inadvisable for persons in advanced stages of congestive heart failure.

Harris, Caspersen, DeFriese, and Estes (1989) maintained that changes in physical activity levels impact risk reduction because inactivity is the most common risk behavior associated with cardiovascular disorders. Even a modest increment in physical activity would yield a significant reduction in the incidence of cardiovascular disease. Currently only about 20% of the adult population exercises on any regular basis).

Only mild to moderate levels of physical activity are necessary (Harris et al., 1989). Previously 30 minutes of vigorous exercise 3 times per week at 80% maximum heart rate was recommended. For older adults, persons with a high-risk profile, persons who have led a sedentary lifestyle, and those recovering from a MI, moderate intensity exercise in small doses over the course of the day that add up to 30 minutes may be the more prudent and realistic routine to follow.

Niemi, Laaksonen, Kotila, and Waltimo (1988) considered psychosocial adjustment in an investigation into the quality of life of stroke survivors. The researchers asked 46 stroke survivors about their work, home, family, and leisure activities. They found that despite an acceptable recovery, the subjects showed deterioration in quality of life in all functional domains questioned, with the most pronounced decrements observed in the leisure activities. Furthermore, deterioration in the quality of life indicators was correlated with subjective reports of depression on the part of the subjects. Clearly this reveals a need for intervention by TR service providers.

Diet

Diet may be addressed indirectly through the TR program as well. If TR activities have food or beverages as part of the activity context (e.g., popcorn served at a movie), proper precautions should be exercised (e.g., butter substitute on the popcorn). More directly, cooking classes delivered by TR Services may impart lessons in healthy food choices (e.g., low fat) and meal preparation alternatives (e.g., not frying foods).

Stress Management

Stress management may be more in line with the skills available to most TR professionals. Assessment of leisure lifestyle serves as a starting point. McGuire et al. (1996) noted that the TR practitioner should not only determine the client's physical activity history and interests, but also detect any risk factors embedded in the context of leisure activities (e.g., smoking at the weekly poker game or drinking beer with the bowling league). The last thing the TRS wants to do is encourage recreational practices that contribute to the disease process.

Following assessment a number of interventions are available to the TRS, although most will require a small amount of further training to practice with competence. McGuire and his associates suggest tai chi, relaxation techniques, yoga, some aquatic therapy techniques, stretching and range of motion exercises, and various mental techniques (e.g., guided imagery) as potential stress reducing interventions.

Stress reduction can also take the form of various paper and pencil exercises to identify the sources of stress. The TR Specialist may help identify stressors at work, home, and leisure. Adjustment and adaptation strategies may then be planned and implemented during the leisure education portion of the TR process. Actual practice of stress management techniques may then be continued following discharge and during the recreation participation phase of the TR process.

Aquatic Therapy

Direct intervention may take the form *aquatic therapy*. Like other potential interventions, research data pertaining to the effectiveness of aquatic programs for persons with cardiopulmonary impairments is scant. The promise of water-based interventions lies in the advantage of the lower physiologic stress placed on aerobic systems because of the buoyant environment for exercise and natural relaxation effect of the water. Another advantage is that of *hydrostatic pressure*—the sheer weight of the ambient water aids in venous return to the heart, temporarily lowering blood pressure and making the heart work more efficiently (Becker & Cole, 1997).

(Green, 1989) exposed 28 older adults (average age 65.8) to an aquatic exercise program twice weekly for 16 weeks. The intervention included a warm-up phase, an exercise phase primarily using calisthenics, and a cool-down phase of flexibility and relaxation exercises. Subjects were asked to periodically monitor their heart rates to assure they were in the age-predicted target range. Results indicated that subjects experienced a significant decrease in diastolic blood pressure, percent body fat, and weight. Keller (1991) replicated Green's study with 36 older adults of about the same age and reported similar results.

TR and Stroke Recovery

MacNeil and Pringnitz (1982) described an inpatient TR program designed to assist the patient in recovering meaningful social and leisure involvement, especially in the home environment, following a stroke. Six program interventions were presented.

The first is an *individual therapy program* designed to adapt past leisure interests and explore new leisure interests. The individualized approach explicit in this program area is necessary to respond to the variations in focus and severity that are encountered when working with patients subsequent to a stroke.

Aquatics was the second program area presented in MacNeil and Pringnitz (1982). This intervention uses exercises and adapted swimming strokes to support patient progress toward the accomplishment of general therapy goals (e.g., prevent muscle atrophy) and specific TR goals (e.g., adopt swimming as an alternative to jogging as a form of exercise). Other activities using water were included, such as boating and fishing. Water safety instruction was part of this area of service as well.

TR services also offered a *unilateral skills class* as a program alternative. TR activities allowed for structured practice of everyday skills necessary to independent living (e.g., daily living skills, dressing skills, community living skills). Community living skills included leisure interests and afforded the clients a relaxed, unstructured time to practice skills necessary to independent function.

Evening programs represented the fourth service area discussed by MacNeil and Pringnitz (1982). The evening activity environment was informal, relaxed, and group-oriented. The objective was to create a safe environment for the practice of social skills, social appropriateness, and daily living skills. Night activities were the first chance the patient had to experiment with adapted and retrained skills in a "normal" environment. Unilateral skills were practiced, coping with deficits

was tested, and muscle strength and endurance were improved within the casual, social context of normal evening recreation.

The fifth program area represented progression from the contrived normal evening recreation program to the real world. *Community integration* included planning, resource identification, and problem solving on the part of the client, TR Specialist, and sometimes the family. Practical experience came from negotiating the real world environment, money management, and use of communication skills necessary to attain desired leisure participation.

Family education was the final TR program area reported. Strokes affect the entire family. Information about the effects of a stroke on leisure lifestyle was provided to family members. More recent research (Niemi et al., 1988) suggests the program described by MacNeil and Pringnitz (1982) is consistent with the notion that leisure lifestyle is the functional area that may suffer the most following a stroke.

Land, Marmer, Mayfield, Gerski, and Murphy (1989) described an existing protocol for persons on a stroke unit at Rancho Los Amigos Hospital. Assessment places the patient into one of three phases of treatment; the patient may enter at any phase. Placement is determined largely on the basis of functional abilities prerequisite to leisure participation. Like the program outlined by MacNeil and Pringnitz (1982), the Rancho protocol is based on a Leisurability approach, but with some latitude for developing individualized goals in response to patient problems. Leisure education is part of the protocol and is directed toward the customary areas: leisure knowledge, leisure attitudes, leisure skills, and leisure resources. Recreation participation provides an opportunity to break with the routine of rehabilitation and hospitalization. The protocol does correlate with other program features identified earlier by MacNeil and Pringnitz (1982)—a community readjustment program and opportunities for participation by family members are available within the context of the Rancho protocol. Discharge planning includes referral to appropriate support groups within the community.

Phase One is for the most severely involved patient. Maximum assistance is assumed and cognitive impairment and aphasia are manifest. Activities for patients in Phase One are restricted to grounds and focus on one-to-one treatment and recreation participation. Phase Two patients require moderate to minimum assistance and present with little cognitive impairment. Phase two patients are eligible for both individualized treatment and recreation participation as well as some group therapy and leisure education. Patients are also introduced to community-based opportunities. The most capable patients are placed into Phase Three programs— they are independent and able to take more responsibility for their own leisure. Patients participate in planning and implementation of community outings and discharge planning. Patients at this level may even provide peer support to those at lower phases of intervention. Visitations to community-based programs, facilities, and resources anticipate discharge and active participation following discharge of the Phase Three patient. Consistent with the Leisurability approach, the therapist takes the least directive role with the Phase Three patient and the most directive role with the Phase One patient. Although Land et al. (1989) do not say so explicitly, the reader assumes that progression is possible from Phases One to Two and Two to Three, if functional abilities and cognitive capabilities improve enough to warrant it.

Insight into further programming for persons with strokes may be found by reviewing the discussion of TR for persons with head injuries. A stroke may be thought of as a type of head injury, although the focal point of damage is different. Several functional impairments associated with strokes are also common to head injuries. For instance, cognitive processing impairments and personality changes may be observed with either disability. Motor impairment is common to both stroke and head injury, although the limitations with a stroke tend to be restricted to one side of the body.

Pulmonary System

Although research pertaining to intervention with persons who have acquired pulmonary dysfunction is scarce, a few recommendations for therapy have been identified in the literature.

Carter et al. (1995) recommend that specific activities can improve the effectiveness of muscles of respiration and abdominal muscles. Sherrill (1986) offers some examples of how this may be accomplished. "Guess who's laughing" is a game in which the object is to identify the peer who is laughing on an audiotape recording. Any game taking advantage of sustained or exaggerated respiratory movements— blowing and forceful expiration, holding one's breath (only for those without secondary cardiovascular impairment), and taking deep breaths—may potentially benefit some persons with pulmonary impairment.

Straightforward exercise programs of mild to moderate intensity may also be feasible for some types of pulmonary disorders (Carter et al., 1995). The TR Specialist should monitor environmental conditions, as pollution, allergens, and secondary cigarette smoke may provoke a adverse reaction on the part of the patient. During the warm-up the TRS can observe the patient's response to exercise and postpone the activity if the patient shows any signs of distress.

The extent of damage and functional impairment should guide the exercise intervention (Carter et al., 1995). Consultation with the primary physician is a usual and customary part of an exercise intervention for the patient with a pulmonary disorder. Unless directed by the physician, exercise and physical activity programs delivered to clients with pulmonary disorders under the auspices of TR Service should be held to mild to moderate recreational level activities; aerobic exercise beyond low stress levels should be avoided by TR professionals. Weight training (with light weights), golf, and bowling are examples of low to moderate intensity physical activities that may be feasible by some clients with pulmonary disabilities.

Horvat and Carlile (1991) used weight training as an intervention with two patents afflicted with cystic fibrosis. A 15-year-old male and a 16-year-old female performed 1 set of each of 15 exercises for the trunk, upper body, and lower limbs with low resistance. During the 12-week intervention program 5 repetitions were added to each exercise every 2 weeks until a complete set of 15 repetitions was achieved, then 10 pounds was added to the exercise. After 1 month, the weight for each exercise was not changed for the duration of the intervention, but the subject worked toward completing 3 sets of 10 repetitions for each exercise.

Both subjects improved grip strength, muscle girth measurements, skin folds, and self-concept from the beginning to the completion of the intervention. One of the subjects also decreased percent body fat. The results are especially encouraging for TR practitioners because they suggest that the exercise intervention does not have to be aggressive or risky to provoke significant improvement in functional abilities and psychosocial variables.

Leisure Education

Leisure education for patients with cardiopulmonary disabilities reflects the therapeutic recreation goals of risk reduction and lifestyle change. Risk reduction focusing on diet, exercise, and stress management remains central. Leisure education for these clients strives to move them toward personal responsibility for the management of their own risk-reducing behaviors. Because much of the general rehabilitation effort following the acute recovery phase takes on an educational theme, the leisure education component of TR is a very promising area of TR involvement with this disability group. In contrast to therapy, leisure education is low risk and consistent with the necessary lifestyle changes that must be adopted by the client to prevent a second MI.

McGuire et al. (1996) maintain that TR may be actively involved with lifestyle change, much of which takes the form of patient education. Carter et al. (1995) add that leisure education can help the person cope with the likely increase in free time, developing meaningful leisure activities that they may participate in safely and on their own. The potential curriculum content is almost unlimited, but certainly some topics are more apt to be common across leisure education initiatives. Educating the patient about the effort requirements of activities seems prerequisite to the patient making informed choices once discharged. Adjustments and adaptations for the post-MI patient can be presented as well, including modifications in frequency, intensity, and duration. Because the intent is to move the subject toward independence patients should be taught how to monitor heart rate and recognize warning signs, as well as how to monitor environmental conditions such as pollution levels, temperature extremes, and humidity.

During the leisure education phase of the comprehensive TR program, the patient may add to the techniques used in therapy to manage stress. While acute interventions bring stress under control during therapy (e.g., relaxation program), the same techniques may be taught to the patient during the leisure education portion of the intervention to advance the person toward self-monitoring and control. Problem-solving strategies, time management techniques, and development of healthy forms of self-expression may be added to relaxation training to round out the leisure education curriculum for the recovering cardiac patient.

The Gushiken et al. (1986) seven-step leisure education model for cardiac patients represents one of the few specific efforts directed toward this disability group. The seven steps can be summarized as follows:

1. Monitor and gradually increase activity level
2. Assess leisure function
3. Match leisure interests with community resources
4. Teach new and adapted skills
5. Develop a leisure time plan
6. Prepare an audiovisual presentation
7. Complete a 6-month follow-up

The first three steps pertain to inpatient interventions, beginning with a closely monitored, gradual

increase in the patient's activity level. TR supports PT and other therapies by keeping the patient active within appropriate limits set by the treatment plan. Assessment of leisure function occurs after the patient is past the acute, crisis stage of recovery. Step three matches the patient's leisure interests with existing community resources, with the community resource guide developed by the TR Specialist. Activity selection matches not only interest with resource, but also recommended exertion level with the treatment plan.

Recent approaches to the development of a leisure resource guide place more responsibility with the client. From a practical standpoint the TR Specialist recognizes that the client will have to do this for himself following discharge. Furthermore, the time and logistic commitment necessary for developing leisure resource guides for all potential communities of discharge for clients is impossible. Steps four through six represent outpatient services. This portion of the leisure education intervention emphasizes problem identification and problem solving. The TRS teaches new skills and adapted skills that represent solutions to problems and help the person overcome barriers to participation. Near the end of the outpatient portion (around 6 weeks post trauma), the patient develops a leisure time plan. An audiovisual presentation completes the outpatient phase, with the emphasis on home-based exercise, appropriate activity selection, self-monitoring, and the value of recreational level exercise. A booklet accompanies the tape and provides resources necessary for activity selection (e.g., MET value chart for activities, wind chill chart, humidity index).

The final step in the leisure education program outlined by Gushiken and his associates (1986) is the 6-month follow-up. The TRS monitors clients for leisure involvement problems. The timing on the follow-up was significant as well for compliance with an exercise program because of the high probability of noncompliance around 3 months (Dishman, 1994).

Gushiken et al. (1986) maintain that leisure education is appropriate when the client has problems with an unexpected increase in free time, often as a result of not being able to return to work. Subjects may become depressed as a result, and depression is more likely among those who are high risk candidates for a MI in the first place—highly competitive, driven, time-urgent individuals. They also identify compliance as a significant problem for clients with cardiac problems, especially after discharge. The poor compliance with exercise after discharge may be caused by boredom associated with limited activity choices. Clearly, the acquisition of additional activity skills and competencies through leisure education can augment the size of the client's leisure repertoire and support perceptions of choice, preventing boredom through cross-training and diversity.

Consistent with Gushiken's observation, most studies of exercise compliance (e.g., Dishman, 1994) suggest that only half of those who begin an exercise program will persist past 3 months. Accordingly, leisure education curricula should not only be concerned with motivation during initial participation, but also teaching strategies for adherence and preventing "relapse" of an inactive lifestyle following discharge. Gushiken et al. note several possible program monitors to evaluate the efficacy of their leisure education model, including adherence with the exercise prescription and improvement in leisure attitudes, awareness, and satisfaction. These variables are consistent with the leisure focus observed throughout the description of the model.

The motivation for maintaining a physically active lifestyle differs from the initial motivation needed to begin an exercise program. This is true whether the person is able-bodied, an older adult, or a person recovering from an MI. Although not specific to the population of persons with cardiopulmonary impairments, Dishman (1994) reviewed the literature on motivating older adults to exercise. One can assume that many older adults are at greater risk for developing cardiopulmonary impairments, or may have latent cardiopulmonary disease. The following outlines common barriers to exercise for older adults, suggests motivational techniques TRS can employ, and reviews a specific program (mail-mediated exercise) that can be used with this population.

Barriers to Exercise

Dishman (1994), Johnson and Heller (1998), and King et al. (1992) enumerate the customary barriers identified by older adults. The barriers—not new to those familiar with the literature on leisure behavior—include access to facilities, fear of injury, lack of support, and negative cultural stereotypes associated with older adults and exercise (e.g., exercise is not appropriate for older adults). Certainly, these barriers need to be addressed to facilitate participation in exercise by older adults and subgroups with cardiopulmonary impairments. But to this usual list of impediments Dishman adds the lack of knowledge of benefits. Specifically, fear of further morbidity (or death) and knowledge of potential benefits of exercise motivate most older adults and cardiac patients to begin an exercise program (King et al., 1992).

Physician's recommendation may also influence exercise adherence (Dishman, 1994). However, even though physicians seem to know that exercise in moderation is useful in preventing cardiopulmonary disorders and assisting in recovery, they often forget to recommend exercise (King et al., 1992) for those patients who might benefit, perhaps because exercise is more preventative than curative.

Motivational Techniques

Dishman (1994) discusses several motivational techniques, including clinical one-to-one, mediated (e.g., self-help kits, mailings), class instruction (e.g., modeling, peer support, supervised and structured), and cost-benefits techniques (e.g., decision balance sheet). Regardless of the technique, the data clearly indicate that for older adults the emphasis should be on continuous moderate exercise rather than vigorous exercise. The older adult (and person recovering from a cardiac event) is more apt to persist with an exercise program of walking or gardening than jogging. Dishman (1994) concluded that if exercise programs for older adults are to succeed (i.e., if clients are going to comply), then flexibility, functional strength, diversity of activity, and prevention and treatment of cardiovascular diseases must be emphasized.

After reviewing the literature, King et al. (1992) discovered that persons who had suffered a MI, had manifest coronary heart disease, or had angina were significantly more likely to adhere to an exercise program than those at risk for a cardiovascular event. This finding supports Dishman's contention that the benefits of exercise motivate initial participation (i.e., one of the benefits is the reduction in risk for a subsequent cardiovascular event). More simply stated, those who have good reason to be apprehensive about their immediate health are fearful, and therefore more motivated to be in an exercise program.

Mail-Mediated Program

A recent study of the effectiveness of a mail-mediated exercise program suggests that after initial adoption of an exercise habit the motivation for continuing to exercise changes. Johnson and Heller (1998) studied adherence to a home-based exercise prescription among 459 patients following an MI or angina. Lack of enjoyment, time, and environmental impediments predicted nonadherence with the exercise program. Conversely, perceived benefits predicted adherence with exercise. The researchers concluded that knowledge of benefits may be enough to motivate people (especially those with cardiovascular impairments) to begin exercise, but enjoyment and perceptions of well-being were necessary for long-term exercise compliance. Johnson and Heller further concluded that the perceived barriers (e.g., lack of enjoyment) and perceived benefits were modifiable. Their findings clearly suggest curriculum content for leisure education during later inpatient and early outpatient stages of recovery from any number of cardiovascular conditions.

The fact that enjoyment seems necessary to continuity of exercise is an added incentive for TR intervention using leisure education. Earlier findings from the Dishman (1994) and Harris et al. (1989) reviews are consistent with the importance of enjoyment in motivating adherence to exercise. Light to moderate physical activity, with an accumulated total of one-half hour of activity per day holds the promise of greater perceived enjoyment than vigorous exercise in single bouts of one-half hour three days per week. The latter exercise protocol may be well-suited to young people, but older adults and those managing cardiovascular conditions seem to respond better to the former.

Cardinal and Sachs (1996) provide further confirmation of the effectiveness of a more relaxed approach to exercise compliance. They studied the effects of two different mail-mediated exercise behavior change strategies on the weekly exercise of 113 healthy female subjects (average age 36.9). The subjects received either a structured exercise packet (promoting a traditional exercise approach of 30 minutes of continuous vigorous exercise 3–5 days per week), a lifestyle exercise packet (emphasizing increases in routine physical activity with an accumulated total of 30 minutes of light to moderate exercise most days of the week), or a control packet (which did not contain any exercise recommendation). The results indicated that the lifestyle exercise group reported significantly more weekly physical activity. The findings support earlier reviews (e.g., Harris et al., 1989) suggesting that if compliance is the desired outcome, then supporting light to moderate exercise is more apt to produce results.

Recreation Participation

A method for addressing the *exercise compliance* problem is to offer more appealing leisure-time exercise options. Schaperclaus and associates (1997) investigated the effectiveness of promoting lifetime sports in encouraging exercise among 74 post-MI subjects. The treatment used was one hour of sports participation per week at a sport and fitness club in the community. The sports program acted as a stimulant to an active lifestyle to maintain the effects of inpatient cardiac rehabilitation. Compared to a nonsports intervention control group of post-MI subjects, the sports group demonstrated significantly better performance on maximum oxygen uptake, risk factors (fewer average risk factors), and perceived well-being. The sports group reported significantly more frequent participation in moderate intensity activities, such as swimming, bicycling, and other sports. The data support the hypothesis that provision of some sporting opportunities in the community can act as a stimulant to further recreational sports participation elsewhere. The data suggest a promising role for community-based TR programs that focus on the recreation participation. A few favorable experiences may stimulate additional self-initiated, self-regulated leisure-time physical activity. Therefore, community TR should be designed to provoke an increment in safe (low to moderate intensity) and enjoyable exercise.

Another significant role for TR is addressing *barriers to recreation participation*. Some of the barriers may be removed or minimized by effective management. Compliance with the Americans with Disabilities Act and the Architectural Barriers Act guidelines for accessibility should minimize access barriers. However, psychological accessibility may be more of a challenge with ageism and other stereotypes prevalent among some community members. Educational initiatives aimed at counteracting stereotypes can make exercise opportunities more psychologically accessible.

Implementation of a sound *risk management program* should reduce genuine risk of injury (and therefore reduce the perceived risk of injury) among older adults and clients with cardiopulmonary problems. Appropriate screening prior to engaging in exercise and sports programs (with physician approval if risk factors or cardiopulmonary symptoms are present) should be a part of a sound risk management program. Leaders directly responsible for structured exercise programs should be properly trained and credentialed. A departmental policy for acceptable exercise intensity may also be indicated, with low to moderate intensity exercise the preferable level for cardiopulmonary clients and for customers with high-risk profiles.

Practical Applications

Screen Clients for Eligibility for Exercise and Physical Activity

Even though low to moderate intensity exercise is the safest investment for the cardiopulmonary client and those with a high-risk profile, key exclusion criteria should be assessed before exercise begins. An easy and effective screening tool is the Physical Activity Readiness Questionnaire (PAR-Q) developed by Shephard, Thomas, and Weller (1991). The PAR-Q asks the subject seven question about critical exclusion criteria. Answering in the affirmative to any of the questions should result in an automatic call to the person's physician for permission to participate. In light of the fact that the PAR-Q is a conservative screening tool (it errors in the side of safety), the TR Specialist should not be discouraged to find that many potential clients will answer "yes" to one or more of the items. This only indicates that additional measures of safety need to be exercised (e.g., calling the physician for permission to participate). Cardinal (1997) found that more than half of his 181 older adult subjects answered at least one item affirmatively. The most frequent problem was high blood pressure. Hence the TRS inclined to use low to moderate intensity exercise or sport activities with cardiopulmonary or high-risk groups should anticipate checking with a physician for clearance in most cases. Developing a short description of the exercise program for the physician to review will often expedite approval. The TRS should anticipate support from most medical professionals because of the compelling and favorable evidence that confirms the usefulness of physical activity with these populations.

Know MET Requirements of Various Activities

McGuire, Young, and Goodwin (1996) remind practitioners to maintain a handy reference of typical energy/effort requirements for activities that may be incorporated into the activity program. Recommendations for exercise and exercise prescriptions that come with the patient after discharge frequently have a maximum desirable amount of exertion that the patient should not exceed. The TR Specialist may request such an estimate while obtaining physician clearance for participants.

Adjustments may be made as the client improves, and consulting the physician periodically to reassess MET limitations on a case-by-case basis may be part of an outpatient protocol for working with those with physical effort restrictions.

Know the Warning Signs of Cardiopulmonary Distress

These include dyspnea (shortness of breath), cyanosis ("bluing" of the digits and lips because of poor oxygenation), unexplained sweating, nausea, pronounced changes in blood pressure (especially elevated diastolic blood pressure), pain in the chest, arm or jaw. Verbal complaints about malaise and discomfort should be taken seriously with this group, and the person should cease activity immediately if discomfort is present. Having a planned protocol for emergencies should be part of any sound risk management plan, and the plan should be rehearsed and reviewed on a regular basis.

Maintain Up-to-Date Certification in CPR and First Aid

Although most curricula and many agencies require CPR and First Aid certification as a condition for employment, often the retention of these skills is not monitored. With a busy schedule, the expiration of CPR certification may be overlooked, and the maintenance of First Aid skills may be forgotten. Risk management and quality assurance programs at many hospitals aggressively monitor periodic maintenance of these certifications; community-based agencies monitor these credentials less often. The TRS should make certification in basic safety procedures a matter of professional responsibility.

Chapter Summary

This chapter examined the cardiopulmonary system and addressed the following key concepts:

- The cardiopulmonary system represents several obvious and subtle systems and structures: blood, heart, blood vessels, respiratory system, and lymphatic system.

- Dysfunction of the cardiopulmonary system accounts for the vast majority of morbidity and mortality in modern society.

- Much of the work of a variety of allied health professions, including TR, is directed at reducing the relative risk of cardiovascular disease by dealing with modifiable risk factors.

- Because of the risk associated with aggressive clinical interventions with these conditions, TR is not often part of clinical treatment. However, TR has the potential to offer a considerable number of services that improve the long-term horizon of persons with cardiopulmonary impairments.

- Leisure education is thought to be a useful strategy for TR involvement with cardiopulmonary impairments in order to assist in transition from clinical settings to community settings and to encourage compliance with lifestyle changes.

- Lifestyle exercise programs have been associated with significantly better compliance among persons with cardiopulmonary disorders than more aggressive traditional approaches.

References

Austin, D. R. (1997). *Therapeutic recreation: Processes and techniques.* Champaign, IL: Sagamore.

Becker, B. E. and Cole, A. J. (1997). *Comprehensive aquatic therapy.* Boston, MA: Butterworth-Heinemann.

Cardinal, B. J. (1997). *Assessing the physical activity readiness of inactive older adults. Adapted Physical Activity Quarterly, 14,* 65–73.

Cardinal, B. J. and Sachs, M. I. (1996). Effects of mail-mediated, stage-matched exercise behavior change strategies on female adults' leisure-time exercise behavior. *Journal of Sports Medicine and Physical Fitness, 36,* 100–107.

Carter, M. J., Van Andel, G. E., and Robb, G. M. (1995). *Therapeutic Recreation: A practical approach* (2nd ed.). Prospect Heights, IL: Waveland.

Dishman, R. K. (1994). Motivating older adults to exercise. *Southern Medical Journal, 87,* S79–S82.

Green, J. S. (1989). Effects of a water aerobics program on blood pressure, percentage of body fat, and resting pulse rate of senior citizens. *Journal of Applied Gerontology, 8,* 132–138.

Gushiken, T. T., Treftz, M. S., Porter, G. H., and Snowberg, R. L. (1986). The development of a leisure education program for cardiac patients. *Journal of Expanding Horizons in Therapeutic Recreation, 1,* 67–72.

Harris, S. S., Caspersen, C. J., DeFriese, G. H., and Estes, H. (1989). Physical activity counseling for healthy adults as a primary preventive intervention in the clinical setting. *Journal of the American Medical Association, 261,* 3590–3598.

Holmes, T. H. and Rahe, R. H. (1967). The social readjustment rating scale. *Journal of Psychosomatic Research, 11,* 213–218.

Horvat, M. and Carlile, J. R. (1991). Effects of progressive resistance exercise on physical functioning and self-concept in cystic fibrosis. *Clinical Kinesiology, 44,* 18–23.

Johnson, N. A. and Heller, R. F. (1998). Prediction of patient nonadherence with home-based exercise for cardiac rehabilitation: The role of perceived barriers and perceived benefits. *Preventative Medicine*, *27*, 56–64.

Keller, M. J. (1991). The impact of a water aerobics program on older adults. *Symposium on Leisure Research Abstracts*, 31.

King, A. C., Blair, S. N., Bild, D. E., Dishman, R. K., Dubbert, P.M., Marcus, B. H., Oldridge, N. B., Paffenbarger, J. R., Powell, K. E. and Yeager, K. K. (1992). Determinants of physical activity and interventions in adults. *Medicine and Science in Sports & Exercise*, *24*, S221–S236.

Land, C., Marmer, A, Mayfield, S., Gerski, M. K., and Murphy, C. (1989). *Protocols in therapeutic recreation*. Alexandria, VA: NRPA.

MacNeil R. D. and Pringnitz, T. D. (1982). The role of therapeutic recreation in stroke rehabilitation. *Therapeutic Recreation Journal*, *16*, 26–34.

McGuire, F. A., Young, J., and Goodwin, L. (1996). Cardiac rehabilitation In D. R. Austin and M. E. Crawford (Eds.), *Therapeutic Recreation: An Introduction* (2nd ed., pp. 258–268). Boston, MA: Allyn & Bacon.

Niemi, M. J, Laaksonen, R., Kotila, M., and Waltimo, O. (1988). Quality of life 4 years after stroke. *Stroke*, *19*, 1101–1107.

Shephard, R. J., Thomas, S., and Weller, I. (1991). The Canadian Home Fitness Test: 1991 update. *Sports Medicine*, *1*, 359.

Sherrill, C. (1986). *Adapted physical education and recreation: A multidisciplinary approach*. Dubuque, IA: Brown.

Schaperclaus, G., de Greef, M., Rispens, P., de Calonne, D., Landsman, M., Lie, K. I., and Oudhof, J. (1997). Participation in sports groups for patients with cardiac problems: An experimental study. *Adapted Physical Activity Quarterly*, *14*, 275–284.

CHAPTER 15
VISCERAL SYSTEMS

The word *visceral* refers to the contents of the ventral body cavity. Hence, some of the systems already covered—the cardiovascular system and the respiratory system, for instance—belong to the visceral category. We elected to separate these systems from the balance of the visceral systems because of the frequency with which Therapeutic Recreation Specialist (TRS) work with cardiovascular and respiratory disorders and the greater presence of diseases and disabilities when compared to the remaining visceral systems.

The visceral systems covered in the present chapter—the urinary, digestive, reproductive, and endocrine systems—share several common attributes. First, all of the visceral systems are tube systems, designed to transport a substance (solid, fluid, gas). Second, all of the tubes systems share a fundamentally similar tissue structure—an inner layer of epithelial tissue, a middle layer of involuntary muscle, and an outer layer of connective tissue. A third similarity among the visceral systems is that each has one or more associated organs. The urinary system has the kidneys and urinary bladder. The digestive system includes the liver, pancreas, and gall bladder. The reproductive system includes testes or ovaries. This chapter also includes the endocrine system, which directly or indirectly controls the work of many of the visceral systems.

Urinary System

Functions

The major function of the *urinary system* is to regulate the balance of water and electrolytes in the body. *Electrolytes* are substances that must be balanced to maintain proper blood chemistry and acid-base balance. Small variations in acid concentrations, for example, can jeopardize the integrity of blood cells.

Secondary functions of the urinary system include the elimination of toxic waste products of some metabolic processes (e.g., urea) and the removal of foreign toxins from the blood stream (e.g., alcohol). Regardless of the source of the waste products, the resultant elimination is accomplished through the formation of urine, combining various waste products with excess water.

Anatomy

The urinary system is composed of two kidneys (in the normal individual), two ureters, a urinary bladder, and a urethra. Blood is filtered through the kidneys where urine is formed. The urine is transported to the urinary bladder by way of two tubes called ureters, one associated with each kidney. The urinary bladder temporarily stores the urine until a sufficient amount has accumulated for voiding. When elimination takes place the urine passes through a short tube called the urethra.

The *kidneys* are two lima bean-shaped structures located against the posterior wall of the abdominal cavity on each side. The functional unit of the kidney is the nephron. Each nephron filters blood and extracts a filtrate similar to plasma. The nephron consists of a long tube with many convolutions. Some of the filtrate that enters the nephron is later reabsorbed. The reabsorbtion process is regulated by internal fluid demands, the presence of certain hormones, and the need for trace elements in the body. Once the fluid has completed its trip through a nephron it is referred to as urine. The urine enters a series of progressively larger tubes within the kidney. It eventually finds its way into the ureters— the tubes that will transport it to the urinary bladder.

The *ureters* and *urinary bladder* are composed of the typical three layers of tissues found in all tube systems of the ventral body cavity. An inner layer of *epithelial tissue* is surrounded by a second layer of *smooth muscle* to help regulate the rate of urine flow. An outer layer of *connective tissue* represents the third layer. The inner, epithelial layer of the urinary bladder consists of an unusual type of epithelium especially designed to stretch and expand to accommodate large amounts of urine. The type of epithelium unique to the urinary bladder is called transitional epithelium. The smooth muscle of the urinary bladder the *detrusor muscle*.

The final tube urine encounters enroute to elimination is the *urethra*. From the urinary bladder the urine enters this three-layer tube. Two sphincters also regulate elimination, one internal and involuntary, the second external and under voluntary control.

Elimination (micturition) begins with filling of the urinary bladder, which stretches the detrusor muscle. Sensory nerve signals are transmitted to the micturition reflex center in the sacral portion of the spinal cord as a result of the stretching. The micturition reflex center then sends motor impulses back to stimulate contraction of the detrusor muscle and release of the internal sphincter. In young children who do not have voluntary control of the external sphincter, or in individuals who have lost control of the external sphincter as a result of injury (e.g., spinal cord lesion), this is sufficient to cause elimination. That is, elimination is simply a reflex act outside of voluntary control.

For children who have learned to control the external sphincter and for adults in normal health, innervation of the skeletal muscle that comprises the external sphincter allows for delay in elimination. Voluntary control of the external sphincter must be acquired through maturation and learning. Inhibitory signals from the cerebral cortex and other parts of the brain are necessary for delay of elimination.

Digestive System

Functions

The second tube system of the ventral body cavity is the *digestive system*. The primary functions of the digestive system are the absorption of nutrients, the absorption of water, and the absorption of minerals and electrolytes. The contents that remain in the digestive system at the end of absorption processes are eliminated. Secondary functions of the digestive system involve several processes designed to prepare food for digestion (mastication) and movement of food through the digestive system (peristalsis). The cumulative effect of the primary and secondary functions of the digestive system is the movement of food in a manner optimal to the extraction of essential nutrients for metabolism. The components necessary to this process include the predictable tube system and several organs dedicated to facilitating digestion.

Anatomy

The tube component of the digestive system is considerably longer than that of the urinary system. It begins with the oral cavity and a tube that connects the mouth to the stomach called the *esophagus*. From the stomach to the rectum the tube comprises the small intestines (about 12 feet) and the large intestines (about 5 feet). Throughout this tube system we again see the characteristic three layers—an inner epithelial layer (the *mucosa*), a middle layer of smooth muscle (the *muscularis*) and an outer layer of connective tissue (the *serosa*).

The small intestines are called so because of their narrower lumen. They are specialized for the absorption of nutrients. The large intestines (the *colon*) have a wider diameter and are specialized to absorb water and

electrolytes. The column-shaped epithelial cells of the mucosa increase the surface area for absorption, especially in the small and large intestines. Mucus secreting cells supply lubrication and lymphatic structures protect against disease throughout the digestive system. The exception to the rule of the middle layer of the tube being composed of smooth muscle in the digestive system lies in the makeup of the esophagus. The superior half of the esophagus contains skeletal muscle to allow for voluntary control of swallowing. Casual observation of swallowing will confirm this fact.

The digestive system contains several important organs interspersed along the length of the tube system, including the stomach, the liver, the gall bladder, and the pancreas. Generally the organs assist with the mechanical or chemical breakdown of food so that it may be absorbed.

The *stomach*, located between the esophagus and the small intestines, is a J-shaped receptacle responsible for preparing food for digestion in the small intestine. The mechanical churning and chemical breakdown of food prepare it for the extraction of nutrients in the small intestines.

The *liver*, the largest internal organ of the body, is situated below the diaphragm on the right side of the upper abdomen. The liver has some functions related directly to digestion. It filters blood from vessels that surround the digestive tract extracting simple sugars (glucose) for storage and removing bacteria and toxins (e.g., alcohol) from the materials digested in the intestines. The liver also stores vitamins and produces bile necessary for the breakdown of fats in the small intestines. The liver removes worn out red blood cells (recycling some components) and synthesizes most of the proteins of blood plasma.

Another accessory digestive organ associated with the liver, the *gall bladder*, is attached to the inferior surface of the liver. The gall bladder stores the bile produced by the liver. Bile produced in the liver and stored in the gall bladder is released into the first part of the small intestines (the duodenum) to help with the breakdown of fats ingested during a meal.

The *pancreas* produces enzymes (pancreatic juice) that assist in digestion. Like the liver, it empties into the first part of the small intestines. The pancreas is part *endocrine gland* (a gland that secretes its hormones into the blood stream) and part *exocrine gland* (a gland that secretes it product onto epithelial tissue).

Food gradually moves through the digestive tract by way of the rhythmic contractions (peristalsis) of the smooth muscle walls of the intestines. After nutrients are extracted by the small intestines and water and electrolytes are extracted by the large intestines, all that remains in the distal end of the digestive tract is the unusable portion of ingested food (called feces). Defecation is a process mediated in a manner similar to micturition. It involves an increase in pressure in the rectum as feces pass into it from the terminal portion of the large intestines. The increase in rectal pressure results in the urge to void. Voluntary control is learned and effected through contraction of the internal sphincter.

Reproductive System

Functions

The function of the reproductive system is perpetuation of the species. Male and female sex organs and accessory glands produce sperm cells and egg cells needed for reproduction. The sex organs also produce hormones required for the production and maturation of sperm cells and egg cells. The sex hormones promote development of secondary sex characteristics—placement of hair, proportion of fat and muscle, stature, voice quality, and others—that distinguish the genders. In this way, the sex hormones are essential to normal growth and development.

Male Anatomy

The male sex organs are the *testes* found in the *scrotum*. The testes are composed of smaller functional units called *seminiferous tubules*. The seminiferous tubules produce *sperm cells*. The sperm cells must mature for a time within the testes and the first part of the tube system leading eventually to the urethra.

Several tubes known collectively as the *spermatic ducts* serve the testes. The first part of the tube system begins on the posterior surface of the testes and is known as the *epididymis*. The epididymis is highly coiled and allows for further maturation of the sperm cell. The second part of the spermatic duct is referred to as the *ductus deferens*. The ductus deferens transports the sperm cells from the epididymis to the *ejaculatory duct*. The ductus deferens ends as a dilated tube called an ampulla. The ejaculatory duct forms when the *ampulla* of the ductus deferens joins with the *seminal vesicle*. The seminal vesicles, which produce about 60% of the total volume of semen, are found at the termination of the ductus deferens and join with the ductus deferens to form the ejaculatory duct. From here the ejaculatory duct passes through the *prostate gland*.

The prostate gland is found superior to the urethra and is responsible for producing the remaining 40% of volume of the semen. The *bulbourethral glands* represent the final accessory reproductive gland. These small glands are located inferior to the prostate, at the point where the urethra begins. The bulbourethral glands secrete a small amount of mucuslike fluid just prior to coitus. The *urethra* is shared by the urinary system and the reproductive system. It represents the final route of exit for the semen with ejaculation.

Sperm cells represent less than 1% of the volume of semen. The seminal vesicles and the prostate gland produce the fluid volume of the semen. Semen suspends the sperm cells is a nutritive environment. It is also alkaline to neutralize the acid environment of the female vagina during coitus. Semen also seems to have a protective value for the sperm cells and plays a role in promoting the motility of the sperm cells.

Female Anatomy

The male and female reproductive systems are very similar. Both develop gonads (sex glands) from a similar portion of the embryo, both secrete sex hormones essential to normal growth and development and maintenance of secondary sex characteristics, and both are involved in the production and maturation of gametes (sperm cells, egg cells).

Unlike the male who produces sperm cells continuously throughout life, the female is born with all the primordial (immature) *egg cells* she will ever produce. The female ceases the capacity to reproduce during *menopause*, whereas the male retains the capacity for reproduction throughout life.

The counterpart to the testes in the male are the *ovaries* in the female. The two ovaries are located in the upper portion of the pelvic cavity. The ovaries contain *follicles*, each of which contains a single egg cell awaiting maturation. Hormones secreted by the *pituitary gland* (located near the brain) cause a single follicle to mature and release its egg cell for potential fertilization. The release of the egg cell by one of the ovaries is referred to as *ovulation*. If fertilization does not occur, then the uterus sloughs its inner lining (known as *menses*) and another egg cell is stimulated to mature and is released via ovulation. The process is repeated about every 28 days.

As is the case in the male, the female sex glands are associated with a tube system that transports the egg cell to a location where fertilization and implantation may occur. The *fallopian tubes* transport the ovulated egg cell toward the uterus, which takes 4–5 days. The egg cell is helped along the way by the peristaltic contractions of the smooth muscle lining the uterine tubes and the *cilia* (hairlike projections) of the epithelial cells lining the inside of the tube.

The destination of the egg cell is the uterus. The egg cell is usually fertilized along its trip down the uterine tube toward the uterus. If fertilized, the rapidly dividing ball of cells (known as a *blastocyst*) implants itself in the vascular and mucous-rich inner wall of the uterus. Here the fetus finds ample nutrients to prosper and develop until maternal-fetal blood supply can be established.

The *uterus* is located superior and posterior to the urinary bladder. It is a very muscular organ shaped like a triangle. It presents an inferior opening (the *cervix*) to the sex organ of the female genitalia, the *vagina*. The vagina is situated between the urethra and the rectum. It is a fibrous/muscular organ that serves as the birth canal in delivery of the infant, a passage for the menses during menstruation, and as a sex organ during coitus. The last of the secondary sex organs covered here are the *mammary glands*. Situated within the breast tissue, the mammary glands serve as an important source of nutrition for the infant should the mother elect to nurse the infant. The process of milk secretion during nursing is referred to as *lactation*.

Endocrine System

Functions

Some glands retain direct association with epithelial tissue by way of a duct (*exocrine glands*). Others do not retain a connection with epithelium and must release their products into the blood stream (*endocrine glands*). The other important difference that serves to distinguish endocrine glands from exocrine glands is the product each secretes. Endocrine glands secrete products known as hormones. Exocrine glands secrete products that are not hormones (e.g., milk from mammary glands).

The *endocrine system*, along with the ANS regulates the internal environment of the body. More specifically, it regulates the production and utilization of energy in the body, the growth and development of the organism, reproductive activity of the individual, and the levels of key minerals in the body (e.g., calcium). Endocrine glands secrete three types of hormones—steroids, proteins, and amines.

Whether naturally produced within the body or derived from an external source, *steroids* enter the target cell (e.g., muscle cell) and alter the protein synthesis mechanism to increase the rate and amount of tissue buildup (recall that the contractile part of a muscle cell is made up of largely protein). The net result on a muscle cell, for instance, is that the cell will increase in size and strength. The sex hormones (e.g., testosterone) are steroid hormones, and they generally have a significant effect on the male and female physique, especially during puberty.

Proteins and *amines* must exert their effects on target cells from the outside. They attach to receptor sites on the cell membrane of the target cell and set in motion a sequence of events that indirectly cause changes in a variety of mechanisms within the target. For instance, insulin secreted by the pancreas is a protein-based hormone. It attaches to the cell membrane of skeletal muscle cells and changes the permeability of the muscle cell membrane to simple sugar or glucose. Hence, the normal effect of insulin is to cause an increase in uptake of glucose by skeletal muscle cells.

Anatomy

The major endocrine glands are illustrated in **Figure 15.1**. The master endocrine gland is the *pituitary gland*. Situated on the inferior surface of the *diencephalon*, the pituitary secretes many hormones that regulate the activities of other endocrine glands, hence the use of the term *master*. Hormones that affect other endocrine glands are referred to as *tropic hormones*. These include thyroid stimulating hormone (TSH), follicle stimulating hormone (FSH), luteinizing hormone (LH), and adrenocortico tropic hormone (ACTH).

The remaining hormones of the pituitary either have more widespread effects (e.g., growth hormone promotes growth in a variety of tissues), or are specific to their target cells (e.g., prolactin stimulates lactation via the mammary glands; melanocyte stimulating hormone stimulates melanocytes to secrete the dark skin pigment melanin). Other pituitary hormones cause the kidneys to reabsorb more water (e.g., antidiuretic hormone) or cause contraction of the uterus at the time of birth (e.g., oxytocin).

The *thyroid gland* is located anterior to the trachea in the neck. It secretes a group of hormones collectively referred to as thyroid hormone (TH). TH accelerates the rate of metabolism. *Metabolism* must be properly calibrated throughout life, but especially during the developmental years to assure proper maturation of organs and systems.

On the posterior surface of the thyroid gland are four *parathyroid glands*. The primary hormone of the parathyroid glands, parathyroid hormone (PTH) increases levels of blood calcium to assure proper function of muscle cells and nerve cells. The human organism is especially sensitive to blood calcium levels and there is little margin for variation. Another hormone of the thyroid gland, calcitonin, has the opposite effect of PTH; it lowers blood calcium. Besides the diet, bone tissue is the most readily available source of calcium; PTH stimulates the breakdown of bone tissue to assure proper blood calcium levels.

The paired *adrenal glands* rest on the superior surface of the kidneys, and are for that reason sometimes called *suprarenal glands*. The adrenal gland is actually two glands in one—an outer cortex and a center medulla. Each gland has its own hormones.

Hormones of the *adrenal cortex* are implicated in several important tasks dedicated to regulation of the internal environment. Some hormones of the adrenal cortex regulate levels of electrolytes (e.g., sodium), while others help regulate metabolism of glucose. Cortisone-type hormones from the adrenal cortex also have an anti-inflammatory effect by suppressing the immune response. Lastly, some hormones of the cortex produce effects similar to the sex hormones secreted by gonads of each gender. All of the hormones of the adrenal cortex are steroid-based hormones.

The medulla of the adrenal gland secretes hormones that mimic the effects of stimulation of the sympathetic division of the ANS. *Epinephrine* and *norepinephrine* cause a series of changes in a variety of tissues that support the "fight or flight" response characteristic of sympathetic stimulation (e.g., increased heart rate, dilation of the pupils).

The *pancreas*, located posterior to the stomach and first part of the small intestines, is part endocrine gland and part exocrine gland. (Its exocrine functions are discussed in the section pertaining to the digestive system.) *Insulin* is the most well-known hormone secreted by the pancreas. It has the effect of lowering blood glucose by facilitating the movement of simple sugar into skeletal muscle cells and liver cells for storage and use. The net effect is to lower blood glucose. This explains why the test for inadequate amounts of insulin (diabetes mellitus) is the presence of excess sugar (glucose) in the blood stream or urine. The pancreas also secretes a second hormone (glucagon) that produces the exact opposite effect of insulin—it raises blood glucose by acting to free stored glucose from liver cells. Together insulin and glucagon have a direct impact on the regulation of glucose in the body, and, therefore, an indirect effect on metabolism and energy production.

Like the hormones of the adrenal cortex, the hormones of the male and female reproductive glands are steroid-type hormones. Testosterone is secreted by the testes and promotes development and maturation of sperm cells. It also supports development of male secondary sex organs (e.g., ducts) and secondary sex characteristics (e.g., male physique). The testes are located in the scrotum.

As indicated in the discussion of the reproductive system, the ovaries are situated in the pelvic cavity. The hormones secreted by the ovaries are estrogen and progesterone. Together these two hormones help regulate menstruation and ovulation. They promote development and maturation of egg cells, and maintain secondary sex organs and secondary sex characteristics. If fertilization occurs, then these same hormones support gestation.

Normal Development

The urinary system is functional in the fetus. Several primordial kidneys develop and regress during gestation. The final kidneys migrate to their position against the posterior abdominal wall and renal blood supply is established early in fetal development. Urine is expelled to become part of the protective, fluid environment that surrounds the growing infant—the amniotic fluid. The urinary bladder and urethra develop from the outer layer of the embryo, the ectoderm; whereas the kidneys develop from the middle layer of the embryo, the mesoderm.

Digestive structures form from all three embryonic germ layers—endoderm, mesoderm, and ectoderm. Oral structures form from the ectoderm, inner layers of the tubes that are part of the digestive system derived

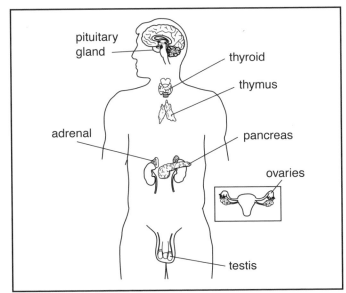

Figure 15.1 Major endocrine glands

from the endoderm. The middle smooth muscle layer and blood vessels that support the digestive system are formed by the mesoderm. Digestive organs such as the liver, gallbladder, and the exocrine portion of the pancreas develop along the tube system as the fetus grows. The primitive gut is the embryonic tube structure that accounts for most of the digestive structures that are derived from the endoderm.

The reproductive systems in both genders begin from the same tissue, with gender distinction largely a function of the influence of hormones. In the male, the primary sex cords differentiate about the fifth week of gestation into the seminiferous tubules of the testes. The testes migrate to their final position in the scrotum by the 28th week of gestation. In the female the primary sex cords differentiate into the ova, although somewhat more slowly than the testes in the male. The female's total allocation of future egg cells is completed during the prenatal period. In contrast, mitosis of sperm cells continues throughout life.

Likewise, the endocrine system develops from all three embryonic germ layers. Different glands develop from different layers, and some glands develop from more than one layer. For example, the thyroid gland and the pancreas (endocrine portion) develop from the inner embryonic layer—the endoderm. The pituitary gland and the adrenal gland develop from more than one layer. The anterior pituitary develops from ectoderm lining the oral cavity, but the posterior pituitary is derived from the same tissue as the brain. Hence, the anterior pituitary is sometimes called the adenohypophysis and the posterior pituitary is sometimes known as the neurohypophysis. Similarly, the adrenal cortex develops from the middle mesoderm layer of the embryo, and the adrenal medulla develops from neurological tissue and during gestation migrates to its final location in the middle of the adrenal gland. Not surprisingly, both the adrenal medulla and posterior pituitary secrete hormones that behave more like neurotransmitter substances.

Primary Disorders of Visceral Systems

Urinary System

Problems with the urinary system are often secondary to primary disorders in other systems. For instance, renal dysfunction may be secondary to hypertension. Likewise, both types of diabetes mellitus are associated

with kidney disease. Steady progression to renal failure is the long-term sequelae in both hypertension and diabetes.

Kidney failure refers to a condition in which the kidneys fail to remove waste products from the blood and concentrate urine. The kidneys are less able to regulate fluid balance, electrolyte concentrations, and pH balance. Together or separately, all of these conditions are life threatening.

Acute renal failure is reversible if the patient can be stabilized. Heart failure or a sudden decrease in blood volume (e.g., as a result of severe, widespread burns) may precipitate renal failure because of the rapid decrease in blood pressure. The lowered blood pressure results in inadequate filtration through the kidneys and an absence in urine formation. Subsequently, waste products fail to clear.

Chronic renal failure is less likely to be reversible and more apt to be associated with chronic conditions such as hypertension. Marked alterations in electrolytes and fluid balance are observed in late stages of the disease process. As a result, abnormally high concentrations of waste products are discovered in the bloodstream.

Once urine is formed it is transported to the urinary bladder from the kidneys through the ureters. Like many of the disorders of the kidneys, problems with the accumulation and elimination of urine are often secondary to other primary lesions. In Chapter 12 we discussed the implications of spinal cord injury (SCI) for the urinary system, with special attention given to the urinary bladder and elimination. Neurogenic bladder may be either spastic or flaccid, depending on the site and etiology of the lesion. SCI above the sacral level tends to be associated with spastic neurogenic bladder, and injury at or below the sacral level (e.g., myelomeningocele spina bifida) tends to result in flaccid neurogenic bladder.

Inability to control retention and elimination of the bladder in the absence of neurological lesions is often related to the aging process, although incontinence is not an inevitable part of aging. Incontinence refers to the involuntary loss of bladder control resulting in elimination in socially undesirable contexts.

One common, nonpathological cause is stress, often resulting from physical effort requiring a valsalva maneuver (i.e., holding one's breath and exerting pressure against the abdomino–pelvic cavity). Women especially are susceptible to stress incontinence because of the loss of muscle tone sometimes associated with childbirth or abdominal surgery (e.g., cesarean section). Obstructions may partially or completely block the urethra resulting in a distended bladder, with small amounts of urine being passed in an unpredictable fashion. In males, an enlarged prostate may cause the obstruction by pressing on the urethra. Various other disorders (e.g., MS, arthritis) or secondary effects of drugs may cause the person not to be able to reach a toilet in time, or prevent detection of urgency in enough time to find a toilet. Incontinence caused by any source is a problem not only because of the associated embarrassment, but also because it contributes to skin lesions and infections. Incontinence is also a leading cause of institutionalization.

Digestive System

Hepatitis refers to an inflammation of the liver. This single symptom has many potential causes, some acute some chronic, some serious and some transient. Drugs, toxins, or infections may cause inflammation of the liver. Mononucleosis is an example of an acute infection that may cause inflammation of the liver, usually without any permanent damage. More serious viral infections are identified by letter—hepatitis A and hepatitis B. The latter is generally regarded as more serious and more likely to convert to a chronic problem. Hepatitis B is transmitted by infected blood and often passed through sexual contact. Universal precautions and vaccination can prevent hepatitis B.

The conversion of healthy liver infrastructures to abnormal, nonfunctional nodules is called cirrhosis. By far, the most common cause of liver cirrhosis is alcoholism, but other diseases (e.g., hepatitis B) may lead to cirrhosis as well. Unfortunately, the liver is a very efficient organ and is known to function with only 10% viable tissue remaining. This means that the alcoholic may remain symptom free of cirrhosis until it is too late. However, if corrected soon enough, the liver has a remarkable ability to regenerate itself.

Alcoholism leads to liver disease because the liver is responsible for filtering out toxins such as alcohol immediately after it is absorbed from the lining of the gastrointestinal tract. The hepatic portal system (see Chapter 14, Cardiopulmonary System) shunts blood rich in absorbed nutrients from the intestines to the liver for filtration. Because alcohol replaces fat for fuel, there is an increase in the accumulation of fat in the liver. Alcohol abuse also causes inflammation of liver cells and tissue death (necrosis). Besides affecting the liver, alcoholism affects the kidneys (to failure), causes bleeding the digestive system (especially in the esophagus), decreases alertness, causes personality changes and violent behavior, increases confusion, and may lead to tremors.

Obesity is one of the leading health problems in the United States. It is frequently associated with several other chronic problems with other visceral systems. Obesity is a risk factor for heart disease, hypertension, diabetes, and some cancers. Obesity is an excess of fat that causes pronounced impairment in health. Although other risk factors are associated with obesity (e.g., heredity, culture, environment, and psychological dependence on eating), poor dietary habits and overeating are the unmistakable contributing causes in most cases of obesity. Coupled with the lack of adequate exercise, diet is the most common cause of obesity. Diet and exercise are also modifiable behaviors; changes in eating patterns and exercise are used in almost all interventions with persons who are obese.

Reproductive System

The rate of sexually transmitted diseases (STDs) is disturbingly high, despite the availability of effective preventive steps. The number of STDs is beyond the scope of this text. Therefore, we discuss only the more common STDs that TRS may encounter during clinical or community practice, including genital herpes, gonorrhea, syphilis, and acquired immunodeficiency syndrome (AIDS).

Genital herpes is an infection of the external genitals. Initial symptoms are itching, pain, and the development of skin lesions in the area of access. The disease advances to systematic symptoms that include fever, muscle ache, headache, and a general decline in energy. The virus grows within the sensory portion of the nervous system, leading to pain over one or more areas of the skin. There is no known cure for genital herpes and it is a resistant virus. Prevention of secondary infections on the host victim and prevention of spread requires attention to conscientious hygiene (e.g., thorough hand washing). Genital herpes is a contact virus, usually spread through sexual relations and direct contact with the lesion or its secretions.

Gonorrhea is a bacteria also spread through sexual contact; it is most frequent among teens and young adults. The bacteria may enter the host through any wet portal, including the eyes if contacted. The latent or sometimes absent symptoms of gonorrhea exacerbate its spread between sexual partners. Untreated cases of gonorrhea can result in the spread of the disease up the urogenital tract to infect secondary sex organs (e.g., prostate gland, uterine tubes). It may enter the bloodstream where it can damage other structures. For instance, gonorrhea may lead to damage of joints, heart valves, and the meninges of the CNS. Treatment with penicillin is effective if the disease is identified early.

Like gonorrhea, syphilis is bacteria commonly transmitted by way of sexual contact with the lesion or a wet area. It is highly contagious, more so than the virus that causes AIDS. Syphilis can even be spread through kissing, or contact with skin abrasions. Initial signs include skin lesions at the site of entry. The initial reaction is followed by more systemic reactions; a widespread rash may develop accompanied by a sore throat and fever. Lesions during the secondary response are highly contagious and exhibit an offensive discharge. The latent period from infection to manifestation of long-term symptoms can number in years. Especially if untreated, long-term morbidity for syphilis includes possible damage to the cardiovascular system (e.g., aortic aneurysm) and the CNS (e.g., dementia, blindness, spinal cord damage). Penicillin is the treatment of choice for syphilis.

First discovered in 1981, AIDS was identified when otherwise healthy people succumbed to afflictions they should normally resist. Shortly after, the virus that causes AIDS, human immunodeficiency virus (HIV) was discovered and labeled. The virus is spread through direct contact with some body fluids—semen, vaginal secretions, and blood. Hence, those at risk for contracting the virus include persons practicing unprotected sex, needle users (e.g., drug abusers), and persons who require transfusions. The virus may be transmitted across the placenta during gestation or during the passage of the infant down the birth canal. Breast milk may also infect the infant during lactation. There is no cure for AIDS and the virus that causes it, making prevention and universal precautions the remaining courses of action.

Once infected, the person with the HIV virus develops flu-like symptoms within a short time. This is followed by a latent period. The person may be unaware that he has HIV during the latent period, which may last many years, dismissing the initial symptoms as the flu. Accordingly, the risk of spreading the disease is greatest during the latent period, usually through unprotected sex with multiple partners. The latency and failure to detect the HIV virus (dismissing symptoms as a cold or flu) leads to spread of the disease more than its ease of transmission.

The HIV virus invades a type of white blood cells (T-lymphocytes) responsible for recognizing foreign microorganisms and infected cells that represent a threat to the individual. The T-lymphocyte next activates other leukocytes responsible for attacking foreign antigens or cancer. Antibodies produced by other leukocytes may also attack the microorganism once it has been identified. When the person manifests a significant decrease in T-lymphocyte count in combination with opportunistic maladies, the HIV is said to convert to full blown AIDS.

The obvious problem for the patient with HIV/AIDS is that his immune system is unable to repel opportunistic infections and cancers that would normally be destroyed. Hence, the usual clinical course for the person with HIV/AIDS is that he succumbs to an infection or cancer that would normally be resisted. Common locations for infections include the respiratory system, the digestive system, and the CNS. The person with HIV/AIDS may expire because of pneumonia, an infection of the esophagus, dementia, or a rare cancer (e.g., Kaposi's sarcoma).

Encouraging results have recently been associated with the use of Azidothymidine (AZT), which is thought to interfere with the transcription of the virus into the T-lymphocyte DNA. In combination with the use of AZT and similar drugs, good health practices have been associated with extended survival and improved quality of life. These health practices include exercise, diet, stress management, avoiding exposure to persons with infections, and avoiding substance abuse. Some of these practices may be part of TRS intervention with HIV/AIDS clients and will be discussed further below. The above treatments must be classified as palliative because at present no cure for HIV/AIDS exists.

Endocrine System

Diabetes mellitus serves to bridge the span between the other visceral systems and the endocrine system. Although diabetes is primarily a disorder of the endocrine system, it has a negative impact on several other systems—primarily cardiovascular, urinary, and digestive. Visual problems and damage to peripheral nerve structures also number among the complications of advanced diabetes mellitus.

Two types of diabetes mellitus have been identified. Type I diabetes mellitus (previously known as juvenile diabetes) is associated with an absolute deficiency in the secretion of insulin from the pancreas. Onset is usually at a younger age, but not all cases of insulin-dependent diabetes mellitus (IDDM) occur during childhood.

Type II diabetes mellitus (non-insulin-dependent diabetes mellitus—NIDDM) is typically the type found among middle-aged and older adults. It is not associated with an absolute reduction in the amount of insulin secreted by the pancreas. Rather, its etiology may be related to impaired insulin secretion, insulin resistance at peripheral structures (e.g., insulin receptor sites on cells), or an increase in the synthesis of glucose in the liver.

Regardless of the type of diabetes, the classic methods of detection reveal the same marker—excess glucose in the blood or in the urine. Insulin normally stimulates the uptake of glucose from the bloodstream into muscle cells, liver cells, and fat cells. Other behaviors are characteristic of the disease as well. Polyphagia (excessive eating) is typical of IDDM but not NIDDM. The aggressive appetite characteristic of IDDM is a subconscious, futile effort to get glucose into cells. "Starvation in the midst of plenty" is a phrase commonly associated with diabetes mellitus because the body has plenty of glucose, but it simply cannot cause enough glucose to be taken up by the cells. Both types of diabetes exhibit unusual thirst (polydipsia) and frequent need to urinate (polyuria). The latter two symptoms relate to the osmotic pressure created by excess glucose in the urine, which attracts fluid into the urinary system instead of being reabsorbed by the kidneys. The thirst perceived by the diabetic is an effort to counter the fluid lost through the kidneys.

Both types of diabetes are associated with long-term complications that have serious implications for the health of the individual. Peripheral nerves may be affected because of the occlusion of blood supply to the nerve fibers. Diabetes may even precipitate demyelination. Vision may be affected because diabetes causes weakness in capillary walls that supply blood to the retina, leading to aneurysms and even small ruptures. Renal failure is often the fatal sequelae for the patient with long standing diabetes. It compromises the blood flow through the kidneys and leads to a progressive loss of function of he kidneys, to eventual kidney failure.

The development of vascular lesions is accelerated by diabetes. With fats more abundant in the circulation of persons with diabetes, this environment likely leads to an increase the accumulation of atherosclerotic plaques on the inside of arterial walls. In turn, atherosclerosis is a risk factor for the development of hypertension, heart disease and compromised peripheral circulation. Blood vessels supplying the heart, brain and lower extremities are especially susceptible to ischemia because of occlusion. Poor vascular perfusion also increases the risk for infections in the feet and lower extremities. Peripheral neuropathy of sensory neurons in the lower extremities is probably a contributing factor—the patient cannot feel the lesion, the infection

remains undetected and untreated. Spread of the infection and poor wound healing among diabetics are leading causes of amputations that result from gangrene.

Other endocrine disorders are fairly rare and usually not seen by TRS. Many of these disorders are congenital and can be managed or corrected today because of early detection and treatment. Earlier, some of these maladies lead to the development of rare forms of mental retardation. In modern countries, few children are seen with mental retardation caused by hypothyroidism. Most disorders of the endocrine system are related to either excess or inadequate secretion of the hormones produced by a gland.

Cancer

Cancer may affect almost any sort of tissue, making its placement in the present chapter somewhat arbitrary. However, manifestation of cancer is more common among tissues represented in the ventral body cavity than others. If not a primary site, cancer often metastasizes to various organs in the viscera. (The liver is a common site of metastases.) Hence, it makes some sense to present cancer here, while acknowledging that it may be manifested elsewhere too.

Cancer refers to the persistent growth of an abnormal cell, a differentiating epithelial cell (carcinoma) or mesenchymal cell (sarcoma). The cancer cell is characteristically aggressive with abnormal and rapid replication. The leading causes of death from cancer in males are lung cancer, prostate cancer, and cancer of the colon/rectum. In females, the leading causes of cancer death are lung cancer, breast cancer, and cancer of the colon/rectum. Even though breast cancer is the most common cancer in women, lung cancer is the most frequent killer, probably because of the increase in smoking among women.

Cancerous growths, or tumors, usually cause their damage in several ways. First, tumors may compress the blood supplying a healthy organ, depriving the organ of essential nutrients. Second, tumors may liberate toxins and other substances that destroy healthy tissue. Third, cancer may compete with healthy cells for the limited number of nutrients, depriving healthy cells of an adequate amount of nutrition to function properly.

Cancer cells may also metastasize. When cells from the primary tumor are shed they may enter the bloodstream, the lymphatic system, or both. These fluid transport systems allow for rapid spread of a cancer, even before the patient presents with any symptoms. Early detection and treatment is the best defense against metastases of cancer.

Many theories about why cancer develops have been presented. The most popular theory suggests that cancer develops when there are mutations in the cell replication process. As cells age they become less accurate in their replications, explaining why cancer is more frequent among older adults.

The data supporting risk factors for cancer derived from epidemiological research are more certain. Heredity is certainly a risk factor for some cancers, because it predisposes the person to be susceptible to some forms of cancer (e.g., breast cancer). The second risk factor for cancer is exposure to carcinogens. Usually the exposure to the carcinogen has to be chronic and long-term. A carcinogen is any agent capable of provoking cancer (e.g., cigarette smoke, asbestos, sunlight, radiation).

Treatment of cancer may be curative or palliative. Therapeutic recreation is almost completely palliative. Surgical intervention, radiation, and chemotherapy are the leading medical interventions for cancer. These methods aim at extracting all or part of the primary site tumor or producing injury in the rapidly growing cancer cells.

Stress

Like cancer, stress is not a problem unique to the visceral systems; it may exert its detrimental influence on any of a number of systems. Stress, while not even a disease in the strict sense, is almost certainly a contributing factor in a number of pathologies, including cancer, heart disease, and hypertension. Visceral systems are often the sites of stress-related disorders (e.g., ulcers in the digestive system).

Stress is not simply muscle tension or nervous tension. Stress is the nonspecific response to any demand according to the noted stress research scientist Hans Selye (1974). It is the part of the human response to illness or crisis that is common across any malady. For instance, the stress response to cancer is the same as the stress response to being startled on a dark night.

When the organism is threatened, it mobilizes resources to prepare to combat the threat—physiological or psychological. Muscle tension is augmented, but the usual stress response is more than simple muscle tension. The ANS is mobilized as a sympathetic fight or flight response. The pituitary gland actively stimulates the adrenal gland to secrete its hormones. However, the repeated exposure to unnecessary stress, often the result of excess emotionality (e.g., anxiety, worry, depression, anger) is especially wearing on the body. The immune system may be depressed and unable to respond to the usual microorganisms. Chronic stress (e.g., type A personality) makes the client more susceptible to opportunistic disorders in the short-term and to chronic conditions in the long-term.

Treatment of stress is largely preventive and palliative, with the TRS potentially involved in several promising interventions. Exercise, biofeedback, relaxation techniques, and guided imagery number among the interventions that fall within the TRS practice borders.

Therapeutic Recreation and Disorders of the Visceral Systems

Among the topics discussed here is terminal illness and the impact TRS can have with persons nearing the end of life. However, we do not assume, nor should the reader assume, that persons with afflictions such as cancer or AIDS are treated as if they will inevitably die. Even though death is a possibility, TRS should distinguish between interventions for persons with AIDS or cancer and those for persons with terminal illnesses.

Making an assumption that all programs for persons with cancer, for instance, are the same as programs for persons who will inevitably die is problematic for several reasons. First, various types of cancers have markedly different survival rates. Second, there may a tendency not to use some potentially beneficial treatments with the idea that the only course of action for the client is palliation. Third, the assumption of the inevitability of death from an affliction may unwittingly discriminate against persons with cancer or AIDS (e.g., members of the healthcare team begin to withdraw because of the assumption of imminent death). Lastly, the assumption shifts the focus of care away from the person and potentially beneficial and satisfying experiences and toward the inevitable event of expiration. Even TRS for terminally ill clients implement quality of life experiences for the present, and not with an eye toward the inevitable demise of the patient.

Related to the relative focus on death is the distinction between interventions for persons with life-threatening illnesses and interventions for persons with terminally illnesses. The distinction here may be one of semantics, one of treatment versus palliation. Coroleo (1988) once maintained that the focus of therapeutic recreation (TR) intervention with persons with HIV/AIDS should not be considered treatment, but he later changed his mind

(Coroleo, 1994) and supported the notion that TRS for persons with HIV/AIDS could be configured as active treatment. The distinction is important for delivery of services and whether a health insurer may cover the services.

Terminal illness as a separate category of persons involved in TR is problematic in its placement along the TR service continuum. TR for persons who are terminally ill may be offered within a clinical setting, which may be acute care or chronic care. But many persons with terminal illness are choosing to spend their last days or months in a hospice setting within the community, often in their own homes (Hodges & Sorenson, 1998). Hence, it is difficult to place TR for this group. We assume palliation is a therapeutic intervention (planned, goal directed, etc.) even though it is not curative. We are also well aware that services for this group are often delivered in the community.

Therapy

HIV/AIDS

Conversion from HIV and various pre-AIDS syndromes requires one of two conditions. First, a significant decrease in the number of T-lymphocytes of a magnitude to make the subject susceptible to opportunistic infections. Second, the manifestation of an opportunistic infection or other common pathology—a compromised immune system and a major complication (LaPerriere et al., 1997). The literature (Coroleo, 1988, 1994; Grossman & Keller, 1994; Mason & Zwiers, 1994) suggests numerous worthwhile goals for intervention prior to the exacerbation of the disease, including interventions aimed at the prevention of secondary problems and health maintenance, stress reduction, enhancing self-worth and empowering the client, countering feelings of loneliness and abandonment.

Coroleo (1994) reported that loneliness and feelings of abandonment are detrimental to the immune system, and may lead the person to practice more risk behaviors, including substance abuse, smoking, and lack of exercise. Unfortunately, little in the way of data-based work has been completed with respect to TR and persons with HIV/AIDS.

Coroleo (1988) described a community-based program in New York patterned after Peterson and Gunn's (1984) Leisure Ability Model of professional intervention. The program offered two of the three interventions articulated on Peterson and Gunn's classic continuum of services—leisure education and recreation participa-

tion. The services were offered through a community-based program for gay men. The variety of services offered were substantial. Some aimed at health maintenance and prevention of secondary problems (e.g., nutrition counseling, stress reduction, exercise) while other interventions focused more on the psychological concomitants of the disease (e.g., support groups, art therapy, leisure counseling). Evaluation of the program (Coroleo, 1988) relied on client and volunteer feedback and program attendance. Feedback proved to be very favorable. Program attendance suggested that the offerings were popular and had increased during the short time the program was offered.

The fact that a model intervention (Coroleo, 1988) was offered through a gay men's program reminds us of the stigma associated with the disease. Even though HIV/AIDS has long ceased to be considered a disease exclusively of gay males, the stigma associated with it remains (Turner & Keller, 1988). In the time since Coroleo's initial report, TRS for persons with HIV/AIDS has diversified into several other service delivery configurations—hospices, home-care, long-term care facilities, day treatment programs, and community outreach (Grossman & Keller, 1994). Because most persons infected with the HIV virus are asymptomatic, in normal health, may have many healthy years ahead, and reside in the community, we conclude that everyday community recreation will have its share of participants who are HIV positive.

Apart from the previous program and setting suggestions, more substantive findings pertaining to the effectiveness of intervention with HIV/AIDS may depend on an older medical model of intervention. Russoniello (1994) has suggested a general pathway for stress-related diseases and psychological problems (e.g., depression) to affect physical health. This model explains the apparently beneficial effects of regular exercise in coping with stress and health maintenance among HIV/AIDS subjects.

Hans Selye (1974) maintained that the stress response set in motion a series of physiological changes that sometimes caused stress-related illnesses (e.g., hypertension). One reaction of the body to excess stress is suppression of the immune system. Although there is not concrete scientific evidence, LaPerriere et al. (1994) argued that it is likely through the same stress-based physiologic pathway (psychoneuroimmunology—psychological stress, nervous system, endocrine system) that intervention with HIV/AIDS clients causes favorable changes in immunity.

Accordingly, authors (LaPerriere et al., 1994; Russoniello, 1994) have identified exercise as a possible mechanism for addressing stress-related disorders and psychological problems (e.g., depression) as well as HIV/AIDS. We are most concerned with the latter application here, although the use of exercise to cope with stress is commonly recommended as an intervention for prevention of secondary disorders related to stress in persons with HIV/AIDS (Coroleo, 1988; Grossman & Keller, 1994; Mason & Zwiers, 1994).

LaPerriere et al. (1997) has reviewed the scientific study of the psychoneuroimmunologic mechanism as a method for keeping HIV-positive people symptom free. Their review focused on the effects of exercise on CD4+ cells (T-lymphocytes) and found that the effectiveness of exercise depended on the stage of the disease. As with many chronic and progressive disorders, the earlier the intervention, the more effective. All but one study reviewed indicated an increase in CD4+ cells (a desirable effect), and no study reported a decline in CD4+ cell counts. Even studies of persons with manifest AIDS showed a maintenance effect for exercise. Some form of aerobic exercise (e.g., stationary bicycle, supervised sports, endurance training) was commonly used.

LaPerriere et al. (1997) maintained that the effect of exercise on the immune systems of HIV/AIDS subjects should be thought of as a return to normal instead of augmentation to a level of hyperimmunity. He further theorized that the stress/psychoneuroimmunologic pathway noted earlier was a probable mechanism for the effectiveness of exercise. Exercise may act in either of two ways—by mitigating the deleterious effects of stress or by neutralizing the decrement to the immune system (LaPerriere et al., 1997).

This interpretation of the results is consistent with the practical observations noted by those implementing programs for persons with HIV/AIDS—stress exacerbates the progression of the illness. Exercise may well be a practical, inexpensive, and therapeutic intervention for persons with HIV/AIDS that diminishes the suppression of the immune system associated with stress and anxiety. LaPerriere and his associates (1997) do caution against making the inference that exercise intervention will necessarily extend life and/or retard the onset other co-morbid conditions. However, LaPerriere et al. (1997) concluded that the use of exercise with persons with HIV/AIDS was an effective intervention, if customary precautions were taken (e.g., usual health screening) and the stage of the illness was taken into consideration. The challenge that awaits the TR profession is to determine if subaerobic intensity, recreational-level exercise is effective in reducing stress if not augmenting host immunity.

Professionals wishing to intervene using exercise with HIV/AIDS clients should heed LaPerriere's recommendation to implement routine health screening with this group. Turner and Keller (1988) remind us that TR for this group is similar to intervention with other disabilities—purposeful intervention using recreational activities. Secondary problems encountered in conjunction with progression of the virus reveal symptoms and secondary problems similar to those seen in other groups—respiratory distress, malnutrition from chronic diarrhea, or some form of cancer. Hence, the TRS should be prepared to address problems associated with related disorders, as well as those unique to the virus—pain, depression, and boredom.

Cancer

Like HIV/AIDS, the practitioner should make a distinction in principle, if not in actual program implementation, between intervention for persons with cancer and persons with terminal illness. Also like HIV/AIDS, because cancer frequently leads to mortality, interventions may overlap to a certain extent. When does stress management change from treatment to palliation? At what moment does the cancer patient become the terminally ill patient? It is best to assume that cancer is being treated until the medical profession and the patient agree that the course of the disease is irretrievably terminal (i.e., always assume the person is trying to recover or reach the highest level of function possible).

Dimeo and associates (Dimeo, Tilmann, Bertz, Kanz, Mertelsmann & Keul, 1997; Dimeo, Fetscher, Lange, Mertelsmann & Keul, 1997) recently published two studies of the effects of exercise on symptoms among persons receiving chemotherapy for cancer. In the first study (Dimeo, Tillman, et al., 1997), subjects in the exercise group walked on a treadmill shortly after completing treatment for 6 weeks. Seven weeks after discharge, the exercise group significantly improved physical performance (treadmill walking speed) and hemoglobin concentration compared to a nonexercise control group. Furthermore, no subjects in the 16-member exercise group reported perceived fatigue, while four persons of the 16 in the control group did report perceived fatigue.

In their second study (Dimeo, Fetscher, et al., 1997b) patients assigned to the experimental group exercised on a stationary bicycle for 30 minutes daily; bicycle seats were positioned in a supine posture. The exercise was completed while the patients were also participating in intensive chemotherapy. The dependent variable was again physical performance (treadmill test) and assessed at admission and discharge. Compared to the control subjects receiving chemotherapy, those in the exercise group scored significantly higher in physical performance at discharge. In addition, subjects in the exercise group experienced less discomfort and complications in association with chemotherapy. In the exercise group reduction in leukocyte cell count was less, severity of diarrhea and pain were reduced, and length of hospital stay was reduced. Based on evidence from both studies, the authors advocated the use of carefully controlled exercise after chemotherapy instead of rest.

Terminal Illness

Medicare covers services that enhance quality of life among persons with terminal illnesses if a patient has a life-limiting malady that cannot be helped via curative means (Hodges & Sorenson, 1998). Hospices offer more a philosophy than a place for the final portion of one's life to be spent—a philosophical locale where the client can exert maximal control over the course of palliative treatments and quality of life. TR figures prominently in this syndrome of dying because it is intimately concerned with the enhancement of quality of life (Hodges & Sorenson, 1998). The actual physical environment for implementation of the hospice philosophy is in the person's own home, though some clinical settings are specialized to serve persons with terminal illnesses (see Sourby, 1998).

Quality of life for the person with terminal illness means two things: pain management and personal (perceived) control. Palliative treatments address symptoms without altering the progression of the disease. Besides self-regulation of pain medications, TR and allied health services can bring a considerable number of pain management techniques to bear. Though many have not been validated scientifically and pain is a different experience for everyone, some interventions for pain seem logical. Diversion and relaxation responses elicited through a variety of activities hold some promise of palliation, including traditional (progressive) relaxation, tai chi, portions of martial arts practice, guided imagery, massage, and aquatic immersion.

Hodges and Sorenson (1998) add two other broad program goals for TR intervention with persons who are terminally ill. Comfort is the next program goal for this group; comfort differs from diversion to manage pain insofar as comfort pertains more to client control. These methods may begin with the assistance of the TR professional and may have to be taught to the client

(technically making them leisure education), but the objective here is to arm the client with personal comfort techniques that he may use to control symptoms. Activities predicated on reminiscence (e.g., genealogy) may also add to perceived comfort.

The third program area described by Hodges and Sorenson (1998) is expression. Offering and facilitating opportunities for self-expression on an individualized basis responds to client needs and interests make activities more meaningful. Several popular means of expression include pet therapy and creative arts.

The latter method for creative expression was implemented during an intervention with a dying man with mental retardation (Harlan & Hawkins, 1992). Goals for the 75-year-old male subject were similar to ones previously described by Hodges and Sorenson: improve sense of control, self-esteem, and ability to communicate feelings. A creative arts intervention was designed to achieve these goals. The client was encouraged to select his own work materials and media throughout the intervention. Previously, the client reported spending most of his time working and watching TV. The authors concluded that the client used creative art to work through feelings about his own death. Further, he was able to attain a sense of mastery by manipulating the materials and artistic representations. In this case study, the use of art as an expressive medium allowed for enjoyment that enhanced the quality of life and provided a sense of accomplishment.

Likewise, Sourby (1998) reported a case study involving a 67-year-old female dying of cancer. The facility was a residential care center that specialized in providing services for persons with terminal illnesses. The author suggested that palliation (pain management, quality of life) was the goal, but decided on socialization as the means instead of a specific creative experience. The subject became progressively more involved in-group activities, and more involved in interacting with group members as time passed. Various games, horticulture therapy, and music were group activities that the subject participated in during her final four months of life. Individualized socialization visits by the TR professional also evidenced attainment of the TR program goal of socialization. Associated benefits inferred from the client's response to treatment included increased sense of accomplishment, reduced depression, increased ability to cope with stress, and decreased social isolation.

Leisure Education

HIV/AIDS

Fear of HIV/AIDS is a strong motive for leisure education. The obvious students for HIV/AIDS education are the professional staff, co-actors, and family. Universal precautions should only mark the beginning of the educational process. Once aware of the facts about HIV/AIDS, the professional may proceed to the more frequent and insidious problem of stigmatization and discrimination experienced by the patient and subtlety practiced by staff and other patients (Turner & Keller, 1988).

Subsequent topics for leisure education include attitude awareness and change. An excellent stimulant for discussion is a fact-finding exercise. Grossman and Coroleo (1992) and Glenn and Dattilo (1993) have used true/false quizzes about HIV/AIDS to evaluate knowledge of TR professionals. These questionnaires are published and available as media for use in leisure education. Knowledge and the facts about HIV/AIDS are the first steps in attitude change. Attitude instruments pertaining to HIV/AIDS are also available (Glenn & Dattilo, 1993).

Coroleo (1988) and Turner and Keller (1988) articulated other topics that may be covered in leisure education. Coroleo suggested that leisure skills, attitudes, and knowledge be taught because of the abundance of free time the subject has. Implementation of these topical areas within a leisure education framework have been suggested as methods for decreasing feelings of loneliness and increasing self-worth (Coroleo, 1988), decreasing isolation and depression (Coroleo, 1988; Grossman & Keller, 1994), and coping with stress (Coroleo, 1988; Grossman & Keller, 1994).

Turner and Keller (1988) advocate instruction in how to exercise properly (see also Mason & Zwiers, 1994). A series of relaxation topics may also be taught, including biofeedback, imagery, and progressive relaxation. Development of personal relationships provides a method for interaction skills to build in both directions (participant and co-actor). Other topics include stress management and proper nutrition.

Oddly enough, some techniques may have to be taught through leisure education before they can be implemented as therapy. This serves to underscore the fact that many times distinctions between leisure education and therapy, and between leisure education and recreation participation, are blurred rather than discrete.

The final leisure education topic is the teaching of safe sex practices. The obvious imperative to this instruction is for the protection of noninfected partners. LaPerriere et al. (1997) identified subsequent exposure to the HIV virus and other viruses by already infected individuals as a stressor with the potential of exacerbating the illness and accelerating the progression of the pathology.

Coroleo's (1988) description of an existing, community-based program offers some practical methods for implementation of some of the leisure education topics suggested above. For example, cooking groups were used to teach proper nutrition, including selection of foods, preparation of foods, and consumption of appropriate amounts of food. Meals and socials also offered an opportunity to practice social interaction skills and to counteract negative attitudes and stereotypes.

Coroleo (1988) also describes stress reduction as an educational topic. Five instructional goals are provided, with each goal statement suggesting one or more educational activities. For instance, relaxation is one goal within the stress reduction education initiative, and the goal statement includes potential activities for inducing relaxation. Activities such as meditation, yoga, tai chi, visualization, martial arts, and massage are suggested.

Terminal Illness

Part of working with persons with terminal illnesses is the unavoidable death of the patient. Leisure education may be used as a forum for the grieving process that naturally follows. Intervention into the natural grieving process is warranted only after about one year or if the person evidences substance abuse as a coping strategy or exhibits persistent depressive symptoms (Cappel & Mathieu, 1997). Grief counseling may be necessary to help the subject work through the grieving process, especially if the death was unexpected and sudden. Education for caregivers, staff, and significant others may begin with a review of Kubler-Ross' (1969) five stages of dying. Cappel and Mathieu (1997) have published five reflective exercises that could easily be incorporated into a leisure education class. They (Cappel & Mathieu, 1997) also mention several coping strategies for persons to use.

Recreation Participation

HIV/AIDS

To no one's surprise, recommendations for investing in quality of life experiences within recreation programs for persons with HIV/AIDS is common (Coroleo, 1988; Mason & Zwiers, 1994; Turner & Keller, 1994). Informal and casual recreation participation environments allow for spontaneous enjoyment. Self-regulated, meaningful use of free time also encourages empowerment (e.g., Turner & Keller, 1988) and the right to leisure (e.g., Mason & Zwiers, 1994). Facilitating enjoyment through recreation participation also responds to the problems of unemployment and underemployment often faced by this population (Turner & Keller, 1988). The excess of free time is all the more aggravating because the client is physically and mentally capable of employment for most of the course of the disease progression, even in a worst case scenario.

Another activity offered by the community-based program for gay men described by Coroleo (1988) is volunteering. Avocational work certainly addresses the problems of unemployment or under employment experienced by persons with HIV/AIDS. Volunteer experiences hold the promise to restore a sense of accomplishment, self-worth, and self-esteem. Volunteering also may assist in the transition from employment as a source of personal identity to a more leisure basis for identity.

Cancer

Quality of life as a personal goal for the client and program goal for TRS is another of the characteristics shared by persons with cancer. Smith (1996) based her discussion of exercise for persons with cancer on the assumption that it enhanced quality of life in a number of ways. However, Smith's (1996) definition of quality of life is quite a bit broader than some: "a person's sense of well-being that stems from satisfaction or dissatisfaction with the areas of life that are important to him/her." Further pursuing quality of life as a critical variable, Smith elaborates several dimensions—physical, functional, psychological, social, and spiritual—and itemizes markers under each of the dimensions that may be improved using exercise as an intervention. The variables that may be improved among clients with cancer following exercise include decreased perceptions of fatigue, improved sleep, and better appetite.

Many differences exist between exercise and quality of life as Smith (1996) discusses it and the manner exercise was used as an intervention by Dimeo, Tilmann, et al. (1997) and Dimeo, Fetscher, et al. (1997). First, the varied benefits associated with the six dimensions of quality of life are primarily nonclinical. Hence, we assume that the outcomes are more likely to occur in nontreatment situations. Second, because many quality of life variables take considerable time to change, short treatment times specific to clinical situations are probably not long enough to see changes. Finally, since Smith is advocating for exercise as a lifestyle change, we assume that most persons with cancer would be eligible for participation, especially at mild to moderate, recreational levels of exercise. Potential clients are then persons with cancer, in remission, or manifest with controlled symptoms, who reside predominantly in the community.

General guidelines for exercise for persons with cancer are sketched by Smith (1996), and closely resemble procedures one would follow for almost any adult interested in beginning an exercise program in a nonclinical setting. Screening is an initial step, with referral to the person's family physician as needed. Physicians should also be consulted if the person is using a medication to manage the disease or control symptoms to avoid potential complications. Recommendations (Smith, 1996) to starting slow and to focus on range of motion and mild to moderate aerobic conditioning are typical of exercise programs for special populations. Light weights using high repetitions may be added later in the sequence. Rest periods may be necessary early in the training prior to adaptation to exercise, or later if the participant changes medications, or must take chemotherapy or some other procedure.

Smith (1996) closes with a list of contraindications (e.g., chest pain, nausea or diarrhea in the previous 24-36 hours=) for exercise for this group. Many of the precautions are common sense, but others are unique to cancer (e.g., low platelet count) and require assessment through laboratory tests.

Obesity/Diabetes

Obesity and diabetes will be treated together in this section because obesity is a risk factor for acquired diabetes (NIDDM), which develops in later adulthood. Furthermore, both conditions are placed in the recreation participation service section for several reasons:

- Most persons reside in the community and are rarely hospitalized exclusively for obesity or diabetes

- Prevention is important in both conditions because each is a risk factor for future morbidity and mortality and

- Day-to-day programs aimed at correction or management are not closely monitored by medical personnel; the client is most often responsible for self-monitoring/self-motivation

In 1996 Epstein, Coleman, and Myers reviewed research on exercise programs for children with obesity. They summarized both the effectiveness of exercise as a treatment and the program methods most effective at inducing favorable changes and weight loss. Most frequently, interventions followed a conventional pattern of three times per week to daily. Other methods less frequently used were additional physical education classes, lifestyle exercise programs, and interventions designed to reduce sedentary behaviors. Two interventions used only exercise without diet and proved to be ineffective. Studies that combined diet and exercise were most effective in improving fitness and reducing weight.

Although few studies compared different exercise programs, two did contrast the effectiveness of a lifestyle intervention program with aerobics methods. Lifestyle exercise programs are popular with older adults because they seek to increase total daily activity at any intensity instead of a structured time for aerobic exercise. In both studies, subjects lost weight regardless of the exercise intervention (plus diet). However, long-term changes favored the lifestyle exercise approach—only the subjects in the lifestyle exercise groups maintained their weight loss for more than 6 months.

A method for increasing exercise related to the lifestyle approach used in one study was to reinforce reduction of sedentary behavior. Compared to reinforcing an increase in physical activity, reinforcing reduction in sedentary behaviors resulted in greater weight loss. Like lifestyle exercise, this method allows for more self-regulation and control, and does not impose a standard for exercise intensity (e.g., 50% maximum heart rate). The objective is to induce an increase in activity of any kind and to continue to adhere to a more active lifestyle for the long-term.

The two major factors found to influence exercise among obese children and adolescents were adherence and diet. Little can be expected of exercise if diet is not included. Improvements will only be transient if exercise habits are not adopted for the long-term. Other less influential factors were also identified (e.g., age, sex, type of exercise).

Marshall and Bouffard (1997) recently reported a community-wide exercise intervention with school-age children. The authors hypothesized that a high quality physical education program (daily participation in a wide range of activities, stressing fitness, and based on the child's growth and development characteristics) implemented in the public school system would improve fitness and enhance development of motor skills in obese children. They reasoned that because obese children were less active they were also had impaired motor development, changes that are also influential in reducing opportunities for social interaction (In fact, an earlier pilot study by the same authors confirmed as much). However, the 1997 intervention demonstrated that a high quality physical education program was successful in improving motor skills in all children who were less movement competent, obese or not.

Lehmann and Spinas (1996) examined the effectiveness of exercise in preventing and managing NIDDM. They concluded that physical activity delays the onset of diabetes mellitus in adults and may even prevent the onset of at risk adults in up to 50% of cases. Regular exercise reliably reduces blood glucose and increase high-density lipoproteins (i.e., good cholesterol). Summative review of studies suggests that an increase in glucose tolerance may result after only one week of exercise, but the favorable effects of exercise may also be lost as quickly if the individual quits. Accordingly, the authors (Lehmann & Spinas, 1996) recommended exercise for at risk and manifest NIDDM at a 60-80% of maximum heart rate, three times a week, and 30–45 minutes per session. If weight loss was also desired, then more frequent exercise (5–7 times per week) and diet should be added to the training regime.

Edwards (1997a, 1997b) completed two small sample studies on the effects of exercise on glucose levels. A single 40-year-old diabetic subject participated in mild (walking) and moderate (slow jogging) exercise, every other day for 16 weeks (Edwards, 1997a). Blood glucose was significantly reduced over the course of the exercise program. In the second study (Edwards, 1997b), six subjects participated in mild or moderate intensity exercise on a stationary bicycle. The encouraging result for the TR profession was that light intensity exercise was more effective in reducing blood glucose than moderate intensity bicycling. However, five of the six subjects reduced blood glucose. Since Edwards work is based on small samples, it must be regarded as suggestive rather than definitive—but the results lend some credibility to the use of low risk, recreational level exercise (i.e., light intensity exercise) with diabetics and those at risk of developing NIDDM.

Polynesian ethnic groups are at more at risk for development of NIDDM. Accordingly, Simmons, Fleming, Cameron, and Leakehe (1996) recruited 108 Polynesian hospital workers to participate in a four-month exercise and diabetes education program. Results were compared with performance of 99 ethnically matched controls. Diabetes awareness was significantly improved in the treatment group, but only two percent reported continuing exercise after completion of the program. This compared to a 9% decrease in exercise in the control group.

Urinary System

Sheldon and Caldwell (1994) reviewed the literature on urinary incontinence and suggested implications for TR intervention. No studies directly used TR interventions to address urinary incontinence. They suggested that realistic goals for TR involvement with persons with urinary incontinence included the following: improvement in self-esteem, increase in social contact, and reduction of social stigma. Review of studies of the effect of urinary incontinence on social and community activities underscored the self-isolation many persons with this problem impose on themselves to avoid embarrassment. Some research identified by Sheldon and Caldwell (1994) found that self-isolation was the most common manner in which persons with urinary incontinence manage their problem.

Based on the literature Sheldon and Caldwell (1994) suggested settings and methods for TR intervention with urinary incontinence problems. Since persons usually reside in the community, services may be delivered by way of a home visitation or community-based programs. Specific methods should be aimed at inducing perceptions of control in experiential domains where control is possible—the obvious candidate here is in recreation. Leisure education, and especially resource identification and planning, should focus on planning activities so that the client can map bathroom locations in frequently visited facilities. Lessons in leisure education curricula can also include teaching abdominal strengthening exercises and Kegel exercises to strengthen muscles of the pelvis. Stigma may also be reduced through planning with the client, including prescheduled bathroom stops on outings, buses with bathrooms, serving beverages that do not include diuretics, and providing disposable pads and containers for discarding. Sheldon and Caldwell (1994) speculate about methods for TR to intervene with these clients in a treatment setting, but usually TR would only be

involved with urinary incontinence if it were a problem secondary to another affliction (e.g., spinal cord injury). In this regard, urinary incontinence would be a variable that would be considered in planning, much in the same manner that it is planned for in community-based programs.

Practical Applications

Know Universal Precautions

Universal precautions intend to prevent HIV infection and Hepatitis B. Plan activities to avoid injuries. Follow appropriate activity precautions and procedures. Equipment should be in good repair, avoid the use of sharp implements in activities, and inspect landing surfaces periodically for safety. Planning to avoid exposure to contaminated fluids should be part of an agency's risk management plan. Second, if an at-risk fluid is present, place an acceptable barrier (e.g., latex gloves) between yourself and the persons you work with. Third, in the event of contact with a potentially infected body fluid, immediately wash the area thoroughly. Also clean surfaces exposed to the fluid, even if the fluid (e.g., blood) is not visible to the naked eye. Small particles of the fluid may still adhere to a surface, but not be immediately visible. A more thorough description of universal precautions should be consulted (e.g., see Turner & Keller, 1988, p. 19, or contact the Center for Disease Control for the most up-to-date precautions). Required training in First Aid and CPR, commonly part of professional preparation, include training in universal precautions for emergency situations. The TR professional should *always assume universal precautions* as a matter of course because of the client's right to confidentiality, and because many HIV-infected individuals do not know that they are carrying the virus.

Confidentiality

Ethical standards adopted by NTRS and ATRA are clear about patient confidentiality. Patients have the right withhold their diagnosis, HIV/AIDS or otherwise. Patients are in control of information about themselves, and even if the therapist knows the diagnosis, he may not reveal it except under dire circumstances (e.g., when the patient or someone else is endangered by withholding the information). Given that the risk of infection with the HIV virus is low when proper precautions are followed, the virus may not be spread through casual contact, and persons with HIV/AIDS are discriminated against and stigmatized, confidentiality is urged.

Change Attitudes through Inservice Education

Knowledge is the catalyst for attitude change, and the place to begin is with the healthcare staff. Grossman and Coroleo (1992) asked 82 TR professionals to identify statements about HIV/AIDS as true or false. The average score was 89%, but the authors believed this was not satisfactory performance. Glenn and Dattilo's (1993) TR practitioners performed significantly poorer on a 25 item, true/false quiz about HIV/AIDS facts. They also found a positive correlation between continuing education and attitude toward persons with HIV/AIDS.

Precautions with Diabetics

Insulin reaction is the most frequent problem among diabetics. It may occur whenever the blood glucose falls below an acceptable level, precipitating a condition referred to as hypoglycemia. Common causes of hypoglycemia include a failure to eat after taking insulin, an alteration of physical activity or exercise habits, or an insulin dose error. Symptoms include acute confusion (brain cells are very sensitive to blood glucose levels) and unusual behavior (sometimes combative), anxiety, tachycardia (rapid heartbeat), cold to clammy skin, and profuse sweating. Quick ingestion of glucose provides almost immediate relief (e.g., orange juice, candy, or honey also works well).

Another problem associated with the balance between insulin and glucose among diabetics is hyperglycemia. Its onset is more gradual than insulin reaction and the conditions are exactly the opposite—there is too much glucose in the bloodstream. The causes may include an excess intake of glucose or an increase in resistance to the effects of insulin. Hyperglycemia creates osmotic pressure and draws water out of cells. Quite logically, the initial symptom is dehydration with polyuria (excess urination) and polydipsia (excess drinking). But if left uncorrected, the condition is accompanied by neurological symptoms, often seizures that may be fatal. Observation of any of these symptoms by the TR professional should result in immediate referral to the medical support staff for attention.

In Type I diabetes, hyperglycemia may lead to a dangerous condition known as acidosis, caused by a mobilization of fats for energy. The excessively acidic environment may overcome the buffering system within the body and lead to coma and even death.

To avoid hyperglycemia or hypoglycemia, the TR professional should always be aware of the patient's diagnosis and if that diagnosis includes diabetes. Dietary restrictions and drug treatment regimes should be followed closely to avoid situations that may lead to either condition (e.g., eating too much birthday cake at a patient party, taking insulin before an outing but not eating promptly, increasing exercise without consulting with the patient's physician).

Chapter Summary

This chapter examined the visceral systems and addressed the following key concepts:

- Common disorders of the visceral systems are often serious and include impairments such as diabetes mellitus, various cancers, sexually transmitted diseases, HIV/AIDS, liver disease, and kidney failure.
- Considerable literature offers programmatic level suggestions about TR programs for persons who are HIV positive, but little research has been completed to date on the effectiveness of these initiatives.
- A person with a serious illness should not be treated as if he has a terminal illness.
- Staff, caregivers, and family should be included in educational programs offered in association with serious and terminal illnesses.
- Lifestyle and/or recreational level exercise have proven to be very effective in the management of some visceral disorders, resulting in physical (e.g., with Type II diabetes mellitus) and psychological (e.g., with stress) improvements.

References

Cappel, M. L. and Mathieu, S. L. (1997). Loss and the grieving process. *Parks & Recreation, 32*, 82–85.

Coroleo, O. O. (1988). AIDS: Meeting the need through therapeutic recreation. *Therapeutic Recreation Journal, 22*, 71–78.

Coroleo, O. O. (1994). Loneliness and anxiety as two of the psychosocial factors associated with HIV illness and their implications for recreation programming. *Leisurability, 21*, 30–36.

Dimeo, F. C., Tilmann, M. H., Bertz, H., Kanz, L., Mertelsmann, R., and Keul, J. (1997). Aerobic exercise in the rehabilitation of cancer patients after high dose chemotherapy and autologous peripheral stem cell transplantation. *Cancer, 79*, 1717–1722.

Dimeo, F. C., Fetscher, S., Lange, W., Mertelsmann, R., and Keul, J. (1997). Effects of aerobic exercise on the physical performance and incidence of treatment-related complications after high dose chemotherapy. *Blood, 90*, 3390–3394.

Edwards, B. G. (1997a). A diabetic's blood glucose response to moderate and low dose exercise requiring similar energy expenditures. *Clinical Kinesiology, 50*, 24.

Edwards, B. G. (1997b). Blood glucose responses to low and moderate intensity exercise requiring the same energy output. *Clinical Kinesiology, 50*, 25.

Epstein, L. H., Coleman, K. J., and Myers, M. D. (1995). Exercise in treating obesity in children and adolescents. *Medicine and Science in Sports and Exercise, 28*, 428–435.

Glenn, C. and Dattilo, J. (1993). Therapeutic recreation professionals' attitudes toward knowledge of AIDS. *Therapeutic Recreation Journal, 27*, 253–261.

Grossman, A. H. and Coroleo O. O. (1992). A study of AIDS risk behavior knowledge among therapeutic recreation specialists in New York state. *Therapeutic Recreation Journal, 26*, 55–60.

Grossman, A. and Keller, J. (1994). Changing trends in the HIV/AIDS epidemic: A new role for therapeutic recreation specialists. *Leisurability, 21*, 3–13.

Harlan, J. E. and Hawkins, B. A. (1992). Terminal illness aging and developmental disability: A therapeutic art intervention. *Therapeutic Recreation Journal, 26*, 49–52.

Hodges, J. S. and Sorenson, B. (1998). Quality during the end of life. *Parks & Recreation, 33*, 72–76.

Kubler-Ross, E. (1969). *On death and dying.* New York, NY: MacMillan.

LaPerriere, A., Ironson, G., Antoni, M. H., Schneiderman, N., Klimas, N., and Fletcher, M. A. (1994). Exercise and psychoneuroimmunology. *Medicine and Science in Sports and Exercise, 26*, 182–190.

LaPerriere, A., Klimas, N., Fletcher, M. A., Perry, A., Ironson, G., Perna, F., and Schneiderman, N. (1997). Change in CD4+ cell enumeration following aerobic exercise training in HIV-1 disease: Possible mechanisms and practical applications. *International Journal of Sports Medicine, 18* S56–S61.

Lehmann, R. and Spinas, G. A. (1996). Role of physical activity in the therapy and prevention of type II diabetes mellitus. *Therapeutische Unschau, 53*, 925–933.

Marshall, J. D. and Bouffard, M. (1997). The effects of quality daily physical education on movement competency in obese versus nonobese children. *Adapted Physical Activity Quarterly, 14*, 222–237.

Mason, L. and Zwiers, A. (1994). The psychosocial impact of HIV disease and implications for the leisure profession. *Leisurability, 21* 23–24.

Peterson, C. A. and Gunn, S. L. (1984). *Therapeutic recreation program design: Principles and procedures.* Englewood Cliffs, NJ: Prentice-Hall.

Russoniello, C. V. (1994). Recreational therapy: A medicine model. In D. Compton and S. E. Iso-Ahola (Eds.), *Leisure and mental health* (pp. 247–257). Park City, UT: Family Development Resources.

Selye, H. (1974). *Stress without distress.* New York, NY: Signet.

Sheldon, K. and Caldwell, L. (1994). Urinary incontinence in women: Implications for therapeutic recreation. *Therapeutic Recreation Journal, 28*, 203–212.

Simmons, D., Fleming, C., Cameron, M., and Leakehe, L. (1996). A pilot diabetes awareness and exercise program in a multiethnic workforce. *New Zealand Medical Journal, 109*, 373–376.

Smith, S. L. (1996). Physical exercise as an oncology nursing intervention to enhance quality of life. *Oncology Nursing Forum, 23*, 771–778.

Sourby, C. (1998). The relationship between therapeutic recreation and palliation in the treatment of the advanced cancer patient. Available online: http://www.recreationtherapy.com

Turner, N. H. and Keller, M. J. (1988). Therapeutic recreation practitioner involvement in the AIDS epidemic. *Therapeutic Recreation Journal, 22*, 12–20.

Books by Venture Publishing

Leisure Services in Canada: An Introduction, Second Edition
by Mark S. Searle and Russell E. Brayley

Leisure Studies: Prospects for the Twenty-First Century
edited by Edgar L. Jackson and Thomas L. Burton

The Lifestory Re-Play Circle: A Manual of Activities and Techniques
by Rosilyn Wilder

Models of Change in Municipal Parks and Recreation: A Book of Innovative Case Studies
edited by Mark E. Havitz

More Than a Game: A New Focus on Senior Activity Services
by Brenda Corbett

Nature and the Human Spirit: Toward an Expanded Land Management Ethic
edited by B. L. Driver, Daniel Dustin, Tony Baltic, Gary Elsner, and George Peterson

Outdoor Recreation Management: Theory and Application, Third Edition
by Alan Jubenville and Ben Twight

Planning Parks for People, Second Edition
by John Hultsman, Richard L. Cottrell, and Wendy Z. Hultsman

The Process of Recreation Programming Theory and Technique, Third Edition
by Patricia Farrell and Herberta M. Lundegren

Programming for Parks, Recreation, and Leisure Services: A Servant Leadership Approach
by Donald G. DeGraaf, Debra J. Jordan, and Kathy H. DeGraaf

Protocols for Recreation Therapy Programs
edited by Jill Kelland, with the Recreation Therapy Staff at Alberta Hospital Edmonton

Quality Management: Applications for Therapeutic Recreation
edited by Bob Riley

A Recovery Workbook: The Road Back from Substance Abuse
by April K. Neal and Michael J. Taleff

Recreation and Leisure: Issues in an Era of Change, Third Edition
edited by Thomas Goodale and Peter A. Witt

Recreation Economic Decisions: Comparing Benefits and Costs, Second Edition
by John B. Loomis and Richard G. Walsh

Recreation for Older Adults: Individual and Group Activities
by Judith A. Elliott and Jerold E. Elliott

Recreation Programming and Activities for Older Adults
by Jerold E. Elliott and Judith A. Sorg-Elliott

Reference Manual for Writing Rehabilitation Therapy Treatment Plans
by Penny Hogberg and Mary Johnson

Research in Therapeutic Recreation: Concepts and Methods
edited by Marjorie J. Malkin and Christine Z. Howe

Simple Expressions: Creative and Therapeutic Arts for the Elderly in Long-Term Care Facilities
by Vicki Parsons

A Social History of Leisure Since 1600
by Gary Cross

A Social Psychology of Leisure
by Roger C. Mannell and Douglas A. Kleiber

Steps to Successful Programming: A Student Handbook to Accompany Programming for Parks, Recreation, and Leisure Services
by Donald G. DeGraaf, Debra J. Jordan, and Kathy H. DeGraaf

Stretch Your Mind and Body: Tai Chi as an Adaptive Activity
by Duane A. Crider and William R. Klinger

Therapeutic Activity Intervention with the Elderly: Foundations and Practices
by Barbara A. Hawkins, Marti E. May, and Nancy Brattain Rogers

Therapeutic Recreation and the Nature of Disabilities
by Kenneth E. Mobily and Richard MacNeil

Therapeutic Recreation: Cases and Exercises, Second Edition
by Barbara C. Wilhite and M. Jean Keller

Therapeutic Recreation in the Nursing Home
by Linda Buettner and Shelley L. Martin

Therapeutic Recreation Protocol for Treatment of Substance Addictions
by Rozanne W. Faulkner

Tourism and Society: A Guide to Problems and Issues
by Robert W. Wyllie

A Training Manual for Americans with Disabilities Act Compliance in Parks and Recreation Settings
by Carol Stensrud

Venture Publishing, Inc.
1999 Cato Avenue
State College, PA 16801
Phone: (814) 234–4561
Fax: (814) 234–1651